The Cardiology Rotation (TCR)

Basic Reading and Board Review

Third Edition
2021

George J. Taylor, M.D.

Professor of Medicine
The Medical University of South Carolina
Charleston, South Carolina

Amanda F. Northup, M.D.

Assistant Professor of Medicine
The Medical University of South Carolina
Charleston, South Carolina

Kindle Direct Publishing

Moment of Conception
Copyright © 2021 by George J. Taylor and
Amanda F. Northup
All Rights Reserved

ISBN: 9798720448363

Dedication:
For Matt, Jesse, and Luke (GJT)
For my mother, Amy, to whom I owe everything (AFN)

Amazon reviews of the second edition:

This is one of the best medical books. It is crystal clear; concepts are solid and easily understood. I wonder why our IM department doesn't give us the book? This book would be great both for medical students on IM rotation, cardiology, etc. and also for interns and residents!

I've been reading this for my cardiology rotation as a fourth year med student. It's been helpful as a good refresher and new content. I like that it's very easy to read and enjoyable.

The right compendium to get back on track and to know what textbooks often don't tell you for clinical practice.

So far impressed with the content of this book…Lots of info for the inquisitive cardiac loving brain cells.

Very good for pathophysiology so that I understand why a med is used for certain diagnoses. I definitely recommend it …

An easy read; it's like a conversation with a friendly and knowledgeable resident.

Preface to the Third Edition, 2021

The Cardiology Rotation (TCR) is for students and house officers on their one month cardiology rotation. It provides an organized curriculum, presented as a broad tutorial that integrates pathophysiology with a practical approach to diagnosis and treatment. It is hard to imagine that all of adult cardiology could be covered in so few pages, but when the object is the big picture it is possible. We cover what we want a resident—or medical student, nurse practitioner, physician's assistant, or pharmacist—to know after a month on our service. This framework for understanding heart disease will allow you to shine on rounds (and find it more enjoyable since learning feels good).

Isn't it aggravating when the attending assumes you know things you couldn't have known before this specialty month? We assume that the reader is starting from scratch, so the approach is basic, focusing on concepts so basic that they often are glossed over on rounds. The plan should be to read TCR cover-to-cover in 10 days. Consider it the cardiology rotation's homework. Reviewers have said that its conversational tone and clear explanations make it an easy read.

TCR also serves as a review for the NBME Medicine Shelf Exam, USMLE Step 3 exam, ECFMG certification exam, and Family Medicine and Internal Medicine board exams. Cardiology has a long history of clinical trials that inform guideline-directed medical therapy (GDMT). TCR emphasizes GDMT, because it is crucial for competent medical practice and for success on boards. But in addition, TCR identifies other board exam favorites. Consider these practical questions:

1. What should I look for if antihypertensive treatment isn't working?
2. Pharmacologic stress testing with adenosine—is it really stress?

3. What am I treating with diuretics? Preload, afterload? What if furosemide doesn't work?
4. Can stress testing be misleading when evaluating stable or unstable angina?
5. How does ventricular afterload affect timing of valve surgery? What is worse, pressure or volume overload valve disease?
6. What workup is needed when a healthy patient's ECG indicates septal infarction?
7. What are the key questions when doing preoperative cardiac risk stratification?
8. What determines whether a patient receives cardiac disability benefits?
9. What congenital heart diseases might I see on the boards?

Look no further—TCR has you covered.

Blackwell Science published the first edition of The Cardiology Rotation in 2001, and updates were published with their permission. Kindle Direct Publishing has not been in the textbook business, so there is no index. The table of contents links to all major and minor section headings, tables and figures. There are practical benefits of online publishing: a 10-month production delay is avoided, and the Kindle edition costs a fraction of the $45 paperback first edition.

TCR is an introductory text, complementary to but not a substitute for clinical knowledge and experience when making medical decisions. The authors and publisher will not be liable for any damages resulting from the use of this book. We have tried to make it clear when we express opinion. If you find errors of commission or omission or have suggestions, please contact us so that updates of TCR will be better.

George J. Taylor, M.D.
Amanda F. Northup, M.D. northup@musc.edu
February 1, 2021

Table of Contents

Chapter 2: Disorders of Ventricular Filling: Heart Failure with Preserved Ejection Fraction, Restrictive Cardiomyopathy, Hypertrophic Obstructive Cardiomyopathy, Pericardial Disease 54

Chapter 1: Congestive Heart Failure, Systolic Dysfunction

Congestive heart failure (CHF) is the clinical syndrome caused by insufficient cardiac output, leading to either pulmonary or systemic congestion (Table 1.1). Extracardiac or valvular heart disease may limit cardiac output, even though ventricular function is normal. This chapter is about CHF caused by ventricular systolic dysfunction. Isolated failure of the right ventricle (RV) causes peripheral edema and splanchnic congestion. Left ventricular (LV) failure causes pulmonary congestion, including exertional dyspnea, orthopnea, paroxysmal nocturnal dyspnea, and eventually pulmonary edema. Easy fatigue and exercise intolerance are early and often subtle manifestations of both left and right heart failure.

There are a half million new cases of CHF in the United States each year. It is the most common admitting diagnosis for elderly people, and the incidence of CHF more than doubles with each decade over age 45. Coronary artery disease is the most common cause of LV systolic dysfunction and CHF (Table 1.1). Hypertension (HTN) was the most common cause in the Framingham study begun in 1949, but more effective treatment of HTN has changed this.

An interesting cause of LV dysfunction is incessant tachycardia (this is now making it to board examinations). Typically, a patient with rapid atrial fibrillation lasting 3 to 4 weeks has a low ejection fraction (EF) on the echocardiogram. After control of the ventricular rate there is gradual improvement in LVEF.

Idiopathic cardiomyopathy is becoming less idiopathic; based on clinical and new genetic evidence most are probably familial diseases. It is complicated. More than 40 genes have implicated at this point, not to mention the fact that the same abnormal genotype can have different phenotypic expression. Detailed discussion is unsuitable for this review. However, there are two practical, clinical implications: 1) it is important to focus on family history, going back three generations, and 2) screening of first degree relatives is now recommended with most cardiomyopathies.

TABLE 1.1. Causes of CHF

Illnesses that inhibit ventricular filling but do not affect ventricular function (result: low cardiac output)

Mitral stenosis (blocks LV filling)

Pericardial tamponade or constriction (blocks RV filling)

Conditions influencing ventricular function, altering either preload or afterload (result: low cardiac output)

Aortic stenosis (high LV afterload)

Aortic regurgitation (LV volume overload + high afterload)

Mitral regurgitation (LV volume overload)

Pulmonic stenosis (high RV afterload)

Tricuspid regurgitation (RV volume overload)

Hypertensive heart disease (high LV afterload)

Primary pulmonary hypertension (high RV afterload)

Obesity (LV volume overload + high afterload due to associated hypertension)

Secondary pulmonary hypertension (high RV afterload caused by lung disease—cor pulmonale—left heart failure, or Eisenmenger's syndrome)

Illnesses primarily affecting LV systolic (contractile) dysfunction (result: low cardiac output)

Myocardial infarction (ischemic cardiomyopathy)

Idiopathic dilated cardiomyopathy

Tachycardia-induced cardiomyopathy (atrial fibrillation, prolonged supraventricular tachycardia, or rarely, ventricular tachycardia)

Viral myocarditis (coxsackie A and B, echovirus, influenza A and B, polio virus, arbovirus, cytomegalovirus, mumps). Covid-19 myocarditis.

LV noncompaction cardiomyopathy (a genetic illness with fluffy appearing muscle on echo)

Acute rheumatic fever (rheumatic myocarditis)

Sepsis (bacterial or fungal)

Toxins (alcohol, cocaine, heroin, amphetamines, ethylene glycol, cobalt, lead, arsenic)

Drugs (adriamycin, cyclophosphamides, sulfonamides, ipecac)

Nutritional deficiencies (protein, thiamine, selenium, L-carnitine)

Electrolyte disorders (low sodium, calcium, magnesium, or phosphate)

Collagen vascular disease (lupus, rheumatoid arthritis, periarteritis nodosa, Reiter's syndrome, systemic sclerosis, Takayasu's syndrome, hypersensitivity vasculitis)

Endocrine disorders (diabetes, hypo/hyperthyroidism, pheochromocytoma, hypoparathyroidism)

Miscellaneous (peripartum cardiomyopathy, sleep apnea, hypereosinophilic syndrome, giant cell myocarditis)

Illnesses causing LV diastolic dysfunction (result: inadequate LV filling and low cardiac output)

Idiopathic diastolic dysfunction (usually elderly women)

Hypertension

Any cardiac condition that increases afterload and induces ventricular hypertrophy

Hypertrophic cardiomyopathy (including hypertrophic subaortic stenosis)

Infiltrative cardiomyopathy or myocardial fibrosis (amyloidosis, sarcoidosis, hemochromatosis, other inflammatory conditions, including collagen vascular disease)

High-output heart failure (in most cases high cardiac output alone does not cause CHF but precipitates it when there is underlying heart disease)

Anemia

Cirrhosis of the liver

Thyrotoxicosis

Arteriovenous fistulas (after trauma, arteriovenous fistula for haemodialysis, Osler-Weber-Rendu disease, rupture of an aortic aneurysm into the inferior vena cava)

Beriberi (thiamine deficiency may contribute to alcoholic heart disease; consider thiamine treatment when the cause of heart failure is obscure or there is an unusual dietary history)

Paget's disease of bone

The natural history of CHF is somewhat difficult to define because of patient selection bias and changes in therapy. The Framingham Study, conducted between 1949 and 1971, included patients with both mild and severe CHF and showed 40% three-year mortality. This study was based on a clinical diagnosis, and few of the patients had documentation of LV function; it probably included patients who did not have CHF. In contrast, a trial conducted by a heart failure research group between 1979 and 1984 focused on patients with proven LV dysfunction and severe CHF and found a 75% three-year mortality.

More recent data (Table 1.2), indicate a mortality rate of about one third during 2 to 4 years of follow-up, and show that the severity of symptoms parallels mortality. A reduction in CHF mortality in recent years can be attributed to modern therapy;

multiple drugs are proven to improve survival (they are guidelines directed medical therapy—GDMT—and you have to know what they are!).   Ventricular fibrillation, a common cause of death in patients with early CHF, can be successfully treated with an implantable cardiac defibrillator (ICD).

TABLE 1.2. Congestive Heart Failure; functional class and survival in placebo groups in large clinical trials

VHeFT I: 642 patients*, Class II-III**, 30 months f/u. Annual mortality = 14%

SOLVD: 2561 patients, Class II-III, 42 months f/u. Annual mortality = 11.4%

CONSENSUS: 253 patients, Class IV, 6 months f/u. Annual mortality > 60%

**Number of patients in the study's placebo group, not on angiotensin converting enzyme inhibitor (ACEI) or beta blocker therapy. So this is the prognosis with untreated heart failure.

**The New York Heart Association (NYHA) functional classification: Class I, no symptoms with physical activity but known disease. Class II, slight limitation of activity and symptoms with normal activity (able to walk 3 blocks). Class III, symptoms with less strenuous exertion that limits normal activity. Class IV, dyspnea at rest or when dressing. The functional class was prespecified by the study; thus, VHeFT I and SOLVD were studies of Class II-III CHF. f/u, follow-up

---

PATHOPHYSIOLOGY

Ventricular Anatomy and Function

The left ventricle is thicker than the right ventricle. It works against higher resistance, or "afterload." You know that weight-lifting builds muscle mass. What is true for the weight lifter's arms is true for heart muscle as well. Because aortic pressure is much higher than pulmonary artery pressure, the left ventricle is more muscular than the right. Raising afterload increases the muscle mass of either of the ventricles, and lowering it allows a regression of hypertrophy.

TABLE 1.3. Determinants of Cardiac Output and Stroke Volume

Cardiac output (mL/min) = Heart rate (beats/min) × Stroke volume (mL/beat)

Stroke volume is augmented (+) or depressed (-) by three factors:

1. (+) Preload = the ventricular load or volume at the end of diastole. (Higher preload augments stroke volume.)

2. (–) Afterload = the load or resistance against which the ventricle empties during systole. (Higher afterload impedes the ventricle's ability to empty, lowering stroke volume.)

3. (+) Contractility = the basic state of ventricular muscle (its innate ability to contract independent of loading conditions—increased contractility means greater ventricular emptying and greater stroke volume).

The labels "right" and "left" ventricle do not accurately describe the position of the heart in the chest. Actually, the right ventricle is anterior to the left ventricle, and the plane of the interventricular septum is almost parallel to the chest wall, positions that are apparent from the echocardiogram. The right ventricular (RV) impulse, when palpable, is felt along the left parasternal border, and the right ventricle is the first chamber punctured by a parasternal needle insertion.

Normally, the interventricular septum acts as a part of the left ventricle. When you think about it, the septum has to choose sides, because it is anatomically a part of both ventricles. It chooses the side that is working hardest, normally the left ventricle. On the echo (or with other imaging studies that show the heart in motion), the septum moves toward the posterior wall of the left ventricle during systole and away from the free wall of the right ventricle. RV overload or failure may lead to a reversal of this normal pattern, with the septum moving toward the right ventricle and away from the left ventricle during systole. This "paradoxical septal motion" is a diagnostic criterion of atrial septal defect (ASD), for example. When an ASD has a 2:1 shunt, it means that the RV is pumping twice as much blood as the LV; in that case the septum changes sides and works with the RV during systole.

Cardiac Output and Ventricular Function

When all is said and done, what the body wants from the pump is blood flow. Output is the product of heart rate and stroke volume, the volume ejected with each heartbeat. The units of measurement are fairly simple (Table 1.3). When output falls, increasing heart rate is an important early compensatory mechanism. With treatment, heart rate should come down. Resting sinus tachycardia is an indicator of persistent decompensation and poor prognosis. It is often ignored by students and house staff, but it is the most important physical finding that predicts survival.

There is a limit on the ability to increase output with increased rate. The duration of ventricular systole—the width of the LV pressure wave—does not change with increased heart rate. Therefore, tachycardia reduces the total diastolic time (e.g. "tachycardia robs diastole"). Because of reduced filling time, at some level of tachycardia output must fall. A normal young person can increase cardiac output until the heart rate reaches 170-180 beats/min; after that, output falls. An elderly person or anyone with a stiff ventricle may have cardiac output fall at rates above 140-150 beats/min.

Three things influence ventricular stroke volume: preload, afterload, and contractility.

FIGURE 1.1. Starling's Observation

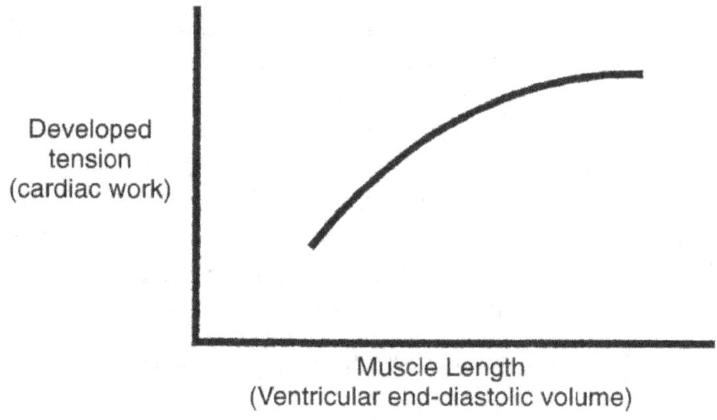

Figure 1.1. Increased muscle fiber length just before contraction (preload) increases strength of contraction. In the intact heart, increased diastolic filling (greater fiber length) increases cardiac output.

Preload

Precisely defined, preload is the length of a muscle fiber *before* contraction. When a strip of muscle is stimulated, it twitches and generates tension that can be measured. Within physiologic limits (meaning that the muscle is not overstretched to the point of injury), increasing the resting length produces a stronger contraction (Fig. 1.1). A century ago, Starling and others showed that this is true for heart muscle as well as for skeletal muscle.

In the intact heart, muscle fiber length is proportional to ventricular volume at the end of diastole. Thus, increased ventricular filling during diastole = increased preload and leads to more forceful contraction when the ventricle is stimulated. That is why volume expansion (salt and water retention) is a basic compensatory mechanism in heart failure. Increased vascular volume → increased venous return to both ventricles, an increase in ventricular diastolic volume, and higher stroke volume.

Because increasing preload increases stroke volume and cardiac output, it would seem that treatments to expand volume would be useful when ventricular function is depressed. The problem with this is that there is a limit to how much volume can be tolerated. When salt and water are retained so that the pulmonary capillary hydrostatic pressure exceeds 25 mm Hg, fluid is pushed into the interstitial space (basically, the oncotic pressure that keeps fluid in the vascular space has been overcome). Pulmonary congestion thus places a limit on the Starling mechanism's capacity to compensate for low cardiac output.

There often is confusion about diastolic function and ventricular compliance. Compliance means the ability to stretch. These terms relate to how easily the ventricle fills during diastole, when it is relaxed. While not quite the case, I think of the LV in diastole as a passive balloon that must be inflated. A compliant ventricle inflates easily, allowing adequate preloading of the ventricle (stretching of muscle fibers) to generate stroke volume. A stiff (noncompliant) ventricle is harder to inflate, and if filling is inadequate stroke volume suffers. Abnormal stiffness, or diastolic dysfunction, may result from hypertrophy, infiltrative cardiomyopathy, or ischemia, and diastolic heart failure is considered in detail in Chapter 2. When describing this to patients, point out that a stiff balloon is harder to blow up; more pressure is needed, and that pressure, shifting back to the body, is the pressure that pushes fluid from the vascular space into the lungs.

Afterload

This is the load the ventricle works against when it contracts. Aortic or pulmonic valve stenosis impedes flow and constitute increased afterload for their respective ventricles, and both induce hypertrophy. Hypertrophy of normal muscle always indicates a high afterload state. In the absence of ventricular outflow tract obstruction, vascular resistance and blood pressure provide rough approximations of afterload. Patients with hypertension have increased afterload, and LV hypertrophy is the basic problem of hypertensive heart disease.

On the other hand, afterload may be reduced without causing a drop in blood pressure. Ohm's law states that *pressure = flow × resistance.* Thus, a vasodilator drug that lowers resistance by20% but allows cardiac output (flow) to increase by 20% causes no change in blood pressure. That is why vasodilator therapy can be used in patients with CHF and low blood pressure.

On the ventricular function curve, a reduction in afterload produces a shift up and to the left (Fig. 1.2). Reducing afterload with vasodilator therapy improves ventricular performance and cardiac output without increasing the myocardium's workload.

Hypertrophy, Wall Tension, and Myocardial Oxygen Demand

The heart responds to increased afterload with an increase in contractility and, eventually, with hypertrophy. Myocardial oxygen demand is proportional to wall tension, and tension is determined by the interplay of ventricular pressure, chamber size, and wall thickness: Laplace's law (Table 1.4). A dilated ventricle thus has higher wall tension than a smaller one and requires more oxygen.

TABLE 1.4. Chamber Size, Wall Tension and Pressure: Laplace's Law
(A Physical Principle that Applies to Many Areas of Medicine)

The law of Laplace describes the determinants of wall stress ("tension") and applies to any "container" of a fluid volume that has measurable pressure. This would include chambers of the heart, blood vessels, airways, loops of bowel & the uterus; when dilated wall tension increases making the chamber more prone to rupture.

Wall tension = (Pressure) (Radius) / 2 (Wall thickness)

When applied to the left ventricle, wall stress (tension) is proportional to myocardial oxygen demand (MVO_2). A dilated left ventricle or one with pressure overload requires more oxygen. Increased LV thickness, hypertrophy, tends to normalize wall stress, and therefore MVO_2, of the pressure overloaded or dilated left ventricle. In this way, hypertrophy is a compensatory response to high afterload. Hypertrophy of the normal ventricle always indicates increased afterload. Patients with dilated cardiomyopathy and paper-thin LV walls do worse than those who maintain normal wall thickness.

This relationship is also important when gauging the possibility of rupture of an aneurysm, dilated loop of bowel, pulmonary bleb, etc. Increased the wall stress raises the chance of rupture. This is why we follow aortic aneurysm size with serial imaging studies.

Contractility

This third determinant of stroke volume is defined as an increase in the force of contraction when both preload and afterload are constant. Another name for contractility is the "inotropic" state. At the cellular level, calcium ions interact with the contractile proteins. Inotropic drugs, catecholamines or digitalis, increase the amount of calcium that enters the myocyte when it is stimulated. Reduced calcium influx depresses contractility (as with the calcium channel blocker, verapamil, and β-adrenergic blockers).

On the ventricular function curve, an increase in contractility leads to a shift in the curve to the left. There is an increase in stroke volume for a given preload (Fig. 1.2).

FIGURE 1.2. Manipulations That Alter the Ventricular Function Curve

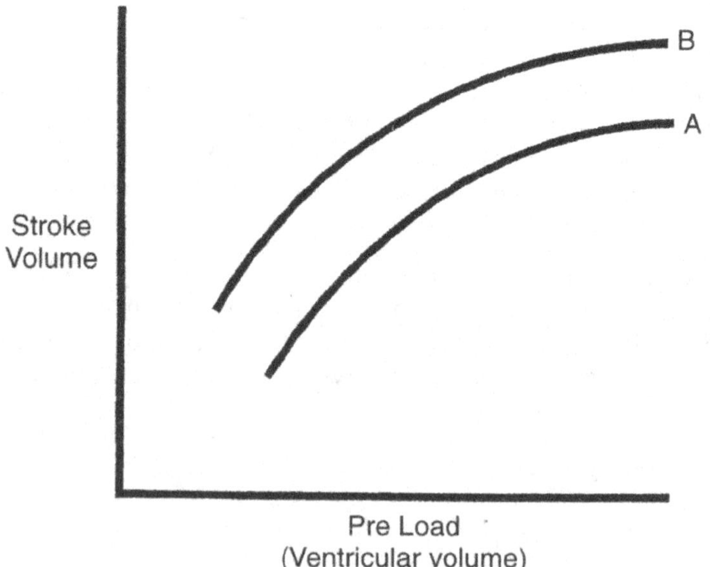

Figure 1.2 Increasing contractility or reducing afterload shift the curve up and to the left, from curve A to curve B. Thus, with either manipulation stroke volume is higher for a given preload. For this reason, drugs that augment contractility or reduce afterload are useful therapies for CHF. What about diuretics? They reduce vascular volume and thus reduce preload; the ventricular function curve does not shift, and the patient moves down and to the left on the same curve. Stroke volume falls, but this is a necessary intervention to reduce pulmonary congestion.

Ejection Fraction (EF)

A common measure of LV systolic function is ejection fraction, or that portion of blood ejected from the ventricle during systole. Thus, if the left ventricle contains 150 mL at the end of diastole and 50 mL at the end of systole, the LVEF is 67% and the stroke volume is 100 mL. It may be calculated by measuring the volume of the left ventricle at end-diastole and again at end-systole using the LV angiogram, echocardiogram, cardiac MRI, or CT angiogram. Because of the quality of newer imaging techniques, we seldom use the radionuclide angiogram (MUGA scan).

EF is a measure of muscle shortening, and like stroke volume, it depends on both contractility and loading conditions. Increased contractility and reduced afterload both increase EF. However, stroke volume and EF cannot be equated. A dilated left ventricle with a diastolic volume of 210 mL and an EF of 33% has a stroke volume of 70 mL. So does a normal ventricle of 140 mL and an EF of 50%. This simple math indicates another way that ventricular dilation compensates for LV dysfunction.

Neurohormonal Response to Low Cardiac Output

The immediate goal is maintenance of cardiac output and flow to vital organs, especially the kidneys which function as the hemodynamic "thermostat." Decreased renal blood flow turns on the renin-angiotensin-aldosterone system. Aldosterone promotes salt and water retention, boosting intravascular volume, ventricular preload and cardiac output. Another immediate response to inadequate cardiac output is an increase in sympathetic tone with elevation of circulating catecholamines. This increases heart rate and contractility. It now appears that a drop parasympathetic/vagal tone with depressed stroke volume is equally important. Activation of the adrenergic and renin-angiotensin systems, and shutting down the vagus nerve all cause vasoconstriction, which helps maintain blood pressure and flow to the kidneys and other vital organs. But a byproduct of increased vascular resistance is elevated LV afterload.

FIGURE 1.3. Ventricular Remodeling

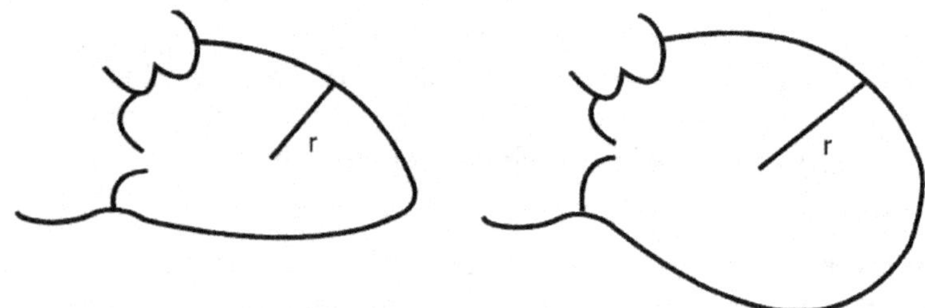

Figure 1.3 The left ventricle is normally an ellipsoid (left). With the development of cardiomyopathy, it enlarges and also changes shape, becoming more spherical (right). Both changes increase the radius of curvature (r), and this increases wall tension (see Table 1.4 for a description of Laplace's law). Wall tension is proportional to myocardial oxygen demand, so the remodeling process aggravates LV dysfunction.

These responses to depressed flow help restore cardiac output, short term. However, over the long run there may be negative consequences. (1) Adverse remodeling: salt and water retention increases total vascular volume leading to LV dilation, and this increases wall tension and therefore myocardial oxygen demand via the Laplace mechanism (Figure 1.3). (2) At persistently high levels the neurohormones appear to have direct cardiac toxicity.

Excessive adrenergic stimulation eventually depresses contractility. Like beating a worn out horse, it may work to improve short-term performance, but cannot long-term. (3) Elevated aldosterone may increase myocardial fibrosis. (4) Recent studies have shown that vagal nerve stimulation may improve function in patients with CHF; this suggests that shutting down the parasympathetic system—the vagus nerve—in response to low output has a negative effect.

HISTORY AND PHYSICAL EXAMINATION

Congestive heart failure is a clinical syndrome, and the diagnosis is based upon clinical findings of congestion. That is to say, a low LVEF is not the same as CHF unless the patient has associated symptoms. (This is a bit of nit-picking, since Class I CHF may be defined as low EF without symptoms—still, the diagnosis of CHF is a clinical syndrome.) Left heart failure causes progressively more severe pulmonary congestion: dyspnea with exertion, then orthopnea, then paroxysmal nocturnal dyspnea, then dyspnea at rest and pulmonary edema. Right heart failure causes peripheral and splanchnic congestion. You hear that LV failure is the most common cause of RV failure, and it is true. Curiously, an occasional patient with biventricular failure has severe peripheral edema and ascites with minimal or no pulmonary congestion. Increased pulmonary lymphatic flow may explain this. CHF in elderly patients may present as fatigue or a change in exercise tolerance, with little congestion.

History taking should include a survey for conditions that may cause or aggravate CHF: myocardial infarction with few or subtle symptoms, viral illnesses, a family history of cardiomyopathy, alcohol use (so often overlooked!), and gastrointestinal symptoms that would suggest blood loss and anemia.

General Examination

Note the overall state of health and vigor. Experienced clinicians know that frailty is not a nebulous physical finding, and its presence indicates a poor cardiac prognosis. When facing a high risk case, an experienced surgeon I know usually asked "how brightly does the fire of life burn in this person?"

Cardiac Cachexia

This is a diagnosis of exclusion. When weight loss develops in a patient with chronic heart failure, you must first exclude another etiology. Remember that occult bacterial endocarditis may cause weight loss in a patient with valvular disease. The pathophysiology of cachexia caused by heart failure is multifactorial. Anorexia is a common symptom of right heart failure because of splanchnic congestion. Rarely, right heart failure may cause protein-losing enteropathy. Severe salt restriction may aggravate anorexia, because food does not taste as good. Digitalis toxicity may contribute to anorexia, and this can be a factor even when the digoxin level is in the therapeutic range. There may also be increased caloric needs. Both increased cardiac work (i.e., with aortic stenosis or regurgitation) and the increased work of breathing with chronic pulmonary congestion raise caloric needs. More recently, patients with chronic heart failure have been found to have higher levels of the proinflammatory cytokine, tumor necrosis factor, and this may contribute to cachexia. Important physical findings include bitemporal and hypothenar wasting.

Vital Signs

Resting tachycardia—usually overlooked by students and house officers—is a powerful sign of decompensation and poor prognosis in a patient with chronic CHF. Hypotension and narrow pulse pressure (the difference between systolic and diastolic pressure) accompany low stroke volume. Wide pulse pressure, on the other hand, is a finding of aortic regurgitation, anemia and thyrotoxicosis.

Jugular Venous Pulse

There are three parts to this examination: estimation of venous pressure, testing for abdominojugular reflux, and assessment of the venous waveform.

Venous Pressure

The sternal angle, or angle of Lewis, is 5 cm above the level of the right atrium. Thus, if the top of the distended vein is 3 cm above the sternal angle, right atrial pressure is 8 cm H_2O. Pressure greater than 7 to 8 cm of water is abnormal. The patient may be examined in any position: With high pressure, you may not see the top of the venous column unless the patient is sitting upright. With low pressure, it may be necessary to have the patient almost flat to see a distended vein.

In most cases, high venous pressure indicates high right atrial pressure. An exception is *superior vena cava obstruction*. In this case, there is no venous pulsation, because the veins are isolated from the heart. Furthermore, the vein fills from above and not from below.

Abdominal Jugular Test (AJT)

Abdominojugular reflux was also called hepatojugular reflux (I admit to using HJR in my write-up). The maneuver is performed with the patient breathing normally (and not holding breath). Push down on the left periumbilical area for 10 seconds. In normal subjects, the venous pressure rises less than 3 cm and only transiently. A greater and more sustained rise occurs with *both right and left heart failure* and with tricuspid regurgitation. Although classically proposed as a test for *right heart* failure, one study found that patients with a positive AJT had elevation of both pulmonary wedge and right atrial pressures (probably because right heart failure is usually caused by left heart failure).

The AJT is especially useful in determining the cause of peripheral edema when there is no jugular venous distension. If the AJT is negative, heart failure is unlikely. The edema must be from some other cause (e.g., amlodipine therapy, veno-occlusive disease, low albumin, lymphatic obstruction—and I recently saw it with hypothyroidism).

The AJT is a go-to physical finding, often used to decide whether or not to increase the diuretic dose.

Jugular Venous Pulse Waveform

Another trick question from the attending: "What valve separates the right atrium from the vena cava?" There is none; it is an open system on both the right and left sides of the heart. Thus, atrial contraction pushes blood back to the veins as well as forward through the open A-V valve. Venous pressure waves are conveniently labeled: The A wave is generated by atrial contraction and the V wave, by ventricular contraction (Fig. 1.4).

To examine the jugular pulse, have the patient breathe normally in a position where you can see venous pulsation through the sternocleidomastoid muscle (the internal jugular pulse) or pulsation of the more easily seen external jugular vein. Feel the brachial pulse while watching the vein to tell systole from diastole. *If the dominant venous pulse is before the brachial pulse (arterial systole), it is an A wave. If the dominant pulse is simultaneous with the arterial pulse, it is a V wave.* On the chart I state what I have observed: "JVP: A > V" (a normal exam) or "V > A" (an abnormal finding).

The V wave is created by ventricular systole, normally by either backward bulging of the tricuspid valve leaflets or slight backward movement of the valve ring during ventricular contraction. The wave is normally quite small. With an incompetent tricuspid valve, the ventricle is no longer isolated from the atrium during systole, and ventricular systolic pressure is transmitted back to the neck veins (Fig. 1.4). A big V wave is not a subtle finding, and you have only to document that the dominant venous pulse wave is systolic (simultaneous with the arterial pulse). Look for a holosystolic murmur that increases with inspiration to confirm tricuspid regurgitation (negative intrathoracic sucks in blood as well as air, so right heart murmurs increase with inspiration).

A giant A wave indicates high RV diastolic pressures. This may occur with pulmonary hypertension (the Eisenmenger syndrome, primary pulmonary hypertension, or recurrent pulmonary emboli) or with pulmonic valve stenosis. RV failure does not cause a giant A wave unless there is also pulmonary hypertension.

FIGURE 1.4. Jugular Venous Tracings

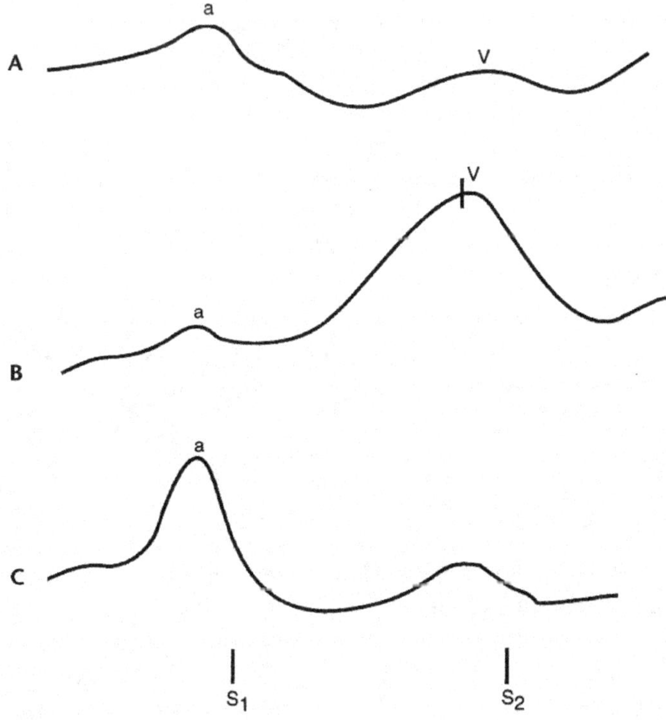

FIGURE 1.4. Jugular venous tracings from three patients. (A) Normal. The A wave is taller than the V wave. (B) Tricuspid regurgitation. There is a giant V wave, with transmission of RV pressure to the jugular veins because of the incompetent tricuspid valve. (C) Pulmonary hypertension. There is a giant A wave caused by elevated RV (and therefore right atrial) diastolic pressure.

Examination of the Chest

Inspection of the chest and the pattern of breathing shows little abnormality when CHF is mild or moderate. *Cheyne-Stokes respiration,* a cyclical breathing pattern with progressively deeper breaths followed by a brief period of apnea, may occur with end-stage heart failure. It is caused, in part, by decreased sensitivity of the respiratory canter of the brain to CO_2 and is more likely to develop in patients with neuropathology. It is aggravated by anything that further depresses the respiratory center, including sleep, narcotics, and some sedatives (particularly barbiturates).

Advanced obstructive lung disease with a barrel-shaped deformity of the chest may point to cor pulmonale as the cause of right heart failure. Kyphoscoliosis may also cause cor pulmonale.

Increased respiratory rate and greater effort of breathing may accompany severe pulmonary congestion and obstructive lung disease. *Patients with emphysema and hyperexpansion may not have audible rales with congestion; a chest x-ray is needed to exclude congestion (a common board question).*

Pleural Effusion

This may be a sign of either right heart or left heart congestion. The pleural space is drained by both the systemic and pulmonary circulations. Physical findings include deviation of the trachea away from the effusion, absence of fremitus (palpable breath sounds), dullness to percussion, and softer or absent breath sounds. Heart failure is the most common cause of effusion; when it is unilateral, it usually occurs on the <u>right side</u>. This seems odd, but isolated left-sided effusion suggests a noncardiac etiology (another board question).

Rales

This may be caused by heart or lung disease. I frequently hear inexperienced examiners describe rales as either "wet" (cardiac) or "dry" (pulmonary). However, when dealing with fine crackles, it is impossible to distinguish between the two based only on the quality of the sounds. More reliable is the *timing* of rales. With heart failure and interstitial congestion, fine crackles occur late in inspiration ("end-inspiratory rales"), and they are best heard at the bases of the lungs. Pulmonary fibrosis also causes fine crackles, but these rales are usually heard throughout inspiration ("pan-inspiratory rales"). Localization of pan-inspiratory rales to one side of the chest or to the upper lung fields further suggests fibrosis, but the rales of fibrosis may be widespread.

It helps to understand the mechanism of rales in heart failure with *interstitial* congestion. You are not hearing bubbles. Instead, opening of collapsed airways causes the crackles. In the absence of congestion, there is little airway closure during normal respiration. But lungs heavy with interstitial congestion have closure of small airways at a higher lung volume than is usual (it is the weight of the interstitium that is the problem). Thus, the airways close during normal expiration. To use the pulmonary physiology term, there is elevated "closing volume." With subsequent inspiration, an even higher lung volume is needed to pop open the collapsed units, and the rales are thus end-inspiratory.

Think of the mechanism of dyspnea. Arterial blood gases and oxygen saturation usually are normal in patients with mild CHF and dyspnea with exertion. It is the increased work of breathing—moving water logged lungs—that probably is responsible for dyspnea and "air hunger." This is usually the case with asthma as well. Try breathing through a drinking straw for 60 seconds; with this increase in airway resistance your blood gases will not change but you will feel terrible—it is the increased work of breathing.

Wheezing

This is usually a sign of airway obstruction. It may develop in a patient with pulmonary congestion ("cardiac asthma'). Occasionally, an acutely ill older patient with wheezing and severe dyspnea may not have audible rales. The absence of a history of asthma points to the cardiac diagnosis, and the chest x-ray readily confirms pulmonary congestion.

For that matter, when in doubt the chest x-ray provides the gold standard for diagnosis of congestion. In clinic, I find that measuring the BNP also helps distinguish between pulmonary disease and poor LV function as the cause of dyspnea.

Abdomen and Extremities

Hepatomegaly and peripheral edema are signs of right heart failure. When it develops rapidly, the swollen liver may be tender. Ascites may develop with chronic congestion, especially when caused by constrictive pericarditis or tricuspid regurgitation. In such cases there may also be splenomegaly. Peripheral edema and jugular venous distension are present when CHF causes hepatomegaly.

Pitting edema is found over the lower legs in the ambulatory patient. The bedridden patient may have edema only in the sacral area. When checking for edema I avoid hard pressure; gentle kneading with a fingertip effectively elicits pitting, and this approach seems more sophisticated than aggressively mashing a patient's swollen leg. Edema caused by heart failure is bilateral, and unilateral edema suggests venous obstruction.

Cardiac Examination

Apical Impulse

The location of the point of maximum impulse (PMI) should be determined with the patient lying flat. Its normal location is the midclavicular line and fifth intercostal space. It is tapping in quality and occupies a space of no more than 2 cm. LVH may not displace the PMI, but it becomes more forceful, like a fist hitting your hand. Systolic dysfunction, volume overload and LV dilation cause displacement of the PMI toward the anterior axillary line and enlargement of the apex beat so that it may be felt in more than one interspace. The volume overload apical impulse is diffuse and rocking in quality.

An RV impulse is not palpable in normal patients. RV pressure or volume overload produces a "lift" along the left parasternal border. When the lift is forceful and sustained, it suggests pressure overload. Volume overload causes a lift that is not sustained through systole.

The parasternal lift may be augmented by left atrial enlargement. The atrium is behind the right ventricle, and pushes it forward when enlarged. A rare patient with severe mitral regurgitation and left atrial enlargement may have a late-systolic parasternal lift in the absence of RV enlargement.

Emphysema

This changes the position of the heart in the chest. There is clockwise rotation, and the left ventricle is more posterior. The heart appears to hang vertically on the chest x-ray. The PMI that is felt in the subxyphoid region comes from the right ventricle, not the left. A forceful and sustained apex beat in this position may reflect RV hypertrophy secondary to pulmonary hypertension (cor pulmonale).

Heart Sounds

CHF usually has little effect on the first or second heart sounds (S_1 and S_2). With advanced heart failure and severely depressed cardiac output, the intensity of both sounds may be diminished. An especially loud S_1 may be an early finding of mitral valve stenosis, pointing to this as a cause of CHF Similarly, an absent A_2 may indicate severe calcific aortic stenosis in an elderly patient. The rigid valve eventually stops moving, and A_2 disappears. To detect this, listen in both the pulmonic and aortic areas. P_2 is audible at the left sternal border but not to the right of the sternum. Thus, an absent S_2 at the right base indicates an immobile and probably stenotic aortic valve.

Gallops

Think for a moment about the significance of gallops and the quality of the apical impulse. They are the physical findings that give you direct information about the diastolic state of the ventricle. Murmurs get a lot of attention, but they do not tell us much about the severity of disease. The gallops do just that: they tell us about ventricular size and compliance (the reverse of stiffness), and provide insight into function.

S_3 Gallop

Big Flabby Ventricle (Volume Overload) The low-pitched vibration in early diastole comes from rapid ventricular filling. The mechanism is related to both high flow and the recipient ventricle being dilated and compliant. Any condition that causes ventricular dilation and low cardiac output (with compensatory volume overload) may cause an S_3. It is the hallmark finding of cardiomyopathy. When an S_3 develops after myocardial infarction, it indicates substantial injury and worse prognosis.

S_4 Gallop

Stiff, Noncompliant Ventricle ("Pressure" Overload) This gallop at the end of diastole corresponds to elevation of the ventricular end-diastolic pressure and the A wave of the precordial impulse (Fig. 1.5). It may be called the "atrial gallop," because the atrium "kicking" the last bit of blood into a stiff ventricle causes vibration and the low-pitched sound. The S_4 is absent when there is no atrial kick (e.g., atrial fibrillation, ventricular pacing, nodal or ventricular rhythms, or complete heart block). Any increase in ventricular stiffness may cause an S_4, including ventricular hypertrophy, infiltrative disease, and ischemia.

FIGURE 1.5, S_4 Gallop

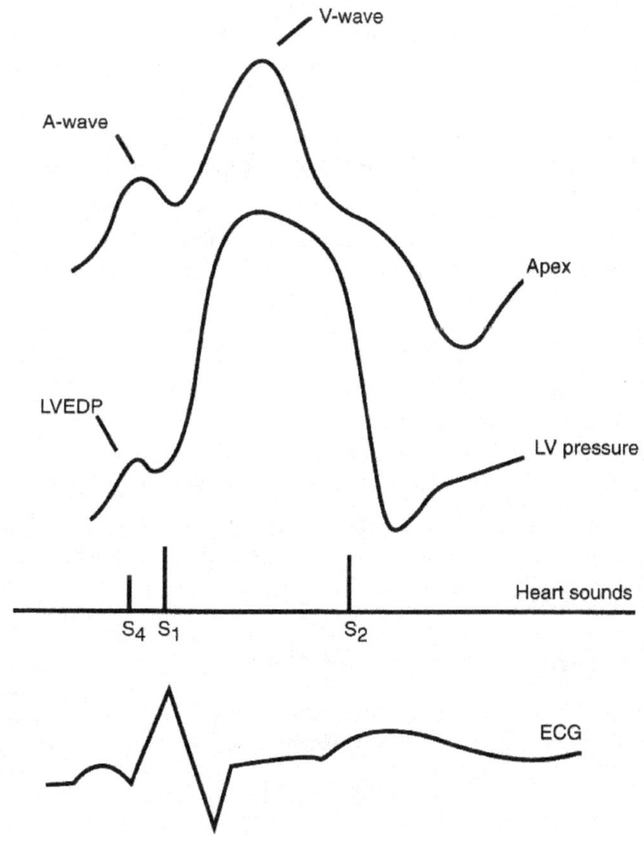

FIGURE 1.5. The contour of the apical impulse (top tracing) mirrors the LV pressure tracing. Just before ventricular systole, atrial contraction causes a small rise in LV pressure that is measured as the LV end diastolic pressure (LVEDP). This is elevated in conditions that increase LV stiffness. It makes sense; the atrium is kicking into a ventricle that has higher pressure during diastole (it is stiff when it should be relaxed). When the apical A wave is greater than 15% of the total apical excursion, it is palpable as a shudder or glitch on the upstroke of the impulse. With practice, it is not difficult to feel, especially with the patient rolled to the left side.

Note that we referred to "ventricular" rather than "left ventricular" gallops. RV disease may produce gallop sounds, best heard over the left parasternal area. They may be subxyphoid in the patient with obstructive lung disease. RV gallops are augmented by inspiration (increased venous return and flow to the right ventricle). I have had little luck hearing the right-sided S_3 gallop; look for it with tricuspid regurgitation and isolated right heart failure. The right-sided S_4 that accompanies pulmonary hypertension is easier to hear (note the parallel with LV disease: Volume overload causes the S_3; pressure overload, the S_4).

When the heart rate is fast, it may be impossible to determine whether the gallop occurs early or late in diastole. An occasional patient with ventricular dilation may also have increased stiffness and thus have both S_3 and S_4 gallops that are fused when heart rate is elevated. In both cases, the patient is said to have a "summation" gallop. A "gallop rhythm" refers to this combination of sounds when the rate is high (it sounds like a galloping horse).

Box 1.1 Gallops Are Difficult to Hear

They are soft, low pitched sounds. A good way to hear a gallop is to concentrate on the segment of the cardiac cycle where it should be found. Thus, to hear an S_3, listen to the space just after S_2, ignoring all other cardiac sounds. Ask yourself, "is anything there?" If there is a soft thud, you are probably hearing the S_3. Occasionally, the gallop is something you feel rather than hear. If you are convinced there is nothing in that space, there is no gallop.

A gallop may be more audible with the patient rolled to the left side. The room must be quiet. Because the sounds are low pitched, use the bell of the stethoscope, taking care not to press too firmly (which would, by tensing the underlying skin, make it work like the diaphragm). The S_3 may be localized, and you must carefully survey the apex and areas close to it. It may be hard to hear gallops in the patient with a thick chest wall. In such cases, the S_4 may be easier to hear over the sternum, aided by bone conduction of sound. The timing of gallops is easier with a hand on the brachial pulse to identify systole. The S_4 is a presystolic sound and the S_3, an early diastolic sound.

Heart Murmurs

A loud murmur may indicate that the cause of heart failure is valvular disease (see Chapter 3). On the other hand, ventricular dilation tends to distort the orientation of the papillary muscles, and this may cause mild tricuspid or mitral regurgitation. The resulting systolic murmur is usually soft. Mitral regurgitation can become substantial with marked dilation, and significant regurgitation indicates a poor prognosis in patients with dilated cardiomyopathy. Mitral valve repair has been the mainstay of heart failure surgery, and is being replaced by the mitraclip procedure.

LABORATORY EXAMINATION

In addition to the history and physical examination, the workup of new CHF would include the studies outlined in Table 1.5. These tests are used to determine causes of CHF or to exclude conditions that may aggravate it, and to define the state of the LV.

If the echocardiogram is technically inadequate (often a problem with large patients or those with emphysema), a *radionuclide angiogram (RNA)*, also called a MUGA scan, may be used to measure LVEF (Box 1.1). This test and the echocardiogram can also be used to assess LV regional wall motion. Coronary artery disease and infarction causes regional dysfunction, whereas global hypokinesis is more consistent with idiopathic dilated cardiomyopathy.

The workup of new CHF with low LV ejection fraction is largely about excluding coronary artery disease. I ask students for a strategy to do this and they usually begin talking about perfusion imaging or cardiac catheterization. However, clinical evaluation helps us decide who needs angiography. A history of heart attack and chest pain (don't forget the history!), Q waves on the ECG and regional wall motion abnormalities with LV imaging suggest ischemic cardiomyopathy; the next step is angiography. With global LV hypokinesis, no Qs and no history to indicate CAD, a perfusion scan may be adequate. CT angiography is a noninvasive approach that reliably excludes stenosis of larger coronary arteries. But with uncertainty, angiography is indicated ("the dye don't lie").

Table 1.5 outlines additional laboratory work-up to consider in special situations.

TABLE 1.5. Evaluation of New-onset Congestive Heart Failure

Procedure/Laboratory Study: Clinical Issue(s)

History: Symptoms of heart failure? Survey for causes of CHF (Table 1.1). History of heart attack? Functional class.

Physical exam: Document congestion (CHF is a clinical diagnosis)

Blood count: Anemia (may aggravate CHF; exclude high output failure)

Serum chemistry profile: Electrolyte disturbances; Diabetes mellitus; Renal insufficiency

Thyroid function tests: Hyper/hypothyroidism (especially with atrial fibrillation and over age 65)

Urinalysis: Proteinuria (nephrotic syndrome, acute glomerulonephritis-both causes of edema)

ECG: Q waves; Ventricular hypertrophy; Incessant tachycardia (arrhythmia)

Chest x-ray: Confirm congestion as the cause of dyspnea (especially important when there is obstructive lung disease); Pulmonary infiltrates/fibrosis; Presence of pleural effusion; Cardiomegaly (although the echocardiogram is more accurate)

Echocardiogram: Differentiate systolic vs. diastolic dysfunction; Wall motion abnormalities (coronary artery disease as etiology); Valvular abnormalities; Pericardial effusion; Intracardiac masses, abnormal muscle morphology

Stress perfusion imaging or coronary angiography? See text.

Ambulatory monitoring in hypertrophic CM and arrythmogenic RV dysplasia (ARVD)

Cardiac MRI: In some cases, better than echo for defining anatomy (i.e., arrhythmogenic RV dysplasia); determines extent and pattern of scarring which may influence therapy.

Less common causes of CHF require other studies. For example, angiotensin converting enzyme (ACE) level may be elevated with sarcoidosis (although cardiac involvement is a later manifestation of the disease), serum iron studies would be needed to diagnose hemochromatosis, toxicology screen may help identify drug abuse or heavy metal intoxication, sedimentation rate and serologies would be needed to diagnose collagen vascular disease, etc.

Endomyocardial Biopsy

The rationale for biopsy is detection of a treatable illness. Abnormal biopsies are uncommon; a histological diagnosis was apparent in just 17% of a series of 673 patients referred with new onset heart failure and low LV ejection fraction. The most common abnormal finding was lymphocytic infiltration suggesting prior or current viral infection.

Unfortunately, the results of immunosuppressive treatment for those with inflammation have been disappointing, so biopsy is not a part of the routine work-up of new onset CHF. Less common causes of cardiomyopathy may be diagnosed by biopsy (Table 1.6). Finding giant cell or sarcoid myocarditis is the best rationale for biopsy in the individual patient, since these conditions may respond to steroid therapy. Wu and colleagues have suggested limiting biopsy to patients with the following characteristics:

Acute CHF refractory to medical therapy
Rapidly deteriorating LV ejection fraction despite therapy and with no clear etiology
CHF plus ventricular tachycardia or heart block
CHF plus rash or eosinophilia or fever
Associated illness that can cause of CHF (i.e., collagen vascular disease, infiltrative diseases such as amyloid, sarcoid or hemochromatosis)

Brain Natriuretic Peptide

BNP is synthesized and released from ventricular myocardium in response to myocyte stretch (it was first isolated from brain, hence the confusing name). It is more than just a biomarker: beneficial actions include natriuresis, sympathetic and renin-angiotensin system blockade, and direct venous and arterial dilation. When the LV fails and there is an increase in LV diastolic pressure and fiber length, there is a rise in BNP; a normal level excludes decompensated heart failure. This is true for both LV systolic and diastolic dysfunction. BNP measurement may prove useful when sorting out the cause of dyspnea for a patient with both heart and lung disease. (A caveat: BNP can be falsely low with obesity.)

Some studies have shown that marked elevation of BNP (above 500 pg/mL) indicates poor prognosis. More useful is the trend in BNP in the individual patient. When it does not fall during hospitalization for CHF exacerbation there is a higher incidence of readmission. Conversely, a BNP below the patient's baseline is a good sign. Having a baseline BNP is a definite aid when making management decisions.

Indicators of Poor Prognosis in CHF

When I ask students about this, they usually begin speculating about LV ejection fraction and laboratory measurements. A better approach to such questions is a more systematic survey beginning with the history and physical examination; that is how we will approach it in Table 1.6.

Table 1.6 Indicators of Prognosis in CHF

Advanced age: True of most illnesses and a good initial answer for the attending while trying to think of other possibilities.

Ischemic etiology

Functional Class: The most important historical marker of prognosis (and more useful than any laboratory finding). Frailty and weight loss are related findings. See Table 1.1. Think about large heart failure trials. The initial criterion for inclusion is functional class.

Comorbidities: Renal insufficiency is the most important, but prognosis is worse with lung disease, diabetes, anemia, uncontrolled hypertension, etc.

Resting tachycardia: Often overlooked by students and house staff, it is a physical finding indicating decompensation and neurohormonal activation (a high circulating catecholamine level, reduced vagal tone).

S3 gallop: Mentioned by some but not all studies, possibly because the finding is difficult to document.

Hyponatremia: Serum sodium is inversely proportional to plasma renin activity; when sodium is low it thus indicates current decompensation (the RAAS is turned on).

Elevated BNP: See text.

Notably absent from this table is LV ejection fraction. In general, low LVEF does indicate poor prognosis, especially in population studies, but it is not as useful as functional class in predicting an individual's future. An occasional patient with LVEF 35% is disabled and does poorly, while another with LVEF 20% continues to work.

PHARMACOLOGIC TREATMENT OF CONGESTIVE HEART FAILURE

The treatment of CHF with reduced LV ejection fraction—HfrEF--involves a variety of approaches:

      Relieve congestion (diuresis)
      Manipulating hemodynamics (preload and afterload)
      Increasing contractility

Blocking neurohormones
(catecholamines and aldosterone)
Preventing sudden death
(implantable defibrillator therapy)
Correcting LV dyssynchrony (biventricular pacing)
Surgery (coronary bypass, mitral valve repair, heart
transplantation)

As you read through the following, pay attention to those therapies found to improve survival. If you choose not to use one of them, the reason should be documented in the medical record.

Nonpharmacologic Measures

These should be adopted in every case. Salt restriction is essential. Most patients benefit from modest fluid restriction, drinking only when thirsty. Our heart failure service advises fluid restriction (<2000 ml per day) for those requiring $\geq$ 80 mg furosemide per day to control congestion, or for patients with serum sodium $\leq$ 140 meq/dL. We recommend continued aerobic exercise even for those with moderate to severe symptoms. Abstinence from alcohol is critical for those with dilated cardiomyopathy, and thiamine can lead to dramatic recovery of LV function for alcoholics with poor nutrition.

Beta Adrenergic Blockade

Patients with CHF have elevated circulating norepinephrine levels. An adrenergic surge is helpful (adaptive) for acute decompensation, but unremitting stimulation is toxic (maladaptive). On the other hand, some beta adrenergic support is needed by the failing heart, and overly aggressive blockade has adverse effects. This may explain the small subset of patients in clinical trials who get worse with beta blockade. The current treatment strategy aims at balance between excessive stimulation and blockade.

Beta blockade is the most potent therapy for systolic CHF. There has been no study directly comparing beta blockade and ACE inhibition, but a review of available trials yields this estimate: the one-year mortality with class II-III CHF is about 13%. With ACE inhibition, it falls by 2.5 percentage points. Adding a beta blocker to the ACE inhibitor lowers it another 4-5 percentage points. Because beta blockade was studied after the efficacy of ACE inhibition was established, most patients in beta blocker trials were on ACE inhibitors.

Our experience in cardiology clinic supports the importance of beta blockade. It is common to witness a dramatic improvement in clinical status. Most have a rise in LV ejection fraction, and a quarter of patients have LVEF increase by more than 15 percentage points. Those with the greatest rise in LVEF have the best prognosis. The number of heart transplantation operations declined after introduction of beta blockade for CHF. One of our transplant specialists commented that "we are just buying the CHF patients time," but that, of course, is what we do with transplantation, and with any life-prolonging treatment.

Most of the beta blockade trials included patients with class II-III CHF, although carvedilol was found useful for those with class IV heart failure. Two beta blockers are commonly used: carvedilol with a target dose of 25 mg twice daily, or long acting metoprolol, 200 mg per day. At this time there is no clear-cut benefit with either drug when treating patients with class II-III CHF. Carvedilol may be preferable for the class IV patient. Clinical trials results have been comparable with bisprolol, bucindolol and nebivolol. Carvedilol and nebivolol are direct vasodilators and are both alpha and beta adrenergic blockers. Because of this combined action, it has been suggested that they may be more effective for black patients.

Like most guidelines directed medical therapy (GDMT) for heart failure, both carvedilol and long-acting metoprolol are available as generics, and are inexpensive.

On the other hand, selection of a drug may be influenced by clinical status. Consider using carvedilol for the black patient with marked blood pressure elevation, since it is a more potent antihypertensive agent than a pure beta blocker. Another special situation is the patient with bronchospasm. We generally avoid beta blockers, but the cardioselective agent, metoprolol, may be tolerated at lower dose by those with obstructive lung disease. Our heart failure clinic considers beta blockade important enough that they routinely try metoprolol for these patients with both CHF and advanced lung disease.

When initiating beta blockade there is myocardial depression (withdrawal of beta adrenergic support), followed by improvement. This should be avoided with decompensated CHF. When the patient is stable, beta blockers are started at one-sixteenth to one-eighth of the target dose. The dose is then increased every 2-3 weeks. I warn patients they will experience fatigue when starting or raising the dose of medicine: "you are used to an elevated adrenaline effect, and when we dial that back, you will experience a temporary set-back until your system adjusts." I emphasize that over the long run, this therapy is their best chance to feel better and live longer, but that patience and perseverance will be needed while adjusting the dose. With frequent follow-up and coaching, 90% can reach the target dose. *The most common error made by primary care providers treating CHF is the failure to uptitrate the beta blocker dose.*

When the patient's heart rate falls to 60 beats per minute, there is adequate beta blockade, and there is no need for a further increase in the dose. Bradycardia is a contraindication to beta blocker therapy, and special care is needed when the systolic blood pressure is under 100 mmHg.

Ivabradine

This is a selective sinus node inhibitor, so it lowers heart rate without an effect on the myocardium. The SHIFT trial documented reduced hospitalization (and thus symptom improvement), with no effect on survival. Consider it for the patients with persistent tachycardia despite maximum dose beta blockade or when beta blockade is contraindicated. Since it works on the sinus node it is of no value for the patient with atrial fibrillation.

Afterload Reduction Therapy

Angiotensin Converting Inhibitors

ACE inhibitors block the conversion of angiotensin I to angiotensin II, which is a potent vasoconstrictor. Afterload reduction is an attractive strategy since cardiac output increases without an increase in cardiac work; the myocardium uses no more oxygen. It is one of those rare times in life that you get something for nothing.

ACE inhibitor therapy is indicated for CHF of all levels of severity, and for those with asymptomatic LV dysfunction (LVEF < 35%). It has been shown to improve survival in patients with severe congestive heart failure as well as to retard the progression of heart failure in patients with less severe disease. Note that patients with advanced aortic stenosis or LV outflow tract obstruction usually do not benefit from ACE inhibition, since their high afterload is structural, and lowering peripheral vascular resistance will not change it (an exception may be the patient with coexisting hypertension).

Though most of the earlier heart failure studies were performed using enalapril or captopril, the benefits of ACE inhibition are felt to be a class effect. Higher dose therapy yields the best results. Our heart failure clinic pushes the dose until the patient has postural dizziness, then backs off.

ACE inhibitors may also prevent CHF. The HOPE trial found that ramapril led to a 23% reduction in the development of heart failure in a population with stable vascular disease. The benefit was greatest in—but not limited to—those with elevated blood pressure, and it was not the result of preventing myocardial infarction.

The most common adverse effect of ACE inhibitors is cough (in as many as 10-15%). It is caused by potentiation of bradykinin and does not resolve with cough suppressants. It is an intolerable side effect and there is an equally effective alternative; any suggestion of ACE inhibitor cough should prompt switching to an angiotensin receptor blocker (ARB). Less common is angioedema, which can be mild or severe; it requires discontinuation of ACE inhibitors with no rechallenge. The risk of recurrent angioedema when switch to and ARB is low (not zero); making that switch is common practice. ACE inhibitors are contraindicated in pregnancy due to fetal and neonatal morbidity and mortality.

Hyponatremia, Renal Dysfunction, and Practical Tips When Starting ACE Inhibitor Therapy

Renal dysfunction may occur with ACE inhibition when there is renal artery stenosis. Maintaining adequate perfusion across the stenosed artery depends on high blood pressure, the result of elevated renin activity. Blocking the renin effect brings blood pressure down, leading to renal ischemia and a rise in creatinine. *Check electrolytes a couple days after starting ACE inhibitors; if creatinine rises by ≥ 0.3 mg/dL stop the drug and evaluate for renal artery stenosis (there is no need to wait longer to check creatinine).*

On the other hand, elevation of creatinine is not a contraindication for use of ACE inhibitors or ARBs. In fact, most kidney diseases—with the exception of renal artery stenosis—benefit from ACE inhibition. But renal dysfunction indicates a need for careful monitoring when starting therapy. Hyperkalemia is another, uncommon side effect of ACE inhibition, and it usually occurs when there is renal dysfunction.

Patients with CHF often have low serum sodium, and hyponatremia is a marker of poor prognosis. Serum sodium is inversely proportional to plasma renin activity (PRA). Those with high PRA are especially sensitive to ACE inhibitors. When there is hyponatremia start with a lower than usual dose to avoid hypotension.

Hypotension may also occur with volume depletion. Remember that volume depletion increases the chance of symptomatic hypotension when starting any vasodilator. A "diuretic holiday"–holding furosemide for a couple days–before starting the ACE inhibitor may help the patient with borderline low blood pressure, or when you feel that the patient is dry. It is particularly useful when the serum sodium is below 140 meq/dl. By the same token, if your patient becomes hypotensive after starting ACE inhibitors, you might try backing off diuretics, then restarting the drug at a lower dose.

Angiotensin II Receptor Blockers (ARBs)

Comparative trials have found that ARBs (irbesartan, candesartan, losartan, valsartan, etc.) are as effective as ACE inhibitors for CHF.

Why not just use an ARB (avoiding the possibility of ACE inhibitor cough and blocking all angiotensin II)? Some of the beneficial effect of ACEI therapy comes from the potentiation of bradykinin and increased production of nitric oxide. ARBs have no effect on this.

Sacubitril/Valsartin (Entresto)

The Paradigm-HF trial showed lower mortality and heart failure hospitalization with the addition of the neprilysin inhibitor to an ARB. Criteria for entry to the study were Class II-III heart failure and LVEF below 40%. When a study documents reduced hospitalization that usually translates to symptomatic improvement, and that has been the experience with Entresto. Note that there should be a 72 hour washout of the ACEI or ARB before starting it.

Afterload Reduction with Other Vasodilators

Hydralazine is a potent vasodilator but is tough to use. A short half-life requires giving it at least three times a day. High doses are needed to achieve a demonstrable hemodynamic effect. In the clinic, I commonly see a patient who is on hydralazine 25 mg twice a day for "afterload reduction." At that dose, do not assume you are doing much good.

Having said that, afterload reduction using the combination of two old drugs, hydralazine and isosorbide dinitrite suggested a particular benefit in black patients. There is a benefit even when BiDil (the combination pill) is added to ACE inhibitors. Among the suggested mechanisms is the antioxidant effect of hydralazine which may prevent nitrate tolerance, making more NO available to improve endothelial function. BiDil has hydralazine 37.5 mg + ISDN 20 mg; begin with 1 thrice daily, and double it if tolerated. The combination is not generic and is expensive.

Increasing Contractility (Inotropic Therapy)

Having raised the awareness of possible toxicity, in practice it seldom is a problem. Decades ago, the standard dose of digoxin was 0.25 mg/day. The DIG trial used 0.125 mg/day, and now that is the standard dose. With normal renal function, toxicity is rare. It can be safely used in patients with renal dysfunction by reducing dosing frequency. Start a patient with modest creatinine elevation on 0.125 mg on a Monday-Wednesday-Friday schedule, and then check a digoxin level in a month.

Recurrent hospitalization, common with end-of-life heart failure, is a definite indication. For the heart failure patient with advanced symptoms and nothing seems to help, it is remarkable how often adding digoxin makes a big difference. It is also remarkable how often this effective therapy is forgotten (in large heart failure trials including class IV patients just 30% of patients are being treated with digoxin).

Inotrope Infusion

This is used for acutely decompensated heart failure, especially for the patient who is hypotensive or who has progressive renal dysfunction with diuretic therapy. This inotropic approach reverses the hemodynamic abnormalities of cardiac decompensation. Cardiac output increases, and pulmonary wedge pressure falls. However, it does not shorten hospital stay, prevent readmission or improve survival. We still use it to control the symptoms of a patient with end-stage disease.

Intravenous *dobutamine* stimulates beta 1 and 2 receptors, raising cardiac output and lowering systemic and pulmonary vascular resistance, usually without raising heart rate. The cardiac selective actions of this and other catecholamines are lost at higher doses. An alternative is *milrinone* which may have less effect on heart rate and ventricular ectopy. Home therapy is possible with either of these drugs with supervision by a visiting nurse—hospice nurses often have experience with it. The dose is determined in hospital either (1) with pulmonary artery pressure monitoring, or (2) by observing heart rate, blood pressure, urine output and symptoms. On the other hand, this is palliative therapy, and we do not feel that you are obligated to transfer a patient with end-stage heart failure to a tertiary center for hemodynamic monitoring in order to use this treatment. Start with a low dose and raise it until there is a slight rise in blood pressure, without an increase in heart rate. Back off if there is increased ventricular ectopy. You should then see improved urine output.

Note that intravenous catecholamine therapy is reserved for the patient with end-stage disease. While it clearly improves symptoms, there have been no large clinical trials that establish safety. Many who work in this area suspect there may be a negative effect on survival, but agree that it is justified for palliation. Dopamine is an alternative to dobutamine, and tradition holds that it favorably affects renal blood flow. When tested, it had no specific renal benefits. Dobutamine is our first choice for chronic infusion therapy because it has less effect on heart rate.

Spironolactone and Eplerenone

Spironolactone will be discussed as a diuretic in the following section. It receives separate attention here because is one of the 4 medicines that have been shown to improve survival with HFrEF (the others are beta blockers, ACEI/ARB's, and Entresto). The Rales Trial found a 30% in all-cause mortality with spironolactone 25 mg/day. At this dose spironolactone is not an effective diuretic. It is thought that persistently elevated aldosterone—common with marginally compensated heart failure—is toxic to myocardium (an effect on myocardial fibrosis has been postulated). Blocking this effect with either spironolactone or the selective aldosterone antagonist, eplerenone (the Ephesus trial), promotes survival.

The aldosterone blocking therapies are contraindicated with renal insufficiency or hyperkalemia.

Preload Reduction: Diuretics

Congestion, either systemic or pulmonary, is the most problematic symptom with advanced CHF. Note that diuresis— a reduction in ventricular preload—does not improve ventricular function. On the contrary, it moves the patient down and to the left on the ventricular function curve, Figure 1.2. Nor does it improve survival—it is not on the list of treatments that will help the patient live longer. It is obvious that the patient with severe pulmonary edema is rescued by diuretic therapy. But prophylactic use of diuretics in the absence of congestion is not indicated.

Loop diuretics are used because of their potency. Furosemide is the cheapest, and we all have extensive experience with it. But bioavailability varies, and furosemide resistance is common. On average, about 50% of an oral dose is absorbed, but the range is 10% to 90%, making it difficult to know how much a particular patient is getting. We solve this by gradually increasing the dose until there is diuresis. The rate of absorption is slowed in heart failure, even more when there is splanchnic edema, so the effective dose may vary with the patient's condition.

The problem of variable absorption is compounded by reduced renal responsiveness to all loop diuretics in patients with advanced CHF, by as much as 70% compared with normals. Renal insufficiency further impairs delivery of Lasix to the site of action; there is reduced secretion of the drug into urine in the proximal tubule, so delivery to the distal tubule is reduced. The net effect is "diuretic resistance."

The maximum effect with Lasix is achieved with a daily intravenous dose of 160-200 mg. Above this there is little increase in natriuresis, and the risk of tinnitus increases. A hospitalized patient with severe pulmonary congestion may need this high intravenous dose several times a day. The maximum effective oral dose is about twice the intravenous dose when renal function is normal, but higher still with renal insufficiency.

When a patient requires high doses of oral Lasix, there may be poor absorption of the drug. That is the time to switch to one of the newer loop diuretics, bumetanide (Bumex) or torsemide (Demadex). Like furosemide they are secreted into the urine in the proximal tubule and act on the distal tubule. The difference is that bioavailability with oral dosing is much better, with at least 80% absorbed even in the presence of splanchnic congestion or renal insufficiency. They are metabolized and excreted by the liver, and the elimination half-life is not affected by renal insufficiency. However, renal insufficiency does reduce the secretion of drug into the proximal tubule, so higher doses are needed.

When treating the patient with intravenous medicines, there is no advantage of Bumex or Demadex over Lasix. However, with oral therapy, more reliable absorption makes the newer drugs almost as effective as intravenous Lasix. When comparing the newer drugs, the major difference is elimination half-life, which is longer for Demadex.

Another issue is whether to give loop diuretics once or twice a day, especially since the half-life is brief. Early in the course of CHF, when congestion is easily controlled, there is no reason for multiple doses. As congestion worsens, twice-daily dosing may be needed. With Lasix or Bumex, morning and noon dosing frees the evening for other activities. Because of its longer half-life, oral doses of Demadex should be separated by 6 hours.

Using Multiple Diuretics

There is synergy between the thiazide and loop diuretics, and adding an oral thiazide is the next step for the unresponsive patient. Thiazides work more distally in the nephron, blocking the absorption of sodium that escapes the loop of Henle (and thus, the action of the loop diuretic). Metolazone (Zaroxolyn) has been marketed for this purpose in the United States. However, hydrochlorothiazide (HCTZ) is more rapidly absorbed, has a shorter half-life (hours rather than 2 days), and is cheaper. For these reasons, HCTZ may be the preferable drug. That said, metolazone is the more commonly used thiazide when a second diuretic is needed.

With the addition of metolazone—a thiazide diuretic--there is an increased risk of hypokalemia.

An occasional patient resistant to loop and thiazide diuretics will respond to a potassium-sparing diuretic, such as spironolactone, that acts on the distal nephron. Clinical responsiveness can be predicted by measuring urine electrolytes. Low urinary sodium and high potassium suggest that potassium is being exchanged for sodium in the distal nephron (the aldosterone mechanism), and spironolactone should help. If urinary potassium is low, spironolactone probably will not be effective. The half-life of spironolactone is sufficient for once-daily dosing (50-200 mg/day). It may take a couple of weeks before diuresis begins. Note that the diuretic dose of spironolactone is higher than the dose recommended for its survival benefit in HFrEF.

Another benefit of spironolactone can be its effect on electrolytes. In addition to its potassium sparing effects, 50 mg spironolactone given daily has been shown to raise serum magnesium 10-15%. With all diuretic therapy, electrolytes must be monitored.

Remember that sudden death is common with CHF; the mechanism is ventricular fibrillation. Either hypokalemia or hypomagnesemia may provoke ventricular arrhythmias in the failing heart. There is loss of potassium and magnesium with loop and thiazide diuretics; the most profound losses seem to occur with thiazides, even though the diuretic effect is less.

Treatment of Anemia

Cardiac output is the product of heart rate and stroke volume, but oxygen carrying capacity is also directly proportional to hematocrit. Lower it from 40% to 30%, and oxygen delivery is reduced by 25%, just as it would be with a 25% reduction in cardiac output. Low-grade anemia, usually the anemia of chronic disease, commonly accompanies heart failure, and is an independent predictor of mortality.

Small pilot studies of patients with poor symptom control despite good medical therapy pushed hemoglobin from a baseline of 10 gm% to about 12 gm% with intravenous iron and/or subcutaneous erythropoietin. In general, functional class and diuretic requirements improved.   There has been no clear survival benefit.

Sodium-Glucose Co-Transporter 2 Inhibitors (SGLT2): Dapagliflozin

This is the most recent addition to HF therapies shown to have a favorable effect on symptoms, hospitalization rate, and mortality with HFrEF. The diabetes drug, dapagliflozin 10 mg/day, was granted FDA approval in May 2020 for treatment of Class II-IV HF for patients with or without diabetes. In the DAPA-HF trial side effects were infrequent and mild. The benefit seemed greater with class II than class II-IV HF. Like other medical therapies for HF, it is likely a class effect.

Biventricular Pacing: Cardiac Resynchronization Therapy (CRT)

The rationale for this new therapy comes from the pattern of LV shortening seen on the echocardiogram. Normally, the interventricular septum and the posterior-lateral walls contract simultaneously, moving toward each other. With left bundle branch block (LBBB) the septum is activated late, and therefore contracts after the lateral wall.

Late septal contraction persists beyond the completion of aortic ejection, and this phase of contraction therefore does not contribute to forward flow. Also, the late contraction continues into diastole, effectively shortening diastole and inhibiting diastolic filling of the LV. The net effect is lower LVEF and stroke volume.

Biventricular (BiV) pacing—that is, pacing from two sites—resynchronizes the LV so that contraction of the septum and lateral walls is simultaneous. One pacing wire is positioned at the RV apex, capturing the septum. The second is threaded into the coronary sinus to the cardiac vein on the back side of the heart where it stimulates the lateral wall. Current technology also calls for an atrial electrode, so that an optimal heart rate and PR interval can be programmed.

BiV pacing works best for the patient with LBBB and a wide QRS (> 150 msec). The hemodynamic effects are impressive, with a reduction in the delay in septal activation and an increase in LVEF. This is accomplished with no increase in myocardial oxygen consumption, since the myocardium is not contracting more forcefully (just more efficiently). Mild to moderate mitral regurgitation (MR), a frequent complication of dilated cardiomyopathy, tends to improve, although severe MR seldom does.

Clinical trials have shown improved exercise tolerance, functional class, and reduced hospitalization for CHF. MADIT-CRT demonstrated a survival benefit.

There are some patients with LBBB who do not improve with BiV pacing. The best predictor of successful therapy is an extremely wide QRS > 150 msec. Paradoxical splitting of S_2 indicates delayed LV emptying, and is a physical sign that allows diagnosis of LBBB at the bedside. Not everyone with LBBB has it, but those with marked widening of the QRS tend to. While not studied, I have wondered if this easily appreciated physical finding is a marker of LV dyssynergy, and might be useful in choosing patients for BiV pacing.

In addition to QRS duration, other predictors of improvement with CRT include female sex, non-ischemic cardiomyopathy, and sinus rhythm (rather than atrial fibrillation). Patients with

severe LV dilation, ischemic cardiomyopathy, and severe MR
are less likely to respond.

Implantable Cardioverter Defibrillators (ICD Therapy)

Sudden death is common in patients with reduced LVEF, and
the usual mechanism is ventricular fibrillation (VF). Clinical
trials have shown a benefit with both ischemic and non-ischemic
cardiomyopathy and LVEF $\leq 35\%$.

Patients with more severe CHF have the greatest benefit,
although trials did not include many with class IV symptoms.
The rate of hospitalization for CHF exacerbation was higher in
the ICD therapy group, suggesting that some patients who
would have died suddenly lived long enough to develop more
severe CHF.

Another interesting finding was a delay in benefit. There was no
separation of the survival curves until about 10 months after
randomization and treatment, indicating little benefit from ICD
treatment in the first year. Because of this, placing and ICD is
not considered a medical emergency. For a borderline patient
(asymptomatic with a borderline LVEF), there is time to
optimize GDMT, especially to up titrate the beta blocker dose,
which can raise LVEF above the 35% cut-off. Another
implication of the delayed benefit relates to the decision not to
treat a high risk, class IV patient. If the expected mortality in the
first year is high from other complications of heart failure, then
ICD therapy would be of little benefit.

It is common for patients to decline ICD therapy, especially
elderly patients. Careful review of clinical trials shows that there
were few octogenarians enrolled in them, so a survival benefit
for those older than 80 years is less certain.

Surgical Therapy

An occasional patient with ischemic cardiomyopathy benefits from revascularization therapy, and that is the rationale for screening for coronary artery disease in the initial evaluation of CHF. The STITCH trial found improved outcome with bypass surgery in patients with low LVEF who had good exercise tolerance, but not for those with advanced symptoms and poor exercise tolerance. In this study, the viability scan was not useful for predicting a benefit.

Mitral regurgitation is a complication of dilated cardiomyopathy that contributes to progression of LV dysfunction. Mitral valve repair—but not replacement—can lead to symptomatic improvement. Mitral valve repair can be accomplished in the cardiac catheterization laboratory using the Mitraclip. At this point, the effect of clipping on mortality is uncertain.

Heart transplantation definitely works. It both relieves symptoms and prolongs survival for the end-stage patient. The young and otherwise healthy person with cardiomyopathy has the best outcome. Contraindications include old age and comorbidities—advanced lung, kidney or liver disease, infection, cancer, obesity etc. A common contraindication is "inadequate social support." Programs are reluctant to transplant a patient who does not have adequate family support; a team is needed to get a person through this complicated and difficult treatment, and equally difficult follow-up. Although partially funded by the state, transplantation and follow-up are expensive, and no program can afford to give it away. A major obstacle is a shortage of donor hearts; there have been about 2,000 transplants per year in the United States for the last few decades.

Device Therapy

Ventricular assist devices (VAD) are the mainstay of advanced heart failure treatment. LVAD was formerly used as a bridge to heart transplantation, but has more lately become a "destination therapy." There are reports of patients living as long as 10 years. Currently the 1-year survival is 80%, and 2-year, 70%.

A Summary of Treatment:

As a rule, it is important to distinguish between treatments that prolong survival and those that just control symptoms. If a symptom controlling medicine is not tolerated or has not worked, then stop it. A common example is nitroglycerin for asymptomatic patients with coronary artery disease; since there is no survival benefit, why take it? On the other hand, I would not want to appear in court to explain why a patient with coronary disease was never offered aspirin or a statin.

That is certainly the case with treatment for HFrEF. The following table summarizes the previous discussion, and provides a simple menu of therapies and what they do.

Table 1.7 A Broad Classification of HF Therapies

Rx to Improve Survival (Also Improves Symptoms)	Rx for Symptom Control (No Survival Benefit)
Medicine	
Beta blockers (carvedilol or metoprolol SA)	Digoxin
ACEI/ARB	Intravenous inotropes
Entresto (instead of ACEI/ARB)	Diuretics
Spironolactone (or Eplerenone)	Ivabridine
Dapagliflozin	
Hydralazine + isosorbide (African American patients)	
Mechanical therapies	
Implantable cardioverter	

defibrillator Cardiac resynchronization therapy Heart transplantation Ventricular assist devices Coronary artery bypass surgery	

This does not mean that every patient has to have everything in the left hand column. There are multiple vasodilator/afterload reducing choices, and the clinician has to make a reasonable choice. But if the choice is to avoid afterload reduction therapy, you need to have a note in the chart explaining why. As mentioned, older patients may not be considered for advanced mechanical therapies, or refuse them.

Furthermore, the table should not imply that therapies with no effect on survival are unimportant. Obviously, congestion or edema has to be treated with diuretics, and it can be argued that failure to control congestion would be fatal. Digoxin is usually the forgotten therapy; it is common to see a patient on iv dobutamine and not digoxin; starting digoxin may allow discontinuation of intravenous treatment.

Disability Evaluation

One of the most useful things we do in practice is help people with the application process. CHF is clearly disabling, and malingering is seldom an issue. My experience is that it is harder to get Social Security Administration (SSA) benefits for heart disease than for other conditions such a back pain or psychiatric disorders. Your letter describing symptoms and documenting illness is critical and worth the effort.

The SSA criteria for disability from heart disease are (1) symptoms that prevent work, and (2) objective evidence for disease. For CHF with systolic dysfunction, the requirement is

LVEF < 30%. For coronary artery disease the objective evidence is an abnormal stress test or angiogram.

There is an occasional problem with the echo report needed for documentation of LVEF. In most cases the EF is an estimate by the reader, and this has been found to be reasonably accurate when tested against other techniques for measuring EF. However, the reader may provide a range, stating that the "LVEF is 25-30%." The SSA has been known to reject an application with that reading. Consider asking the echo reader to look at the echo again, and if the LVEF is low, to change the estimate to "25-29%."

A problem that should not be overlooked in the disability letter is the likelihood of missing work. People with advanced heart disease often have bad days, and cannot work. This makes holding a job difficult, even when it is part time.

Treatment of End-Stage CHF

All of our therapies for CHF may be considered palliative; they relieve symptoms as well as prolong survival. None of the standard medical treatments for CHF is withdrawn from the patient with end-stage disease.

When all else fails to control severe pulmonary congestion, morphine usually provides relief. It is a venodilator, reducing blood return to the heart. Pulmonary capillary pressure and symptoms of congestion are quickly reduced. In addition, it blunts the anxiety that comes with severe dyspnea.

Morphine is safe for patients with pulmonary congestion or the dyspnea of advanced lung disease. Despite widespread concern, respiratory depression is rare short of extremely high doses. Regular oral dosing is useful (Roxanol starting at 2.5-5 mg at 2-4 hour intervals). It may be preferable to use the medicine as needed rather than throughout the day, especially if attacks of dyspnea are intermittent. Within reason, there is no maximum allowable dose, and the dose may be increased at 4-12 hour intervals as needed to control symptoms.

Consider hospice care for those with end stage CHF. The hospice nurse monitors salt and water intake, and regulates diuretics and other drugs. Patients often improve dramatically. There is no doubt that physicians are qualified to manage patients on opioids. But there are practical advantages to having hospice involvement. The first is that "narcotics" may not appear to be "usual treatment" for CHF; hospice care avoids any suggestion of abuse. Another is that hospice nurses are competent regulate the opioid dose and monitor its use at home.

What to do with the implanted defibrillator (ICD) is an important end-of-life issue. In the last stage of CHF there is little survival benefit; the patient is dying from pump failure, and the ICD cannot change the trajectory of the disease. Furthermore, at end-of-life frequent ICD discharge can add to suffering. Most patients elect to have the ICD turned off.

Extreme Symptoms in the Terminally Ill Patient

Some with CHF have ventricular fibrillation and die suddenly. Our experience with cardiac hospice showed that many die with "dry pump failure." This happens when congestion is well controlled and the heart fails. The patient becomes progressively hypotensive, then drifts into coma and dies peacefully.

A minority come to the emergency room with pulmonary edema at end-of-life, and it may be refractory to intravenous diuretics. In such cases it is unfortunate when the emergency department doctor tells the patient and family that intubation and mechanical ventilation is the only hope for relieving symptoms. Despite an earlier decision to avoid ventilator therapy, a desperate patient and family may have a change of mind, when told this is the only chance for relief.

An effective alternative that should be considered is higher dose morphine, titrated to relieve dyspnea. There may be depression of respiration with a dose sufficient to relieve symptoms. In this case the moral imperative is to provide relief of suffering for the dying patient, even if high-dose morphine contributes to more rapid death. There is no culpability. This is not considered assisted suicide or euthanasia, but rather, necessary therapy for extreme symptoms.

Chapter 2: Disorders of Ventricular Filling: Heart Failure with Preserved Ejection Fraction, Restrictive Cardiomyopathy, Hypertrophic Obstructive Cardiomyopathy, Pericardial Disease

Abbreviations

ACE, angiotensin converting enzyme
AF, atrial fibrillation
AS, aortic stenosis
ASH, asymmetric (ventricular) septal hypertrophy
AV, atrioventricular
BNP, brain natriuretic peptide
CHF, congestive heart failure
DHF, diastolic heart failure
ECG, electrocardiogram
EF, ejection fraction
Echo, echocardiogram
HFpEF, heart failure with preserved ejection fraction
HCM, hypertrophic cardiomyopathy
HOCM, hypertrophic obstructive cardiomyopathy
ICD, implantable cardioverter-defibrillator
IHSS, idiopathic hypertrophic subaortic stenosis
LV, left ventricle (ventricular)
LVEDP, LV end diastolic pressure
LVEF, LV ejection fraction
LVH, LV hypertrophy
RV, right ventricle
SAM, systolic anterior motion (of the mitral valve)
SCD, sudden cardiac death
TTR amyloid, transthyretin amyloid cardiomyopathy (ATTR-CM)

HEART FAILURE WITH PRESERVED EJECTION FRACTION: HFpEF

The Greek word *diastole* means to dilate, expand, or in the case of a balloon, to inflate. Diastolic dysfunction is an inability to inflate the ventricle to a normal end-diastolic volume without an excessive increase in end-diastolic pressure (EDP). Excessive EDP is the problem. Remember that when the mitral valve is open it is an open system; left ventricular EDP is also the pressure in the left atrium, the pulmonary veins, and at the capillary-alveolar interface. Capillary pressure exceeding oncotic pressure, normally 25mg Hg, forces fluid into the interstitium.

Diastolic dysfunction is like trying to blow up a stiff, thick-walled balloon. A patient with diastolic CHF usually has normal contractility and left ventricular ejection fraction (LVEF), but has elevated LVEDP. The condition is now called HFpEF.

Etiology and Natural History

Cardiac illnesses that provoke LV hypertrophy (LVH) result in increased LV stiffness and may cause diastolic heart failure. The most common of these is hypertension, a comorbidity in more than half of those with DHF. Aortic stenosis with associated LVH causes obvious problems with diastolic filling, although the reduction in stroke volume is primarily the result of LV outflow obstruction.

Myocardial relaxation is an energy-requiring process, so ischemia also causes diastolic dysfunction. Recall that the usual gallop heard in patients with ischemic heart disease is the S_4, reflecting the atrial "kick" into a stiff ventricle. An occasional patient with coronary artery disease presents without chest discomfort but instead with exertional dyspnea as a manifestation of ischemia. Transient diastolic dysfunction is the mechanism of this "anginal equivalent," pulmonary congestion but no chest discomfort. In others with chronic diastolic dysfunction, transient ischemia may aggravate symptoms.

HFpEF is frequently a condition of advanced age. Old people get stiff hearts as well as stiff joints. It is more common in women as well—a majority of patients in large studies of DHF are women. Both hypertension and diabetes confer a greater risk of heart failure for women compared with men, suggesting a fundamentally different biologic response. In nursing homes, where the ratio of women to men is seven to one, most of those with new heart failure have DHF.

In general, the best predictor of survival in adults with heart disease, particularly coronary artery disease, is LVEF. However, the 5-year survival with HFrEF and HFpEF is similar, about 50%. The mortality risk with both forms of CHF is higher with advanced age and coronary artery disease.

Pathophysiology

Diastolic Function

When considering ventricular function, it is natural to think primarily of the contractile process. There often is confusion about diastolic function and ventricular compliance. These terms relate to how easily the ventricle fills during diastole, when it is relaxed, and have little to do with contraction. But diastolic compliance of the ventricle determines *preload* and therefore affects stroke volume (Figure 2.1)

Figure 2.1 Effect of Changing LV Stiffness on LV Function

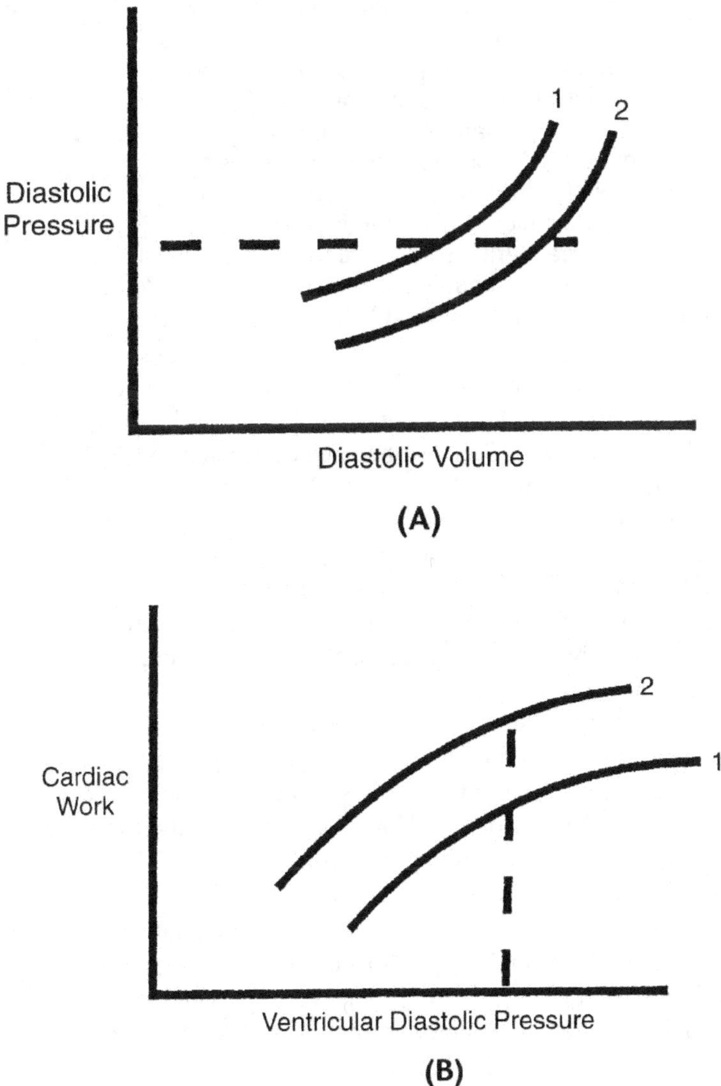

Figure 2.1 (A) Compliance of the ventricle during diastole influences ventricular filling. At a given ventricular diastolic

57

pressue, Patient 1 has a lower ventricular volume (and therefore muscle fiber length) than Patient 2. Patient 1 has a stiffer, less compliant ventricle. (B) In practice, it is easier to measure ventricular diastolic pressure than volume. Because the two are roughly proportional, pressure is substituted for volume on the ventricular function (Starling) curve. Patient 1 appears to have worse ventricular function than Patient 2, and that would be the case if diastolic compliance is the same for both. But if Patient 1 has a stiffer ventricle (as in A), end-diastolic volume may be lower than it is for Patient 2. In this case, at equal ventricular volumes, the two might have identical systolic function, and therefore identical ventricular function curves. This illustrates the potential problem of substituting diastolic pressure for diastolic volume on the abscissa of the LV function curve.

Students are often confused by preload, because we describe it using two different measurements. In reality, preload is the length of the muscle fiber just before contraction, or in the case of the intact heart, the volume of the LV at the end of diastole. Unfortunately, it is hard to measure LV volume precisely; a 20 to 30 ml increase in diastolic volume provides enough extra stretch to increase stroke volume, but the echocardiogram is not precise enough to measure that difference. Also, volume is impossible to monitor continuously. For this reason, you do not see end-diastolic volume on the x axis of the LV function (Starling) curve (Figure 2.1B). Instead, we substitute the more easily monitored pulmonary capillary wedge pressure which is the same as the LVEDP (again, it's an open system in diastole, with the mitral valve open). That works most of the time since diastolic pressure and volume are proportional.

A compliant ventricle fills easily, allowing adequate preloading of the ventricle (stretching of muscle fibers) to generate stroke volume. A stiff (e.g., noncompliant) ventricle does not allow adequate ventricular filling, and with less myocyte stretch, stroke volume suffers (Figure 2.2). Abnormal stiffness, or diastolic dysfunction, may result from hypertrophy, fibrosis, ischemia, or infiltrative disorder (amyloidosis, sarcoidosis, hemochromatosis).

The problem is that fall in LV compliance (diastolic dysfunction) changes the pressure-volume relation. Higher pressure is needed to inflate the LV to an adequate volume (or preload). The ventricle must operate with a much higher than normal diastolic pressure to maintain stroke volume and cardiac output. Higher LV diastolic pressure is accomplished by volume expansion, the same neurohormonal and renal responses to low cardiac output that occur with systolic heart failure (HFpEF). Remember that during diastole, with the mitral valve open, there is no valve separating the LV from the pulmonary capillary bed. Thus, high LV diastolic pressure is transmitted to the left atrium and pulmonary capillary bed, leading to pulmonary congestion.

(Forgive the redundancy. I had to see this information many times and presented in different ways to get it. It seemed I had to dream about diastole to get it.)

Figure 2.2 Increased LV Stiffness, Steeper Pressure-Volume Curve

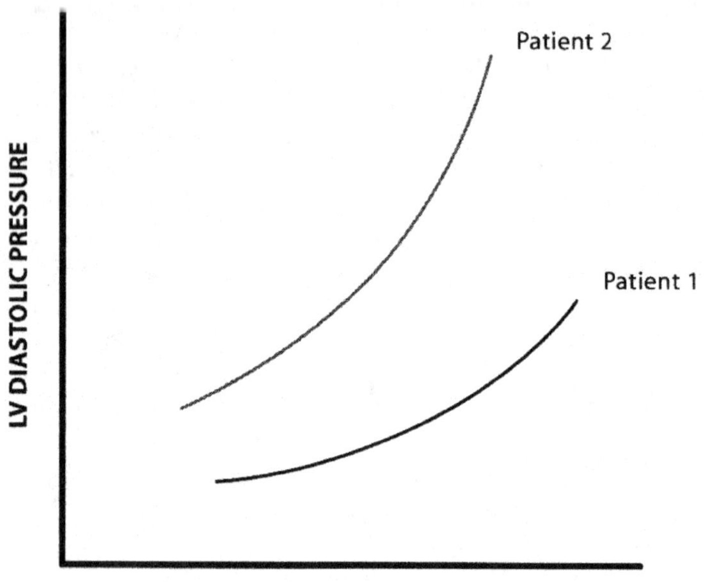

Figure 2.2 LV diastolic presuure–volume curves from two patients. Patient 1, normal. Patient 2, hypertensive heart disease with LV diastolic dysfunction. For a given volume, Patient 2 has higher diastolic pressure (the balloon is stiffer). Furthermore, the curve is steeper, as is usually the case with diastolic dysfunction. For this reason, small changes in diastolic volume lead to much greater changes in pressure. (And the LV diastolic pressure is transmitted to the left atrium and pulmonary capillary bed, leading to congestion.)

The Steeper Pressure-Volume Curve

Increased stiffness means that the pressure-volume curve is shifted up and to the left (Figure 2.2). With HFpEF, the curve is steeper, so that a small increase in volume leads to much greater increases in LV diastolic pressure. This is the explanation for "flash pulmonary edema," or the rapid development of pulmonary congestion after a relatively modest increase in salt intake (i.e., the nursing home resident who has a couple beers with chips when watching the Super Bowl with her chums).

The reverse is true as well, and over-diuresis may cause hypotension. Consider a patient with hypertensive and coronary heart disease who has had cardiac catheterization. The patient has had little to drink, and the contrast agent functions as an osmotic diuretic. Because the ventricle is stiff, hypotension may develop in the hours after angiography with volume depletion. In such cases, we pay careful attention to hydration after the procedure.

Atrial Contraction

Contraction of the atria—the atrial kick—at the end of diastole provides the last increment of ventricular filling, increasing preload and, therefore, stroke volume.

The simple and interesting experiment that defined the contribution of atrial contraction to cardiac output is illustrated in Figure 2.3. A person with normal diastolic function may have a 10% drop in cardiac output when atrial contraction is bypassed with ventricular pacing. But another with diastolic dysfunction may have cardiac output fall 25% or more with loss of the atrial kick.

Patients with stiff ventricles are said to be preload dependent, and are especially susceptible to loss of atrial contraction or volume depletion.

Many who have atrial fibrillation (AF) are asymptomatic, and the irregular rhythm is discovered on routine examination. However, a person with hypertensive heart disease and LVH is more prone to experience fatigue and dyspnea with the onset of AF.

Figure 2.3 Atrial Contraction and Cardiac Output

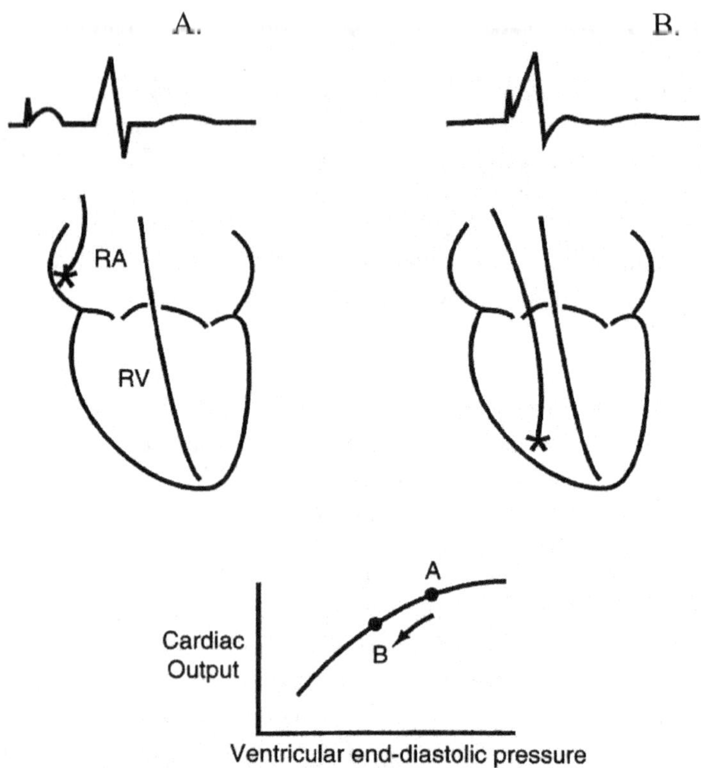

Figure 2.3 This simple study is easily repeated in the cardiac catheterization laboratory. The heart is paced at a rate just above its baseline, and cardiac output is measured. (A) When the pacemaker is in the right atrium, atrial contraction is preserved (a P wave follows the pacing spike.) (B) Pacing from the right ventricle leads to a loss of the P wave and atrial contraction. Ventricular diastolic pressure and volume decline–a drop in preload–and LV stroke volume and cardiac output fall. On the LV function curve, the patient shifts from point A to point B (bottom).

Pacemaker Syndrome

This is also the explanation for the *pacemaker syndrome*, an abrupt onset of fatigue when a ventricular pacemaker turns on. It is avoided with dual chamber, atrio-ventricular pacing, which maintains atrial contraction.

Heart Rate

"Tachycardia robs diastole." The duration of systole on the LV pressure tracing is constant, regardless of the heart rate. With an increase in heart rate, the total duration of diastole declines, and there is less time for ventricular filling. Those with stiff ventricles need as much time in diastole as possible for ventricular filling.

Consider a patient with aortic stenosis and LVH who develops rapid atrial fibrillation and has a drop in blood pressure. There is a double insult to LV filling and stroke volume: loss of atrial contraction plus tachycardia. If hypotension is severe enough that the patient appears to be in shock, the atrial fibrillation is a medical emergency and requires immediate electrical cardioversion. Do not wait for a cardiology consultation or take time to administer rate-lowering drugs. You must act promptly to resuscitate the patient when any tachyarrhythmia causes hemodynamic compromise, even when it is an atrial tachyarrhythmia.

History and Physical Examination

Diastolic heart failure may be mild, with only effort intolerance or dyspnea with exertion. Diastolic dysfunction is often diagnosed from the echocardiogram in asymptomatic patients with hypertension, but the heart failure syndrome is needed to call it diastolic DHF.

At the other end of the spectrum is the syndrome called "flash pulmonary edema" mentioned above. This may occur in a person with no prior history of heart disease, and who has no history of gradually increasing exertional dyspnea or orthopnea. In contrast, CHF from systolic dysfunction typically develops slowly and progressively. Flash pulmonary edema illustrates an important clinical feature of diastolic heart failure, the narrow window between volume overload (congestion), and depletion (hypotension). Small changes in volume produce either dyspnea on exertion or postural hypotension. Juggling diuretics and salt intake can be tricky for the elderly patient with HFpEF. On days when dyspnea is the problem, take furosemide; but when dizziness on standing is the problem, omit a furosemide dose and drink Gatorade.

Features of the history that suggest diastolic dysfunction as the cause of CHF include advanced age, hypertension, and female sex. Both the history and physical exam should screen for other conditions that may cause LVH such as aortic stenosis or hypertrophic subaortic stenosis. Look carefully for any evidence of coronary artery disease. Myocardial relaxation is an active, energy requiring process, and ischemia has an immediate negative effect on diastolic function. Those with ischemic cardiomyopathy have an element of diastolic dysfunction, although low LVEF is the predominant mechanism.

Most patients with HFpEF have just pulmonary congestion. Right heart failure may occur, and jugular venous distension and peripheral edema can be present. The physical findings of left heart congestion are typical.

Box 2.1 Pseudo-Isolated Right Heart Failure:

The most common cause of right heart failure is left heart failure. We commonly admit patients with advanced CHF and anasarca, but not much pulmonary congestion. If left heart failure—systolic or diastolic—is responsible, then why isn't the patient in pulmonary edema? The probable mechanism is that lymphatic drainage of the lungs is effective enough to prevent pulmonary congestion for that particular patient.

The cardiac examination may allow you to differentiate diastolic from systolic failure at the bedside. With diastolic CHF the heart is usually small, so the PMI is in the mid-clavicular line. It is not diffuse and sustained. If there is LVH, it may be forceful. There is no S_3 gallop. Instead, increased LV diastolic stiffness causes an S_4 gallop, the result of the atrium forcing blood into the stiff ventricle at the end of diastole.

An especially useful physical finding is a palpable S_4, the *apical A wave* (Figure 2.4). To detect the A wave, have the patient roll to the left and carefully feel the apex impulse. Normally its upstroke is smooth. The A wave is felt as a glitch or shudder. Practice feeling for it in those with hypertension and LVH; it is not that subtle a finding. Describing an apical A wave indicates advanced understanding and physical diagnosis skills (and is very cool). More importantly, the A wave is the most specific physical finding for increased LV stiffness, and its presence reliably indicates elevated LV diastolic pressure. Remember that the A wave and S_4 gallop disappear with atrial fibrillation and the loss of atrial contraction (medical residents *always* ask students if they hear the S_4 in patients with atrial fibrillation).

We have become accustomed to using brain natriuretic peptide (BNP) as an indicator of heart failure. It is less sensitive in patients with diastolic than in those with systolic failure. However, it is still useful. Patients with LVH and CHF have elevation of BNP, while others with LVH and no heart failure may not.

Figure 2.4 S_4 Gallop and Apical A Wave

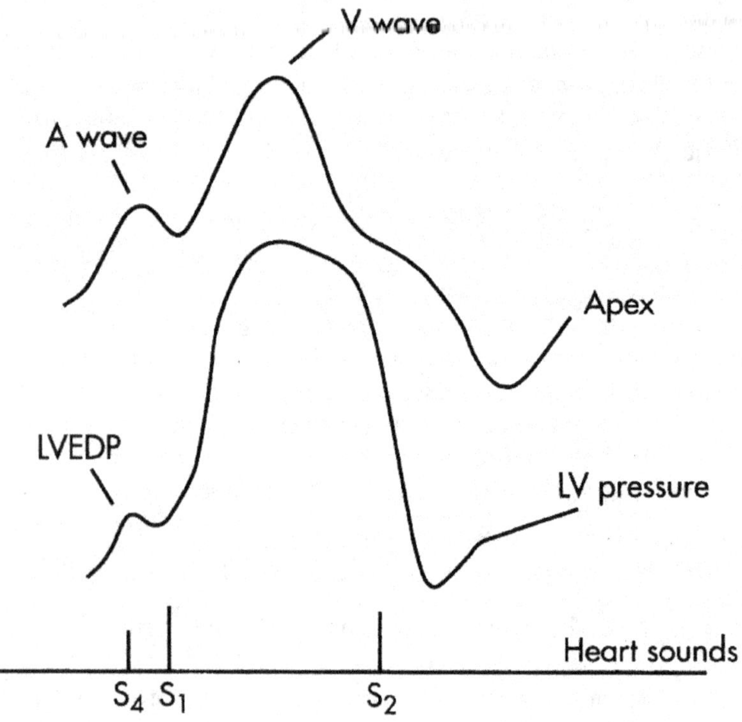

Figure 2.4 The contour of the apical impulse (top tracing) mirrors the LV pressure tracing. Just before ventricular systole, atrial contraction causes a small rise in LV pressure that is measured as the LV end-diastolic pressure (LVEDP). This is elevated in conditions that increase LV stiffness. When the apical A wave is greater than 15% of the total apical excursion, it is palpable as a shudder or glitch on the upstroke of the impulse. This is a reliable indicator of elevated LVEDP and is audible as the S_4 gallop.

Laboratory Examination

There are just two things needed to make the diagnosis of diastolic failure. The first is to establish the diagnosis of CHF. A chest x-ray showing congestion that subsequently responds to diuresis is adequate evidence. BNP is elevated with diastolic failure, but less so than with systolic heart failure where there is more LV stretch.

The second step is documentation of LV ejection fraction, usually with an echocardiogram. If the LVEF is above 50%, then it is DHF. Some studies use 40% as the criterion for diastolic dysfunction; in practice, most patients have normal or even hyperdynamic LV contraction, and the ventricle is small. LV hypertrophy supports the diagnosis, but many with HFpEF have normal LV thickness.

Left atrial size: this is the canary in the coal mine for HFpEF, and may trump complex Doppler measures of diastolic function. HFpEF is unlikely when LA size is normal, and it is an easy and reliable echo measurement. (When I suspect HFpEF, LA enlargement is the first thing I look for on the echo report.)

Diastolic dysfunction is about abnormal LV filling, and the echo-Doppler study allows assessment of flow across the mitral valve during diastole (Figure 2.5). Normally flow into the ventricle is highest in early diastole—the E wave—but with increased LV stiffness the velocity of flow following atrial contraction increases—the A wave. A Doppler study showing an abnormally low E/A confirms abnormal LV relaxation, but is not necessary for making the diagnosis.

The echocardiogram may not be technically adequate to assess LA size, or LV size and function (this can be the case with obesity or emphysema). Cardiac MRI is a reliable alternative.

Figure 2.5 Doppler Measure of Diastolic Dysfunction

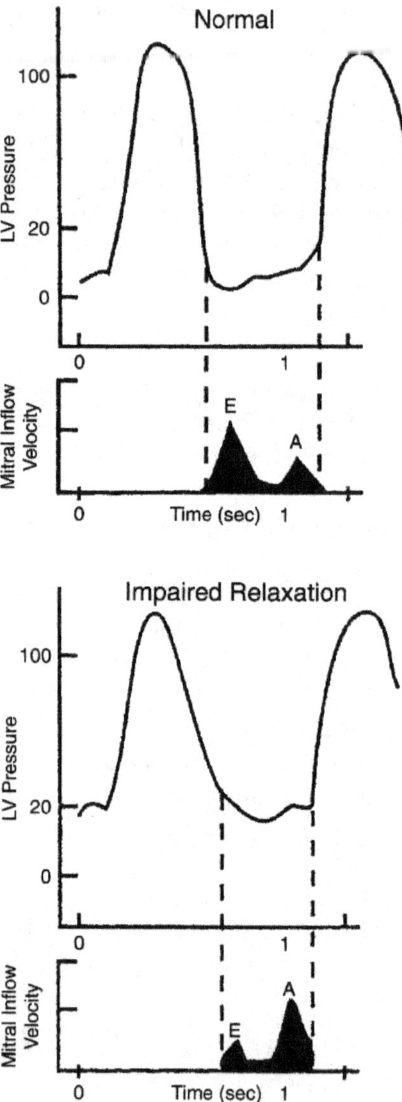

Figure 2.5 The effect of impaired LV relaxation on LV pressure (measured at cardiac catheterization) and flow across the mitral valve (measured from the echo–Doppler study). Normally,

maximal flow into the ventricle occurs in early diastole (the E wave). With impaired relaxation in early diastole, atrial contraction produces a higher flow velocity, and the A wave is larger than the E wave. Note that with the stiffer ventricle, the LV diastolic pressure is higher.

As with the work-up of systolic heart failure, it is important to exclude ischemic heart disease, especially for a younger patient. Heart failure is an indication for revascularization. In the absence of a history or ECG evidence for MI, a stress perfusion study may be adequate. If the clinical picture is suggestive, consider coronary angiography or CT angiography.

When the cause of dyspnea remains uncertain—a common problem—exercise testing with right heart catheterization may help. Pulmonary capillary wedge pressure (LV filling pressure) rises with exercise when there is diastolic dysfunction.

Treatment of Diastolic Heart Failure

Unlike systolic heart failure, there have been few clinical trials to guide therapy for DHF. The strategy outlined in Table 2.1 is a reasonable approach based upon experience and the pathophysiology of the illness.

Table 2.1. A Treatment Strategy for Diastolic CHF

1. Treat congestion. Because of the steep pressure-volume curve, low dose diuretics usually work (see text; this is a useful concept to understand). Although this reduces preload—which has a negative effect on LV function—pulmonary and peripheral congestion must be corrected.
2. Treat hypertension. Short term, lower afterload favorably affects LV relaxation. Long term, there may be regression of LVH.
3. Treat ischemia; revascularization when possible. Dyspnea as an angina equivalent is from increased diastolic stiffness during ischemia.

4. Lower heart rate. At increased heart rate, total diastolic time is reduced, so there is less time for LV filling.

5. Maintain atrial function; prevent, or correct, atrial fibrillation. The stiff LV is preload dependent, and atrial contraction is about preload.

6. Spironolactone

Congestion is relieved by lowering preload. Small doses of furosemide are usually sufficient, as the pressure volume curve is steep (Figure 2.1), and there is a small difference between congestion and volume depletion; a resident described this as "a narrow euvolemic window." It is common to overshoot with diuretics. We usually begin with 20 mg furosemide daily, and carefully up-titrate the dose. Stable patients may be controlled with thiazides. Nitrates may also be used to reduce preload, especially when there is ischemia. Again, start with a low dose, 15-30 mg isosorbide mononitrate (Imdur).

Reducing blood pressure has an immediate benefit, since the excessive afterload of hypertension slows relaxation. Over the long run, control of blood pressure can lead to regression of LVH and improved diastolic function. Angiotensin converting enzyme inhibitors and receptor blockers appear to be the most effective for regression of hypertrophy, and they may have a direct myocardial effect. Calcium channel blockers, beta blockers, and centrally acting sympatholytic agents also work.

As noted, tachycardia is a major problem when there is diastolic disease. Drugs that lower the sinus rate (beta blockers, verapamil or diltiazem), or control the ventricular rate with atrial fibrillation will improve exercise tolerance. This is the only indication for digoxin in diastolic heart failure. When using arterial dilators—including ACE inhibition, angiotensin receptor blockers, and calcium blockers—watch for reflex tachycardia.

Atrial contraction is critical for the patient with a stiff LV. Unfortunately, atrial fibrillation is a common complication of HFpEF, since there is elevation of the left atrial pressure. The preload dependent patient with diastolic dysfunction is often symptomatic, and every effort should be made to restore sinus rhythm.

Spironolactone is the only drug that has been found to have a specific benefit for HFpEF.

HYPERTROPHIC CARDIOMYOPATHY (HCM)

HCM is a unifying diagnosis for illnesses with a common pathophysiology: LVH in the absence of pressure overload. About 60% of the cases are inherited with the remainder sporadic. Several genetic defects may contribute to the pool of patients with familial HCM.

The most common HCM is a familial disorder, and includes obstruction of the LV outflow tract: hypertrophic obstructive cardiomyopathy (HOCM). It has also been called idiopathic hypertrophic subaortic stenosis (IHSS). The anatomical defect is hypertrophy of the interventricular septum; a thickened lump of septal muscle just below the aortic valve that obstructs flow. Diastolic dysfunction is one of four mechanisms that contribute to symptoms in HOCM. The others are aortic outflow tract obstruction, myocardial ischemia, and arrhythmias.

Pathophysiology and Physical Examination
Valvular aortic stenosis causes a pressure gradient across the valve; systolic pressure in the LV is higher than aortic pressure. With HOCM the level of obstruction—the level of the pressure gradient—is subvalvular (Figure 2.6). The lump of septal muscle crowding the outflow tract causes high velocity and a Venturi effect, sucking the anterior mitral leaflet into the outflow tract toward the interventricular septum. This is seen on the echocardiogram as systolic anterior motion (SAM) of the

mitral valve. The displaced mitral leaflet, into the outflow tract, contributes to the obstruction, and when there is no SAM on the echocardiogram, there usually is no pressure gradient. The semantics of this condition may be confusing, and without a gradient it may be described as asymmetric septal hypertrophy—ASH—rather than HOCM.

Figure 2.6 HOCM, LV Pressure Gradient

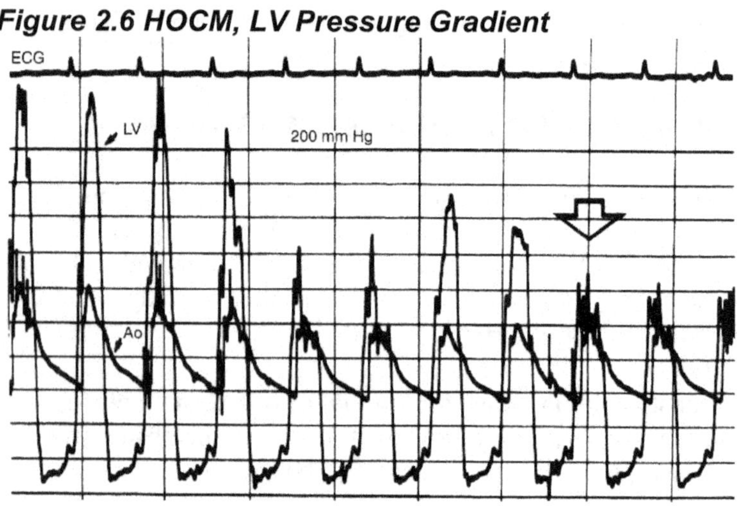

Figure 2.6 Hypertrophic cardiomyopathy with left ventricular outflow tract obstruction. These are simultaneous pressures from the left ventricle (LV) and aorta (Ao). Left ventricular pressure is initially measured at the LV apex, the left side of the tracing. As the catheter is withdrawn toward the aortic valve (right side of the tracing), a point is reached just below the valve (arrow) where there is no difference, or gradient, between left ventricular and aortic pressure. This indicates that the level of obstruction is subvalvular, in the body of the ventricle, rather than valvular.

The outflow tract gradient and murmur increase with lower LV volume. It is a matter of geometry. Less filling of the ventricle means that the outflow tract is narrower, flow velocity and the Venturi effect are heightened, and there is more SAM. Standing after squatting and the strain phase of the Valsalva maneuver lower venous return and accentuate the systolic murmur. In the echo laboratory, amyl nitrite, a venodilator, does the same thing, provoking SAM, the gradient and murmur.

The systolic murmur is a key diagnostic finding. Unlike valvular aortic stenosis (AS), there is little radiation of the murmur to the neck. The peripheral pulse also helps differentiate HOCM and AS. With HOCM, initial LV emptying is normal since obstruction to outflow worsens in mid-systole, as the ventricle empties and is smaller. Thus, the pulse upstroke is brisk; with valvular AS, the pulse upstroke is delayed. The stiff ventricle produces both an S_4 gallop and an apical A wave.

The diagnosis is made by the echocardiogram-Doppler study. The pattern of hypertrophy is easily visualized on the transthoracic echo, and the muscle may appear qualitatively abnormal. The Doppler examination allows measurement of flow velocity across the outflow tract and calculation of the pressure gradient between the LV and aorta.

Box 2.2 Tetralogy of Fallot

Another outflow tract geometry condition: the right ventricular outflow tract, the infundibulum, is narrowed in tetralogy, creating sub-pulmonic valve stenosis. It's comparable to the subvalvular stenosis in the LV caused by HOCM. By reducing RV contractility and relieving crowding, beta blockade reduces the subvalvular pulmonic stenosis in infants with tetralogy.

Treatment

None of the treatments for HOCM has been shown to improve survival, though many relieve symptoms. The principles of treating diastolic dysfunction apply (Table 2.1). In addition, medical therapy is directed at increasing space in the outflow tract. Drugs that reduce contractility (verapamil, beta-blockers, and disopyramide) cause ventricular dilatation, widening the outflow tract and reducing flow velocity, which minimizes SAM. The outflow tract pressure gradient is thus reduced.

Pacemaker therapy has been tried, and is worth mentioning because it illustrates the interesting physiology. Pacing the right ventricle creates a left bundle branch block pattern on the electrocardiogram. Septal activation is thus later in systole, and this septal dyskinesis has been shown to reduce the outflow tract gradient. It is the reverse of resynchronization therapy for systolic heart failure (Chapter 1). One small trial showed no long-term benefit with pacing, but there are small series that described symptomatic benefits.

A more effective therapy is ablation of septal muscle with local infusion of alcohol through a coronary catheter positioned in a small septal perforating artery. This kills septal muscle, and the septum shrinks. This technique has replaced surgical resection of septal muscle for patients whose symptoms are not adequately controlled with medical therapy. Septal ablation reduces the LV outflow tract gradient and results in improved symptoms and exercise capacity. Heart block requiring pacemaker therapy is a possible complication. Septal ablation has not been shown to have a survival benefit.

Box 2.3 Septal Infarction—a Misnomer—and ECG Changes with Alcohol Septal Ablation

The ECG computer often reads "septal infarction" when there is a Q wave in V_2 (it is normal to see it in V_1). Anatomically this makes little sense; it would require occlusion of a septal perforating branch of the left anterior descending artery (LAD), but plaque is never seen in these small, intramural branches. To lose flow to a septal branch would require occlusion of the LAD, and this would cause more extensive ECG changes. Alcohol septal ablation further supports this: the common ECG change after ablation is right bundle branch block, occasionally with left anterior fascicular block (never a Q wave in V_2). The usual cause of a Q in lead V_2 is lead misplacement, often an

> intercostal space too high. In this case, the tip-off may be a P
> wave in V_2 that is not positive.

Sudden Cardiac Death (SCD)

Annual mortality with HCM is relatively low, estimated at 2-
3%. About half the deaths are sudden and unexpected, and SCD
may be the initial symptom. Risk factors for sudden death
include extreme LVH, family history of sudden death, prior
history of ventricular tachycardia or syncope, and failure of
blood pressure to rise during exercise. An evaluation of a large
cohort (1101 patients) found that a resting outflow tract gradient
$\geq$ 30 mm Hg is a predictor of progression to severe symptoms of
heart failure and of death. On the other hand, therapies that
lower the outflow gradient and relieve symptoms have not been
shown to prevent SCD, and that includes septal ablation.

Because sudden cardiac death may be a presenting symptom of
HCM, screening echocardiograms in first-degree relatives is
justified.

Antiarrhythmic drug therapy is of no benefit, although
amiodarone has been suggested. The implantable cardioverter-
defibrillator (ICD) is indicated for secondary prevention—that is
to say, as treatment for one who has experienced syncope caused
by ventricular tachycardia or fibrillation. ICD therapy has been
recommended for primary prevention in patients with a family
history of HOCM and SCD.

Sudden Death in Young Athletes

HOCM is the most common cause of sudden cardiac death in
young athletes in the United States, a consideration when doing
pre-sports physical examinations. If you hear a soft murmur,
have the person stand then squat for a couple minutes, then
stand again. You should listen in both positions (the examiner
squats and stands with the patient). A murmur that is louder
after squatting or with Valsalva is typical for HOCM and is an

indication for an echocardiogram. This is a go-to physical finding—a murmur that does not intensify with this maneuver is not HOCM (my opinion). HOCM is rare enough that a screening echocardiogram is not currently recommended in the US for young athletes with no family history and a normal physical examination.

RESTRICTIVE CARDIOMYOPATHY

Restrictive cardiomyopathies may or may not lead to reduction in LV ejection fraction. All of them cause an increase in LV stiffness, and diastolic dysfunction contributes to the CHF syndrome. The general principles of treatment are those outlined for other forms of HFpEF (Table 2.1). In addition, some of the conditions respond to disease-specific therapy.

The restrictive illnesses have a characteristic LV ventricular filling pressure. Initial filling is rapid, but filling quickly "hits the wall" of the restrictive process. This leads to the square root sign: an early dip in LV diastolic pressure followed by a plateau, without the gradual rise in pressure that is normally observed through the rest of diastole.

Amyloidosis

Primary—now called AL—amyloidosis is the most common cause of restrictive cardiomyopathy. It is caused by plasma cell disorders like multiple myeloma. Senile amyloidosis may involve the heart, but usually causes dilated cardiomyopathy and systolic heart failure.

The other common form of amyloidosis is transthyretin amyloid cardiomyopathy (ATTR-CM). Making this diagnosis has become more important, because effective new therapies are available.

Hypertrophy on an echocardiogram is the finding that usually initiates consideration of amyloid. Table 2.2 is a list of "red flags" that heightens suspicion.

Table 2.2 Red flags for Amyloid Cardiomyopathy

1. LV hypertrophy on echo but low voltage on the ECG (a common board question)
2. LV hypertrophy without a history of LV pressure overload (e.g., HTN)
3. Atrio-ventricular block in the presence of LVH
4. Diffuse infiltration on the echo, including hypertrophy of the RV, atrial septum, and A-V valves. Muscle may have sparkling pattern on the echo.
5. Polyneuropathy beginning in the feet (sensory and motor), autonomic neuropathy
6. Bilateral carpal tunnel syndrome
7. Persistent, mild troponin and BNP increase
8. Male predominance and advanced age

Amyloidosis is more common in men, presents as HFpEF, and often with atrial or ventricular arrhythmia. Carpal tunnel syndrome may accompany it. The fibrillar protein is deposited throughout the myocardium, leading to a rubbery consistency and concentric hypertrophy. Both the right and left ventricles are thickened, an infrequent finding with the usual causes of LVH.

Laboratory evaluation includes a search for plasma cell dyscrasia, serum protein electrophoresis (looking for light chains).

A useful diagnostic clinical finding—and it is nifty enough that it makes it to board exams—is the absence of high QRS voltage on the ECG even though the left ventricle is thick. The amyloid infiltrate is not muscle and therefore does not generate voltage (thick ventricle + low voltage = amyloid).

The diagnosis of amyloid heart disease is supported by fat pad aspirate or rectal biopsy indicating systemic amyloidosis. Endomyocardial biopsy is required for a definite diagnosis. In addition to concentric hypertrophy with normal or reduced chamber size, the echocardiogram often shows a qualitative abnormality of muscle described as granular or sparkling. LVEF may or may not be reduced, and there is usually evidence for diastolic dysfunction.

The prognosis with amyloid heart disease is poor; the severity of LV hypertrophy predicts mortality. Doppler measures of diastolic dysfunction also indicate early mortality. Systemic amyloidosis has been considered a contraindication for heart transplantation, primarily because of disease progression in other organ systems. It is not certain whether the transplanted heart is at risk.

Transthyretin (TTR) amyloid is caused by variant forms of TTR. Making the diagnosis is important because it is a cause of amyloid heart disease that can be treated (with TTR stabilizers). Myocardia scintography with technetium-99 pyrophospate—the isotope used for bone scans—is diagnostic; sensitivity and specificity is high.

HEMOCHROMATOSIS

This iron storage disorder primarily affects the liver, and should be considered with the clinical triad of diabetes, hyperpigmentation and liver disease. Iron deposition in the heart is in the myocardial cells, not interstitial. It tends to affect the subepicardium primarily, with less subendocardial involvement. The heart is dilated, with or without hypertrophy (distinguishing it from amyloid heart disease). LVEF is reduced, and there usually is diastolic dysfunction. Endomyocardial biopsy is needed to make the diagnosis of cardiac hemochromatosis. Most patients die from liver failure, not from heart disease.

LOEFFLER'S ENDOCARDITIS

The illness begins with eosinophilia, either idiopathic or in response to chronic infection. About 80% of those with chronic eosinophilia develop myocardial fibrosis within 5 years. Eosinophils invade the subendocardium, degranulate and provoke tissue damage, necrosis and then fibrosis. Mural thrombus often forms over the necrotic myocardium, and systemic or pulmonary embolism is a feature of the illness.

The ventricular inflow tracts and apices are preferentially involved, and this may include tricuspid and mitral valves leading to regurgitation. It affects both right and left ventricles, so right and left heart failure are common.

Suspect the diagnosis when there is heart failure with peripheral eosinophilia. About 20% of patients do not have eosinophilia at the time of diagnosis; presumably, they had it at one point. When eosinophilia is present, prednisone and hydroxyurea may be effective. Anticoagulation should be considered, especially when there is suspicion of mural thrombus.

PERICARDIAL EFFUSION, TAMPONADE AND CONSTRICTION

Although the pericardium is external to the heart, tamponade and constriction compress the heart and limit cardiac filling. This inadequate preload—since that is what it is—results in reduced stroke volume.

Pericardial Tamponade

Clinically, acute tamponade causes a precipitous fall in blood pressure. Think of it when there is low blood pressure unresponsive to intravenous fluids plus jugular venous distension.

Tamponade occurs when pericardial fluid accumulates quickly and the pericardium has no time to stretch. Slowly accumulating effusions (most commonly hypothyroidism) allow time for the pericardium to expand with no increase in pericardial pressure. Causes of effusion are reviewed in Table 2.3, and most of them can cause tamponade. However, the most common cause of tamponade is malignancy (more than half the cases), followed by viral and uremic pericarditis. Anticoagulation increases the risk.

Table 2.3 Causes of Pericardial Effusion

1. Idiopathic
2. Viral (coxsackie, adenovirus, HIV, mononucleosis)
3. Bacterial (tuberculosis, staphylococcus, pneumococcus, brucella, salmonella, mycoplasma)
4. Neoplastic (breast and lung cancer)
5. Collagen vascular disease (systemic lupus erythematosis, rheumatoid arthritis)
6. Drugs (procainamide, hydralazine)
7. Hypothyroidism*
8. Uremia
9. Early post-myocardial infarction (bruised epicardium, local irritation)
10. Late post-myocardial infarction (Dressler's syndrome)
11. Post heart surgery (postcardiotomy syndrome, similar to Dressler's syndrome; high sed rate)
12. After radiation exposure
13. Aortic dissection

*Any of these may cause tamponade, but this may not be a not be a complication of an effusion that accumulates slowly, as is common with hypothyroidism.

Inflation of the atria and ventricles is determined by transmural pressure, or the difference between the internal (inflating) pressure and external (deflating) pressure. Normally, the pericardial pressure is zero, and the diastolic inflating pressure within the cardiac chambers is unopposed. Rapidly accumulating effusion increases pericardial pressure, so the transmural pressure declines. This limits diastolic filling. With tamponade, pericardial pressure is so high that it exceeds intracardiac diastolic pressure. This leads to the key diagnostic feature of both tamponade and constrictive pericarditis: equalization of the diastolic pressure in all four cardiac chambers (Figure 2.7). Normally the thicker LV has a higher diastolic pressure than the RV. Diastolic pressures in the atria and RV are higher than usual because of the external pressure, not because of increased filling of the chambers. Filling is actually lower, and the echocardiogram may show collapse of the atria and/or right ventricle.

Figure 2.7 Tamponade, Physiology

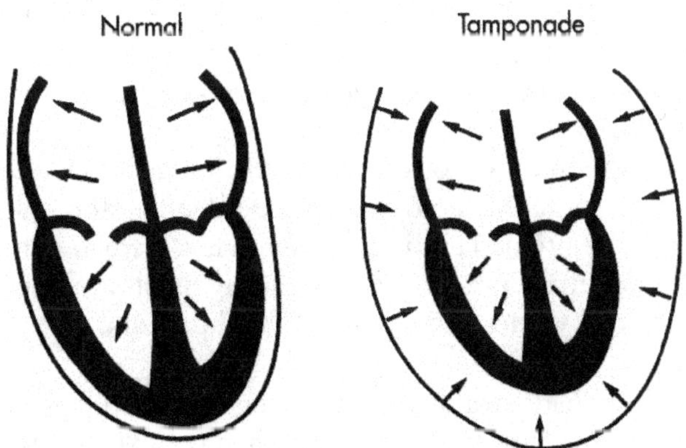

Figure 2.7 In the normal state, pericardial pressure is near zero and intracardiac pressures, in effect, inflate the cardiac chambers. With tamponade, pericardial pressure increases and tends to compress the heart. Intracardiac pressure is the sum of pericardial pressure plus the pressure generated by volume

within the cardiac chambers. During diastole, the pericardial pressure is sufficiently high to be the major determinant of intracardiac pressure, and pressures in the four chambers tend to equalize. External compression of the atria also retards venous return to the heart, lowering cardiac output and blood pressure.

The external pressure blocks blood return to the heart. With reduced cardiac filling stroke volume and cardiac output fall. The consequence is hypotension. The key findings on physical examination are jugular venous distension and pulsus paradoxus.

There isn't much that is paradoxical about pulsus paradoxus, and the term misleading. Normally, the systolic blood pressure falls during inspiration, by less than 10 mmHg. With pulsus paradoxus it falls more; if severe, there may be an appreciable diminution of the arterial pulse with inspiration.

The mechanism may seem complex, but like most of cardiology, it is easily understood. Normally intrathoracic and intrapericardial pressures become negative during inspiration; this sucks blood (as well as air) into the chest and increases venous return to the right heart. Right ventricular volume increases. The expanded right ventricle pushes the interventricular septum toward the LV, reducing LV volume. In addition, pulmonary venous return to the left atrium is decreased during inspiration. Physiologists speak of "respiratory preload variation," RV preload (filling) rises and LV preload (filling) falls. The net effect is a smaller LV during inspiration, leading to lower stroke volume and systolic blood pressure.

Cardiac tamponade exaggerates these changes. Both ventricles are smaller than usual because of elevated pericardial pressure. With inspiration, there is still an increase in flow to the RV. Bowing of the septum toward the LV has an even greater effect on LV stroke volume, because the LV is already small—and systolic blood pressure falls by more than 10 mmHg.

Pulsus paradoxus is measured with the patient breathing normally. The best method is to inflate the blood pressure cuff and then have it deflate very, very, very slowly. You will initially hear the Korotkoff sounds during expiration but not during inspiration; record that blood pressure as Pressure-1. As the cuff continues to deflate slowly, at some point you will hear the sounds during both inspiration and expiration. Record that as Pressure-2. The difference between Pressures 1 and 2 is the pulsus paradoxus. When there is a large pulsus, there may be an appreciable reduction in the arterial pulse volume with inspiration.

Laboratory Diagnosis and Treatment or Pericardial Effusion

The ECG may show ST segment elevation and PR segment depression with acute pericarditis, but in most cases of effusion and tamponade, these changes are absent. With large effusions, QRS voltage may be low. Electrical alternans, a rise and fall in QRS voltage, may occur with the heart swinging in the enlarged pericardial space (and is referred to as the "swinging heart syndrome"). The echocardiogram is quite accurate and detects even small effusions.

With tamponade, there may be apparent collapse of the atria or right ventricle. Hemodynamic instability is an indication for urgent pericardiocentesis. When done at the bedside as an emergency procedure, the complication rate is about 20%. With echocardiographic guidance, usually in the catheterization laboratory, the complication rate is less than 5%.

It is possible to have a large effusion without tamponade. This occurs when the accumulation of fluid is slow enough for the pericardium to expand, and intrapericardial pressure does not rise. This is often the case with hypothyroidism (a board question).

Diagnostic pericardiocentesis is of little use when viral pericarditis is likely. It is not usually needed to make a diagnosis for those with collagen vascular disease. On the other hand, pericardiocentesis may be diagnostic in a patient with suspected malignancy. This usually involves an older person with no history indicating pericarditis (no fever or pain, and a normal sedimentation rate). The effusion may be an incidental finding on chest x-ray or echocardiogram. A bloody pericardial effusion in the absence of anticoagulant therapy points to tumor, and cytology is usually diagnostic.

Constrictive Pericarditis

Chronic inflammation and thickening of the pericardium may lead to constriction, which limits diastolic filling. The usual clinical presentation is isolated right heart failure. Hepatomegaly and ascites are common, and constriction is one of the causes of cryptogenic cirrhosis. We see one or two cases each year as part of the evaluation for liver transplantation, and surgical correction of constriction leads to a cure of the liver disease.

Like tamponade, there is equalization of right and left heart diastolic pressures. Unlike tamponade, early diastolic filling is normal, but it is limited in later diastole. This leads to the characteristic dip-and-plateau, or "square-root" wave form of the ventricular pressure tracing (Figure 2.8). This may be similar to the pressure waveform of restrictive cardiomyopathy. One way to differentiate the two is to infuse saline; with restrictive myopathy the LV diastolic pressure rises more than RV pressure, but with constriction equalization of diastolic pressures persists.

There is elevation of jugular venous pressure, but constriction prevents a fall with inspiration. Instead, venous pressure may rise with inspiration (Kussmaul's sign). Elevated pulsus paradoxus is uncommon with constriction, and is always present with tamponade. A rare patient with constriction has an extra heart sound in early diastole, a pericardial knock.

Pericardial calcification on an over-penetrated chest x-ray supports the diagnosis, and may be the best noninvasive evidence. MRI is able to measure pericardial thickness, but normal thickness does not exclude the diagnosis.

Figure 2.8 Constriction, LV and RV Pressure

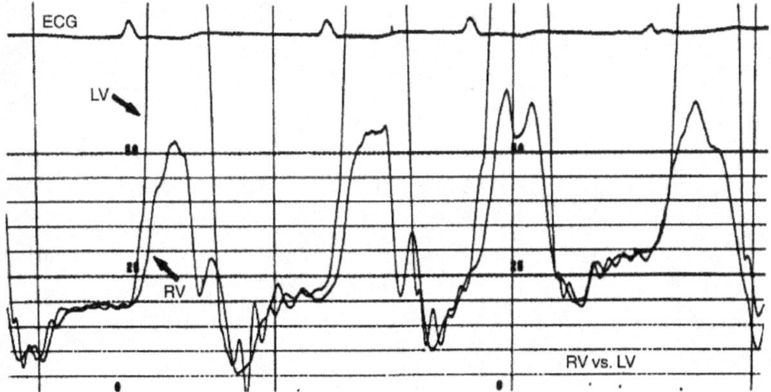

Figure 2.8 Simultaneous left and right ventricular (LV and RV) pressures in a patient with constrictive pericarditis. Normally, the left ventricular pressure is much higher than right ventricular pressure during diastole, and identical pressure during diastole is a hallmark of both constriction and pericardial tamponade. In addition, this patient has the early diastolic pressure dip and then plateau that is typical of constriction (best seen in the first and last beats).

When suspected, left and right heart catheterization is needed to make a diagnosis. Equalization of pressures, which persists after a fluid challenge, is the usual indication for surgical stripping of the pericardium. But this is a tough diagnosis to make. Even when all studies point to constriction, a fair number of patients are found to have no pericardial disease at operation. I tell patients this before surgery, indicating that the procedure is, in a sense, an exploratory operation. The possibility of a surgical cure justifies it.

Effusive-Constrictive Pericarditis

Concomitant tamponade and constriction may occur. In this case, constriction comes from a thickened visceral pericardium (the layer of pericardium that is attached to the epicardial surface). Measuring pericardial pressure at the time of pericardiocentesis, and at the same time measuring RA, RV, and LV pressure makes the diagnosis. As the fluid is drained, pericardial pressure falls, but there is little if any fall in intracardiac diastolic pressure. The dip and plateau morphology of the ventricular diastolic pressure persists.

Effusive-constrictive disease is possible with all types of pericarditis, but it is more common with radiation and neoplasia. Effective therapy requires both pericardiocentesis and surgical removal of the visceral pericardium. Consider this if draining the pericardium does not relieve the patient's symptoms.

Chapter 3: Valvular Heart Disease

Abbreviations

A_2, aortic second heart sound
ACEI, angiotensin converting enzyme inhibitors
AF, atrial fibrillation
AR, aortic regurgitation
AS, aortic stenosis
ASD, atrial septal defect
CHF, congestive heart failure
ECG, electrocardiogram
FDA, Food and Drug Administration
IE, infective endocarditis
LA, left atrium
LV, left ventricle (ventricular)
LVEF, LV ejection fraction
LVH, LV hypertrophy
MI, myocardial infarction
MR, mitral regurgitation
MS, mitral stenosis
MVP, mitral valve prolapse
OS, opening snap
P_2, pulmonic second heart sound
PA, pulmonary artery
PCW, pulmonary capillary wedge pressure
RHD, rheumatic heart disease
RV, right ventricle
SCD, sudden cardiac death
TR, tricuspid regurgitation

Inexperienced clinicians tend to believe that managing valvular heart disease is more complicated than it is. Taking a logical, physiologic approach simplifies it. Evaluate the patient's heart murmur with the following questions in mind:

1. What cardiac chamber is most affected by the valve lesion (Table 3.1)?

2. What is the effect? Does the lesion change left ventricular (LV) preload, afterload, or contractility, and is there hypertrophy or dilation?
3. What changes in LV size and function necessitate valve surgery, and how will surgery affect function? If LV function is not jeopardized, what is the indication for surgery?

Table 3.1. Overview of Valvular Heart Disease: Usual Causes, Pathophysiology, and Timing of Surgery

Mitral Stenosis (always rheumatic heart disease)
<u>Chamber effect:</u> LA overload with sparing of the LV (normal preload and afterload)
<u>Surgery:</u> since the LV is unaffected, wait for symptoms

Chronic Mitral Regurgitation (mitral prolapse syndrome, IE)
<u>Chamber/effect:</u> LA and LV volume overload, LV afterload is low because of emptying into the low pressure LA making the LV look better than it is (see text)

<u>Surgery:</u> there is LV injury by the time symptoms develop so surgery is needed sooner, with any evidence of LV dysfunction or dilation (serial echocardiograms needed). Volume overload is harder on the LV than pressure overload, and injury from volume overload usually does not resolve with valve repair.

Acute Mitral Regurgitation (rupture of chordae tendineae or papillary muscle, IE)
<u>Chamber/effect:</u> abrupt volume overload of LA and LV; since the LA has no time to stretch, pressure is transmitted to the lungs

Surgery: pulmonary edema necessitates early surgery in most cases

Aortic Stenosis (bicuspid valve or a calcific, degenerative process of old age)
Chamber/effect: increased LV afterload leading to concentric hypertrophy

Surgery: because surgery lowers afterload, LV function improves. Plus, pressure overload does not injure the LV as much as volume overload. For that reason, onset of symptoms has been the indication for surgery. New guidelines suggest earlier surgery based on echo/Doppler measures of stenosis.

Aortic Regurgitation (Marfan's and related syndromes, IE)
Chamber/effect: LV volume overload with increased afterload as well, so there is both dilation and hypertrophy of the LV (eccentric hypertrophy).

Surgery: as with mitral regurgitation, volume overload can cause LV injury before symptoms develop. Early LV dysfunction detected by serial echo is the indication for surgical repair (preferred over valve replacement).

Acute Aortic Regurgitation (rapid destruction of the valve with staph endocarditis in an intravenous (IV) drug user; also possible with gonococcal endocarditis)

Chamber/effect: abrupt LV volume overload and pulmonary edema. With elevated LV diastolic pressure, and low aortic diastolic pressure (basically a nonfunctioning valve with no diastolic gradient), the AR murmur may not be audible.

Surgery: usually an emergency. Think of this in a young person with unexplained, overwhelming pulmonary edema, and a history of IV drug use (a common board exam question).

Tricuspid Regurgitation (as a complication of left heart failure, or mitral valve disease; other causes of pulmonary hypertension; IE with iv drug use)

<u>Chamber/effect:</u> RA and RV volume overload. With inspiration the murmur intensifies.

<u>Surgery:</u> tricuspid valve repair is occasionally needed at the time of mitral valve surgery. Isolated tricuspid regurgitation seldom requires surgery (rather, treat the cause of pulmonary hypertension).

IE, infective endocarditis; LA, left atrium; LV, left ventricle; LVH, LV hypertrophy; LVEF, LV ejection fraction; RA, right atrium; RV, right ventricle.

MITRAL STENOSIS

Mitral stenosis (MS), for practical purposes, can be equated with rheumatic heart disease (RHD). All patients with RHD have scarring of the mitral valve apparatus. This has a typical appearance on the echocardiogram, and you may therefore use the echo to diagnose or exclude RHD. Isolated aortic valve disease, with a normal mitral valve, is not caused by rheumatic fever.

Treatment of strep throat with antibiotics makes RHD rare in western countries; a primary care doctor in the US might never encounter a case. It remains a common illness in lesser-developed countries. In rural Latin America or India, RHD often has a more aggressive course, with symptomatic MS appearing at an earlier age. In developed countries, the usual history is rheumatic fever in the early teens and then onset of symptomatic MS or atrial fibrillation when the patient reaches early-middle age.

Pathophysiology, History, and Physical Examination

One of my teachers told us "mitral stenosis is a disease of the lungs." The blocked valve causes pressure overload of the left atrium (LA), and LA dilation (Table 3.1). The increased pressure in the LA is transmitted to the pulmonary capillary bed. Dyspnea on exertion, fatigue (due to limited cardiac output), and winter bronchitis are the usual symptoms, and they may be insidious in onset. A middle-aged nurse with known MS for years called this winter to get an antibiotic for a "chest cold she couldn't shake." She and her family doctor were concerned she might be developing asthma. But with questioning she admitted that her exercise tolerance had gradually worsened over the previous 4 to 6 months. This is the typical, slowly evolving story. Patients are often unaware just how bad they feel until symptoms are relieved by valve surgery.

With time, most patients with LA enlargement caused by mitral valve disease develop atrial fibrillation (AF). A minority with advanced disease develop pulmonary hypertension, and with it symptoms of right heart failure: edema, ascites, and fatigue.

Most of the symptoms of MS are common to other forms of heart failure. Hemoptysis is more specific for mitral stenosis, and is caused by the rupture of small bronchial veins. It may be substantial, with cough producing a few ounces of blood—more than just blood-streaked sputum. With bleeding, the veins decompress and the bleeding stops. Hemoptysis is rarely a fatal complication of MS.

The LV is unaffected by MS. LV afterload is normal. The stenosed valve inhibits LV filling, and a poorly compensated patient with low cardiac output has a low preload. But the asymptomatic patient does not; adequate LV filling is accomplished by raising LA pressure, thus forcing blood across the stenosed valve. This pressure gradient across the valve is the definitive hemodynamic finding in MS (Figure 3.1).

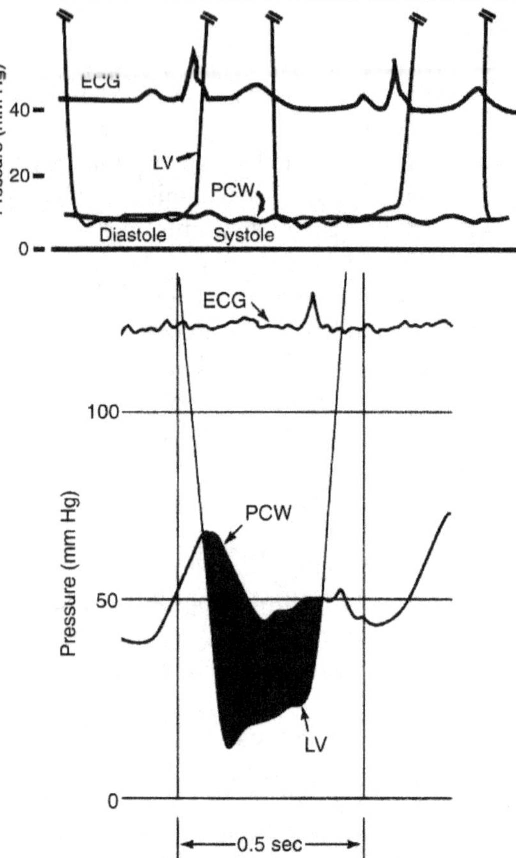

FIGURE 3.1 (Top) Normal: the mitral valve is wide open during diastole, and there is no pressure difference, or gradient, between left atrial and LV diastolic pressure. (Bottom) Mitral stenosis: there is obstruction during diastole, and a pressure gradient (shaded area).

The LV is usually small and contracts normally. The high LA pressure and limited cardiac output can lead to the congestive heart failure syndrome, mimicking the effects of cardiomyopathy. The neurohumoral response to low cardiac output is the same (Chapter 1).

On physical examination the apical impulse is normal. With pulmonary hypertension, there may be a right ventricular lift. Since LV loading is normal, there is no gallop. Recall that gallops occur during diastole and reflect LV filling abnormalities: rapid early diastolic filling of a big, flabby LV causes the S_3, and atrial contraction at the end of diastole forcing a column of blood against a stiff ventricle causes the S_4. With MS the LV is neither dilated and flabby, nor hypertrophied and stiff.

The earliest physical finding is a loud S_1, and this physical finding is easier to detect than the soft murmur. With time the valve stiffens and becomes less mobile, and S_1 softens. The diastolic murmur is low pitched, probably because flow velocity across the stenosed valve is relatively low given a pressure gradient of 10-15 mmHg (compared with the higher flow rate and pressure gradient across a stenosed aortic valve). Listen for it over the apex impulse using the bell of the stethoscope (the diaphragm is better for higher pitched sounds). The murmur is much easier to hear with the patient rolled to the left side.

The opening snap (OS) is an interesting physical finding, created by the movement of the calcified valve. It is high-pitched, and that distinguishes it from the much lower pitch of the S_3 gallop—both are heard best at the apex. Opening of the mitral valve occurs shortly after closure of the aortic valve, so the OS follows S_2. With more severe stenosis, the OS occurs earlier, and an S_2-OS interval less than 0.11 seconds indicates severe stenosis. Measuring this interval using the phonocardiogram was the best noninvasive test for gauging MS severity in the days before echocardiography. That test is no longer used, but you can estimate the S_2-OS interval at the bedside using an old-fashioned diagnostic trick: When you say the words, the interval between the letters b and l in *blah* is 0.10 seconds, and between the b and t in *butter* is 0.14 seconds. Admittedly low-tech, but this works, and using physical diagnosis to determine the severity of a valvular lesion is still

great sport for clinicians.   (You can probably guess the age of
the writer!)

Diagnostic Studies

The electrocardiogram (ECG) shows left atrial enlargement,
usually with a P mitrale pattern (Figure 3.2). Another common
finding is AF. On chest x-ray, LA enlargement straightens the
left heart border and creates a double density at the right heart
border.

Figure 3.2 Two Patients with Left Atrial Abnormality

Patient 1

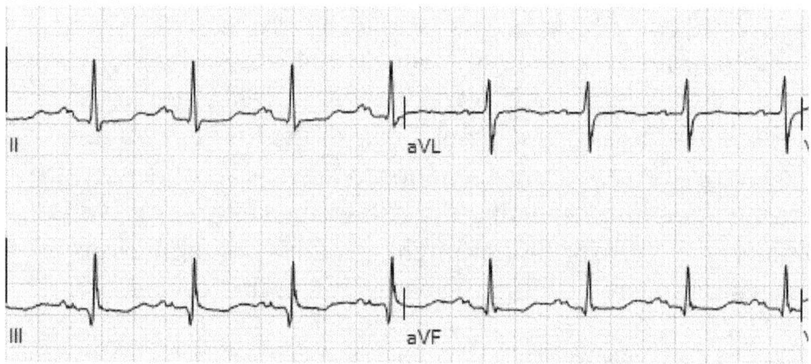

Patient 2

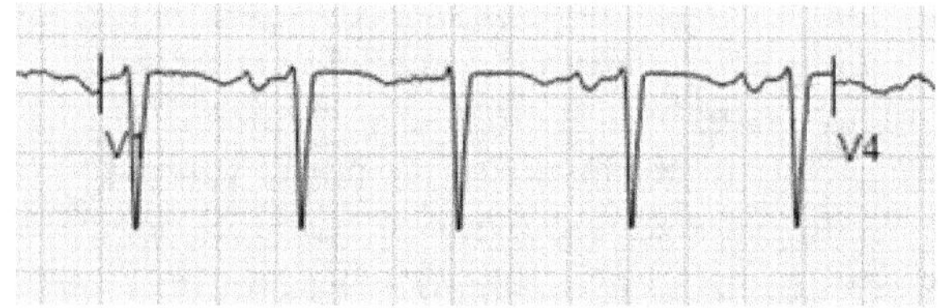

FIGURE 3.2. Left atrial abnormality. Two ECG findings may be
used to make the diagnosis. Patient 1: broad notched P wave in
one of the limb leads, most commonly II, III, or aVF (the P wave
vector is aimed inferiorly). The notched P wave—conveniently M
shaped—is often seen with mitral valve disease ("P mitrale").
Patient 2: biphasic P wave in lead V_1; the negative deflection
should be 1 mm deep and wide. This pattern is more common
with hypertensive heart disease. Occasionally patients have
both patterns.

The echocardiogram demonstrates the typical rheumatic deformity of the valve, reduced leaflet mobility and calcification. All patients have LA enlargement. There are three methods for measuring the severity of MS with the echo-Doppler study. The first is visualization of the valve in cross-section and measuring the size of the opening. Two Doppler measures of severity come from flow velocity across the valve. First, flow velocity in meters per second is proportional to the valve gradient. This is analogous to increased flow velocity at the end of a garden hose as the nozzle is tightened. Second, the flow velocity remains high for a longer time with more severe stenosis, decaying at the very end of diastole. The "pressure half-time" is a measure of the time to decay of the flow velocity curve, and it is proportional to the pressure gradient.

Cardiac catheterization is seldom needed to make the diagnosis of MS, and symptomatic young people have mitral valve surgery without it. Older patients usually have coronary angiography before surgery, so that coronary bypass can be accomplished during the operation. In the cath lab, the definitive measurement is the pressure gradient across the valve (using catheters in the pulmonary artery and the LV, Figure 3.1).

Timing of Surgery

As a consultant, we are rarely asked if the patient has MS (or another valve problem). That is usually obvious from the physical examination and noninvasive studies. Rather, the patient is sent to the cardiologist to determine whether surgical repair is needed. The timing of surgery is the issue you face in clinic, and will encounter on board exams.

The key issue in timing surgery is the state of the LV, just as LV function is a fundamental issue with most of the adult cardiac illnesses. With MS, the LV is unaffected; there is no abnormal loading that could lead to muscle injury. Thus, surgery is not required prophylactically to save the LV. For this reason, the indication for surgery is the onset of symptoms. Prognosis also tends to worsen when there is pulmonary hypertension, and this is a second indication for surgery. Pulmonary artery pressure can be estimated from echo-Doppler measurement.

Some have recommended surgery when AF develops. Correction of MS may allow the LA to shrink, restoring sinus rhythm. At present, this is not a standard indication for open surgery. But it is now a soft indication for mitral valve balloon repair.

When the valve is mobile and there is little calcification—often the case with young patients—repair is possible. Closed balloon valvulotomy in the catheterization laboratory works well, with an average doubling of the valve area that is maintained long-term. Associated mitral regurgitation (MR), thrombus in the LA, and valve calcification are contraindications to balloon repair, and indicate a need for surgery.

(As an aside, there is little experience with this procedure in the US. If I needed it, I would look for a center doing a large number of cases, probably in Mexico or India.)

Medical Therapy

The asymptomatic patient in sinus rhythm requires only antibiotic prophylaxis for infective endocarditis (IE), and to prevent recurrent rheumatic fever. When symptoms develop, surgery is needed. If surgery is not to be done, for whatever reason, diuretic therapy lowers LA pressure and relieves congestion. There is no role for measures to lower LV afterload or increase contractility. The only rationale for digoxin therapy or beta blockade is the control of ventricular rate in the patient with AF.

AF is common. Reduced flow across the mitral valve and the enlarged LA make the risk of thromboembolism much higher than it is with other causes of AF. Anticoagulation with warfarin or a thrombin inhibitor is indicated. The control of ventricular rate with digoxin, beta blockers or calcium blockers is especially important for control of symptoms. Tachycardia reduces total diastolic time, a big problem for the patient with LV inflow obstruction; the LV needs time to fill.

MITRAL REGURGITATION

The mitral valve prolapse (MVP) syndrome—not RHD—is the most common cause of primary mitral regurgitation (MR). Isolated MR may also be caused by ischemic injury of papillary muscles, endocarditis, or LV dilation, which changes the orientation of the papillary muscles and slightly dilates the valve ring.

Chronic Mitral Regurgitation

Pathophysiology, History and Physical Examination

There is volume overload of the LA and LV, and both chambers dilate slowly. The large, flabby LA gives, absorbing the shock of the regurgitant jet. For this reason, LA pressure remains fairly normal, and the ventricular pressure wave (V wave) is not transmitted directly to the lungs.

LV afterload is low (Figure 3.3). Normally, systemic arterial resistance constitutes the impedance to LV ejection (afterload). With MR, the ventricle is able to unload into both the low-pressure LA and the higher-pressure aorta. Net impedance to ejection—a.k.a., afterload—is thus low. The lower the afterload, the easier it is for LV muscle to shorten. With easier shortening, LV ejection fraction (LVEF) is high, artificially so. But what happens when the mitral valve is repaired and the LV can no longer dump its load into the low-pressure LA? There is a net increase in afterload.

Figure 3.3 LV Afterload with Mitral Regurgitation

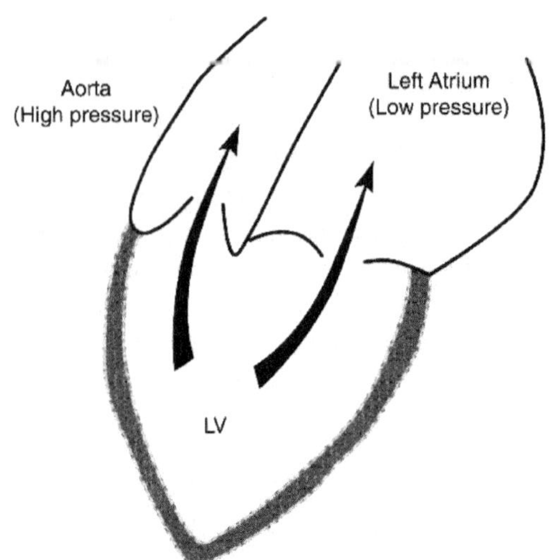

Figure 3.3 In the absence of MR, the ventricle empties into the aorta, a high-pressure system. But with MR, the left ventricle (LV) can also empty into the low-pressure left atrium. The net afterload, or impedance to injection, is therefore low. Replacing the valve may be expected to increase net afterload, and left ventricular function suffers.

Afterload *increasing* therapy? That doesn't sound good for the LV, and it is not. In fact, LVEF often declines following surgery for MR. For this reason, the risk of surgery for chronic MR was high when the operation was new; they waited too long to operate.

The eventual symptoms of MR are those of left heart (pulmonary) congestion and low cardiac output. On exam the apical impulse is displaced and has a volume-overload quality; it is "rocking" and occupies more than one rib interspace. There may be an S_3 gallop caused by the rapid filling wave early in diastole.

The murmur is holosystolic, extending to S_2, and is audible at the apex and axilla. The plane of the valve is perpendicular to a line from the apex impulse to the axilla, and a "fish-mouth," fixed orifice would direct the murmur in that direction. On the other hand, a dysfunctional lateral leaflet may prolapse and serve as a baffle, directing the jet—and murmur—toward the base of the heart along the sternum. It may be audible at the right base rather than at the axilla. Thus, a loud systolic murmur at the base of the heart that does not radiate to the neck may be MR rather than aortic stenosis. Furthermore, MR from papillary muscle dysfunction may generate a diamond-shaped murmur (crescendo-decrescendo), since peak dysfunction occurs at peak LV systolic pressure.

Diagnostic Studies and Timing of Surgery

The echocardiogram is the key study. It identifies the source of the systolic murmur (mitral vs. aortic valve), defines the valvular anatomy (prolapse, chordal rupture and flail leaflet, vegetation, calcification, etc.), and provides critical LV size and function data. Preoperative cardiac catheterization examines coronary anatomy and measures pulmonary artery pressure, but it is seldom needed to determine a need for surgery.

Many patients with MR are asymptomatic and tolerate it for years. But waiting for symptoms to develop is a disaster, since symptoms may not occur until the LV is irreversibly damaged. The basic problem is overestimation of the quality of the LV preoperatively, because of low afterload.

Because LVEF is expected to decline with repair, a preoperative LVEF <50% is a poor prognostic sign. Dilation of the LV during diastole is not a problem if the ventricle contracts down to a normal volume at end-systole. This, of course, also indicates a normal LVEF. With volume overload disease, both MR and aortic regurgitation, an elevated end-systolic volume predicts higher operative mortality, more postoperative heart failure, and persistent LV enlargement after surgery.

The LV end-systolic dimension is easily and accurately measured with the transthoracic echocardiogram, and it is a good substitute for end-systolic volume. This is the measurement that we follow when monitoring patients with volume overload valvular disease. An LV end-systolic dimension >4.5 cm indicates a higher risk of surgery.

Best surgical results are obtained when the LV end-systolic dimension is < 4.5 cm, or the LVEF is ≥60%, even when there are no symptoms. Asymptomatic patients have serial echocardiograms to follow these LV measurements. Surgery is indicated when LV size and function approach these levels. Follow-up Doppler studies are unnecessary, as the diagnosis of MR is established. If you can order the cheaper "echo without Doppler," you will get the data you need. Some patients are difficult to study, but the technician should be aware that measurement of LV dimensions is critical.

Repair of the mitral valve is better than replacement with a prosthesis. It is now clear that the mitral valve supporting structures contribute to LV function. Physiologists speak of the papillary muscles and chordae "tethering" the ventricle on its long axis, contributing to stroke volume by preserving normal LV shape during contraction. One study found a decline in LVEF from 55% to 35% with mitral valve replacement but no significant decline with valve repair and salvage of chordal structures. Most patients with mitral prolapse are candidates for repair.

Advanced LV Dysfunction

Is it ever too late to attempt to correct MR? Mitral valve *replacement* with loss of the chordae tendenae and papillary muscles usually leads to catastrophe in patients with LVEF <30%.

On the other hand, mitral valve *repair* has been successfully performed in patients with low LVEF. Preservation of papillary muscle function makes it possible, and if that is not likely, most surgeons will not operate.

Transcatheter mitral valve repair (TMVR) is now a reality. It is based upon the operation developed by Alfieri. He found that tethering the anterior and posterior leaflets together with a single stitch to the middle of the leaflets corrects MR. During diastole, the midpoint of the leaflets cannot open, but there is opening to either side of the stitch—it becomes a "double barreled valve." The single stitch is enough to correct regurgitation, and it does not cause stenosis. A catheter delivered clip is used to stitch the mid-point of the mitral leaflets without surgery—the Mitraclip.

Medical Therapy

Vasodilator therapy has been found to be helpful in patients with aortic regurgitation, and it seems that afterload reduction would "promote forward flow" in patients with MR. Angiotensin converting enzyme (ACE) inhibition has been found to reduce LV size in patients with *symptomatic* MR. However, the standard therapy for such patients is surgical correction, and vasodilator therapy is no substitute.

The more common question is whether to treat *asymptomatic* patients with afterload reduction therapy, hoping to delay a need for surgery. Recall that LV afterload is already low with MR. A further reduction with drug therapy has not been supported by clinical trials. Small studies found no reduction in LV size with vasodilator therapy in the absence of clinical heart failure.

Symptomatic patients with MR who are not candidates for surgery benefit from standard therapy for HFrEF including diuretics, vasodilators, and digoxin (Chapter 1). The role of beta blockade is uncertain.

Cardiomyopathy and Mitral Regurgitation

Marked LV dilatation changes the orientation of the papillary muscles and chordae, and it stretches the annulus slightly. It is common to see MR in patients with dilated cardiomyopathy, and significant MR indicates worse prognosis. The Everest II trial found that Mitraclip repair reduced MR severity and symptoms, and there was improved LV size and function. At this time there are no data indicating a survival benefit, but the procedure is still in its early stages of development.

Acute Mitral Regurgitation

MR after acute myocardial infarction is reviewed in Chapter 5. Think of it when acute pulmonary edema develops after a relatively small MI, since little injury is required to disrupt papillary muscle function.

Spontaneous rupture of chordae may occur in the absence of coronary artery disease, most commonly in middle-aged men with MVP. The history often includes a single, brief episode of non-anginal chest pain at the time of rupture. Over the next few days there is progressive dyspnea, and severe pulmonary congestion is apparent at the time of initial evaluation.

Because of the abrupt onset of symptomatic MR, there is insufficient time for the LA and LV to dilate. Therefore, the apical impulse is not displaced. Since the LV is not large and flabby, there is no S_3 gallop. In fact, the large volume of blood hitting the relatively small LV at end-diastole may cause an S_4 gallop even though the LV is not stiff.

The normal LA has no time to stretch and is too stiff to expand with the regurgitant wave, so there is a marked rise in LA pressure during ventricular systole. This V wave is transmitted to the pulmonary capillary bed, aggravating congestive symptoms (Figure 3.4). It is also an important finding in the cath lab, supporting the diagnosis of acute rather than chronic MR. (There is a low amplitude V wave with chronic MR; the dilated,

flabby LA gives with the regurgitant jet and transmits little
pressure to the pulmonary circulation.)

Figure 3.4 Hemodynamics of Acute Mitral Regurgitation

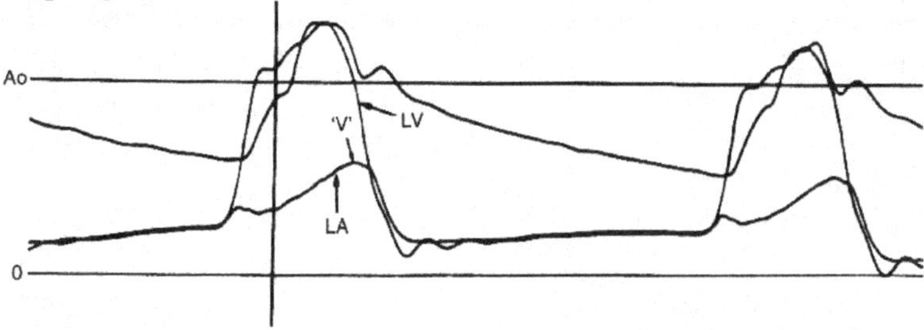

Figure 3.4 This is simultaneous left atrial (LA), LV, and aortic
(Ao) pressure tracings from a patient with *acute* MR. During LV
systole, the LV pressure wave is transmitted back to the LA
through the defective mitral valve and measured as a V wave. In
the absence of MR there is a tiny V wave caused by the slight
posterior bowing of the mitral valve. With chronic MR the large,
flaccid left atrium absorbs the pressure wave, and the V wave is
not as prominent.

The systolic murmur is usually loud. As noted above, it may
radiate medially, rather than to the axilla (the mitral leaflet
working as a baffle). A patient with severe pulmonary
congestion may have a soft or inaudible murmur. The
echocardiogram shows the MR jet, and may also identify
marked prolapse of the untethered leaflet edge, a flail leaflet.

Acute MR with associated pulmonary edema requires urgent
surgery. Most patients have damage to valve support structures,
yet valve repair is possible. As noted above, this is preferable to
replacement as anticoagulation is not required, and LV function
is better preserved.

Mitral Valve Prolapse (MVP)

MVP has been over-diagnosed. Thin young girls have stretchy
connective tissue, and their chordae tendenae and mitral leaflets

are as flexible as their joints. It is common to see a small amount
of mitral valve prolapse on their echocardiogram. But they do
not have myxomatous degeneration of the valve, e.g. pathologic
MVP.

The diagnostic criteria have been refined in recent years.
Pathologic MVP includes posterior motion of the valve beyond
the plane of the mitral ring plus a thickened and redundant
valve, the typical "floppy" or "parachute" valve. The presence
of a mid-systolic click on examination is considered diagnostic,
even when the echocardiographic findings are unimpressive.

Primary MVP can be inherited. It commonly accompanies other
connective tissue disorders such as Marfan's syndrome. In fact,
MVP could be considered one of the diagnostic criteria for
Marfan's syndrome. In such cases other features suggest
abnormal connective tissue, including pectus excavatum,
straight back, high arched palate and an enlarged aortic root.

Although serious complications are possible (Table 3.2), they
are uncommon. Recent studies suggest that a diagnosis of MVP
does not convey an increased mortality risk. Advanced age,
more severe MR and atrial fibrillation predict cardiovascular
death. It often surprises students that the demographic group
most commonly needing valve repair is middle-aged men (it is
common to see this illness at the VA hospital, less so at the
university hospital).

Table 3.2 Complications of Mitral Valve Prolapse (MVP)

Infective endocarditis: 1% by age 75, higher if there is MR or a
thickened valve

Mitral regurgitation: 5% of men by age 75 (just 1% of
women), higher with obesity or hypertension

Sudden death: about 1 in 200 with MR (1 in 5,000 without MR). Long QT = higher risk

Embolic stroke: Rare, and probably no risk with mild MVP. Higher risk with atrial fibrillation, large LA, thickened valve.

The excursion of the prolapsing valve is increased when the LV is smaller. Thus, the findings of MVP are magnified by maneuvers that reduce venous return and LV size, such as standing. Amyl nitrate, a venodilator, is used for this purpose in the echo laboratory.

The click is mid-systolic and the murmur follows it. When you hear a mid to late systolic murmur, the usual cause is MVP. Listen carefully for the click; it may be localized to a small area near the lower sternum or apex.

Diagnosis and Treatment

Avoid over-diagnosis. Healthy young people often have vague symptoms, including chest pain and palpitations. Do not assign a diagnosis of MVP and "heart disease" when the physical exam is normal, and the echocardiogram shows trivial prolapse but normal mitral valve morphology. Population studies have shown that the prognosis is good for those with mild prolapse, with little risk of stroke, sudden death or progression to severe MR.

On the other hand, serious illness is possible for those with pathologic MVP (Table 3.2). Interestingly, it is not the thin young woman who is at risk for developing severe MR, but the middle-aged man with hypertension (a fact that has appeared on the medicine boards). Antibiotic prophylaxis to prevent endocarditis is no longer recommended with MVP. Although untested, many prescribe aspirin for those with severe prolapse to prevent thromboembolic stroke. It is not indicated for mild MVP.

While uncommon, it is possible for severe MVP to cause angina. The parachute valve increases papillary muscle tension, creating ischemia. This can lead to an abnormal stress ECG, with a perfusion abnormality in the region of the papillary muscle. In such cases, beta blockade may help.

A common management issue is the patient with mild MVP and vague, nonanginal chest pain or palpitations. Monitoring usually shows no arrhythmia during symptoms. Treating either symptom with beta blockers rarely helps. In the absence of convincing angina, I try to avoid stress testing; false positives are common and add to the confusion. Most believe that anxiety is the usual cause of these symptoms. One randomized study showed improvement with prescribed aerobic exercise. That seems a sensible approach; exercise helps relieve stress and is not bad for the heart. Such symptoms tend to resolve with time.

AORTIC STENOSIS (AS)

Etiology, Pathophysiology and History

About 1-2% of the population has a bicuspid aortic valve and may develop AS. Most who do are men, and they become symptomatic in the fourth or fifth decades of life. It is inherited, affecting about 10% of a patient's family. Typically, a murmur is present from childhood reflecting increased turbulence, and with turbulence the valve degenerates prematurely. The degenerative process in vascular structures—including cardiac valves—involves the deposition of calcium. I tell patients that it is like a carpenter's hand developing callus after years of using a hammer.

Bicuspid aortic valve stenosis has been associated with aneurysm of the ascending aorta, with a risk of dissection, and with coarctation of the aorta.

Most adult patients with AS have tricuspid valves. A minor abnormality of valve shape is the probable cause of increased turbulence (and a murmur). This turbulence leads to "premature" stiffening of the valve and stenosis in the seventh or eighth decades of life. Those with a normally streamlined valve and no murmur could go a few decades longer before the aortic valve wears out. This degenerative model of senile AS is consistent with the usual history of a heart murmur present since early adulthood.

Inflammation of valve leaflets is largely responsible for the progression of AS. The early valve lesion is histologically similar to early atherosclerotic plaque, and atherosclerosis is now considered an inflammatory process. That said, statin therapy to reduce vascular inflammation has not been found to slow the progression of AS.

While it is a critical mechanism, I do not buy inflammation as the sole cause of AS. There are many people who develop advanced coronary artery disease with associated inflammation, but never have valvular disease. Conversely, many with senile AS have no vascular disease. Finally, the common history of a murmur earlier in life suggests that longstanding turbulence—and a structural abnormality—contributed to premature degeneration of the valve. Turbulence around the valve may promote inflammation, which then contributes to progression of the disease. As with other medical conditions, the etiology of senile AS probably is multifactorial.

The term aortic "sclerosis" is commonly used to describe the asymptomatic patient with a murmur and reduced valve mobility on the echocardiogram. The natural history of this condition is benign. Progression to AS occurred in 16% in one study, and only 2.5% developed severe AS. In this small subset, the average time for progression to severe AS was 8 years.

AS primarily affects the LV. It is pure afterload, and the echocardiogram documents concentric LV hypertrophy (LVH). The earliest symptoms are those of left heart failure, including dyspnea on exertion or easy fatigue. A patient usually describes a nonspecific decline in exercise tolerance, and probing for changes is important when taking a history.

The second of the triad of symptoms is angina pectoris. This may occur without associated coronary artery disease; the hypertrophied LV has outrun its blood supply. However, about half of those with AS and angina are found to have a significant coronary stenosis at the time of catheterization.

Syncope is the last of the triad of symptoms. When syncope occurs at rest, it may be the result of a transient tachyarrhythmia, either ventricular tachycardia or atrial fibrillation (with severe diastolic dysfunction, either can lead to a drop in blood pressure and cerebral perfusion, Chapter 2). Syncope during exercise suggests another mechanism: cardiac output is fixed because of AS, and thus fails to increase with exercise. Yet there is peripheral arterial dilation with exercise, and the result is hypotension. An abnormal baroreceptor response of the hypertrophied LV, similar to that seen with neurocardiogenic syncope, may also contribute (Chapter 6).

Physical Examination

AS is easy to diagnose; a loud systolic murmur that radiates to the neck cannot be much else. The critical issue is whether it is severe. The physical examination usually provides an answer, and the expected findings of severe stenosis may be deduced from the pathophysiology of AS (Figure 3.5)

Figure 3.5 Physical Findings with Aortic Stenosis

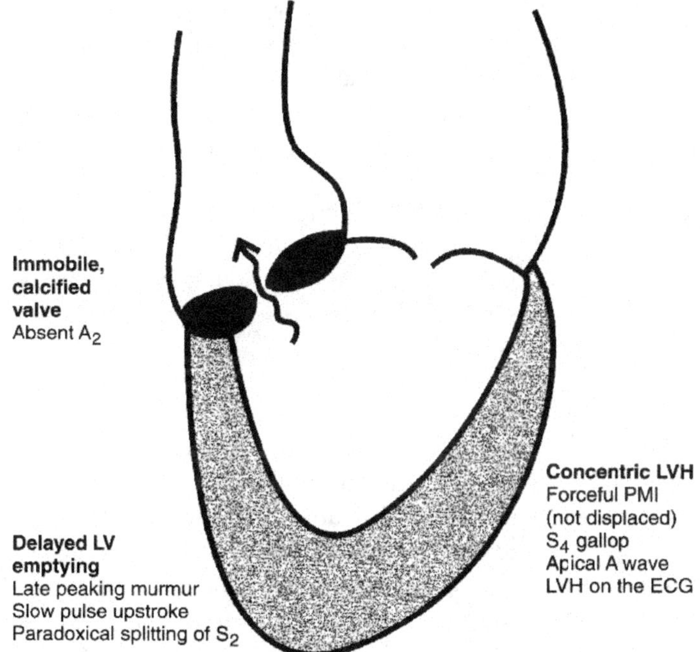

Figure 3.5 This is calcific (senile) aortic stenosis. The physical findings that indicate severe AS reflect LVH, delayed LV emptying, and a heavily calcified, immobile valve. PMI, point of maximum impulse.

1. LVH. The apex impulse is forceful, yet still in the midclavicular line, since hypertrophy is concentric (e.g. from the outside in, so the LV cavity is small). If there is a gallop, it would be the stiff ventricle gallop, and S_4 (see Figure 2.4)

2. The quality and length of the murmur. A mid-systolic, diamond-shaped murmur is typical with mild AS. With more severe disease, ejection is delayed and the murmur peaks later. Eventually the murmur is loud and occupies most of systole, without the crescendo-decrescendo pattern. A palpable murmur (thrill) indicates severe stenosis.

3. Evidence for a calcified valve. My go-to physical sign in elderly patients is the quality of the aortic second sound, A_2. When the valve is heavily calcified, as is usual with senile AS, it becomes immobile; A_2 softens, and then disappears. An audible A_2 means the valve is mobile and is evidence against clinically significant AS. How do you tell the difference between A_2 and the pulmonic second sound, P_2? In the absence of pulmonary hypertension P_2 is relatively soft, and can only be heard to the left of the upper sternum. AS rarely causes severe pulmonary hypertension. If you hear a second heart sound over the aortic area, you are hearing A_2. If the second sound is absent at the right base, A_2 is missing.

4. Evidence for delayed LV emptying. In addition to a longer murmur, prolonged ejection causes a delay in the carotid upstroke. This is a reliable finding in younger patients. It is less so in the elderly who have stiffer arteries, which can mask the delay in the upstroke. I am cautious about mashing on the carotid arteries of elderly patients. There are stories of inexperienced and aggressive examiners provoking stroke. Paradoxical splitting of S_2 is another sign of delayed emptying. It is a useful finding in a young person with a bicuspid valve that is still mobile. On the other hand, if A_2 is absent or too soft to hear to the left of the sternum—usually the case with calcific AS—there will be no audible splitting of S_2.

When these physical findings are present you may count on a high gradient across the aortic valve (Figure 3.6), and on a small valve area (less than 0.8 sq cm).

Figure 3.6 Pressure Measurements with Aortic Stenosis

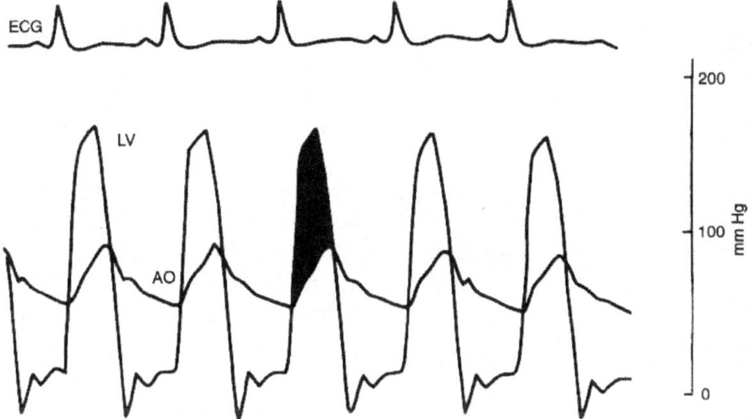

Figure 3.6 Simultaneous LV and aortic (AO) recordings show a pressure gradient across the valve (shaded area). That is the excess pressure that the left ventricle must generate to maintain stroke volume.

Diagnostic Studies and Timing of Surgery

Echo-Doppler study provides an accurate diagnosis for most patients. It also excludes idiopathic hypertrophic subaortic stenosis or mitral regurgitation, although neither causes a murmur that radiates to the neck. The flow velocity across the aortic valve may be an especially important finding; 70% of asymptomatic patients with a jet velocity above 4 m per second (corresponding to a peak gradient of 64 mm Hg) become symptomatic and require valve replacement within 2 years.

Exercise testing is contraindicated for those with symptomatic AS. It is being used more frequently to evaluate asymptomatic patients with borderline echo findings. Exercise induced symptoms or a drop in blood pressure are indications for surgery. In one study, a third of those tested had symptoms for the first time with treadmill testing. This makes sense, since older patients with valvular disease tend to attribute a gradual decline in exercise tolerance to aging, and have learned to avoid activities that provoke symptoms.

Cardiac catheterization allows accurate measurement of the valve gradient (Figure 3.6). Given a technically adequate echocardiogram, this usually is not needed. Coronary angiography is required before surgery.

Symptomatic AS

The onset of symptoms is the indication for surgery, since the mortality risk increases following their appearance (Figure 3.7). As noted, symptoms may be subtle, and it is important to ask carefully about changes in exercise tolerance.

Figure 3.7 Natural History of Aortic Stenosis

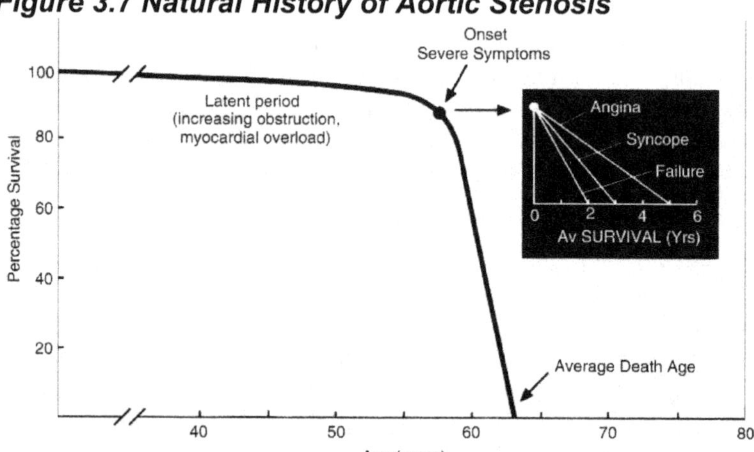

Figure 3.7 In the absence of symptoms, survival is normal. However, once the symptoms of angina, syncope, or congestive heart failure develop, the survival curve plummets. As seen in the inset, average survival is 5 years after developing angina, 3 years with syncope, and just 2 years with heart failure.

One reason that new symptoms have traditionally been the indication for surgery is that sudden cardiac death (SCD) is seldom the initial symptom. It is usually preceded by heart failure, including pulmonary congestion. An early British study found that 16 of 135 patients with tight AS died during a 6-month wait for surgery. All of those with SCD had symptomatic congestive heart failure. Because the risk of SCD increases after the onset of other symptoms, a recommendation that surgical repair should be accomplished within a month is sensible.

Asymptomatic AS with a High Gradient

The prognosis is excellent in the absence of symptoms, even when AS is severe. Nevertheless, when flow velocity across the valve is >4 m per sec, there is rapid progression of disease, so this is now an indication for surgery. Thus, we now have an indication for serial echocardiograms in patients with severe AS.

Low gradient AS Plus Low LV Ejection Fraction

The question is whether a patient's symptoms are from the valve or sick muscle. A gradient below 40 mm Hg is considered nonsignificant AS. But the gradient can be low because of low cardiac output. That is a possibility with advanced AS; high afterload depresses the LV, so that EF is low, cardiac output is low, and the gradient and calculated valve area are low. In this case, fixing the valve lowers the afterload. LVEF and cardiac output rise, and there is clinical improvement.

On the other hand, it is possible that LVEF is low because of coexisting cardiomyopathy. In this case a low calculated valve area is the result of low cardiac output. Afterload is relatively normal, and the LV fails to improve after surgery. As a group, those with a transvalvular gradient below 30 mmHg plus low LVEF have a 20% operative mortality, and less than half are alive 4 years later.

What we would like to do is identify the patient whose low LVEF and gradient are the result of high afterload (bad AS), but who has an intrinsically good LV. This can be tested in the catheterization laboratory by increasing cardiac output with dobutamine. With aortic pseudostenosis the aortic valve gradient changes little as cardiac output increases. With severe AS, the cardiac output and valve gradient both increase. Nitroprusside as also been used: with arterial vasodilatation, downstream resistance falls but there is little change in cardiac output if AS is severe (e.g., all the afterload is in the valve). With cardiomyopathy, cardiac output rises with vasodilation and afterload reduction.

Dobutamine stress echo may also sort it out, and has emerged as the key diagnostic study. Dobutamine increases ejection fraction and cardiac output. The valve gradient will increase when there is true AS. If AS is mild and the patient has a cardiomyopathy, the ejection fraction increases with little change in the valve gradient.

Elderly and High Risk Patients

There is no age limit for correction of AS in the absence of comorbid conditions. Surgical correction increases an 80-year-old person's life expectancy about 6 years, and they are good years with fair exercise tolerance and few symptoms. Coronary artery disease, other valvular heart disease, advanced renal and neurological diseases all increase the risk of surgery and must be considered.

An occasional older person declines surgery, most commonly one with poor general health. With the onset of symptoms, survival with AS can be as long as 2-5 years. It is probably less than that for a frail octogenarian.

Transcatheter aortic valve repair, TAVR, is a viable option. Initial trials were limited to high-risk patients, most of them elderly, and the results have been good. The indications have expanded to intermediate risk AS, and I am telling patients with early AS that it may become an alternative to surgery when the time comes.

Medical Therapy

Mechanical conditions require mechanical solutions, and medical therapy is no substitute for surgery. Asymptomatic, presurgical AS requires no therapy to improve cardiac function. AS is no longer an indication for antibiotic prophylaxis before dental and other invasive procedures. It is reserved for those with prosthetic valves.

Medical therapy does little to affect survival for those who are not to have surgery (for whatever reason). Symptomatic congestion should be managed with diuretics. Raising cardiac output with digoxin may help. The use of afterload reducers has been reported and is of clear benefit for those with aortic pseudostenosis (whose real illness is cardiomyopathy). However, with pure valvular AS, vasodilation has little effect on cardiac output.

AORTIC REGURGITATION (AR)

Etiology, Pathophysiology and History

AR is caused by diseases of the aortic root (Marfan's syndrome, ankylosing spondylitis, syphilis, or the annuloaortic ectasia of aging), or by conditions affecting the valve leaflets (infective endocarditis, rheumatic fever, congenital biscuspid valve, or collagen vascular disease).

Chronic AR

The LV responds to the volume overload with dilation but also with eccentric hypertrophy. In contrast, MR—a pure volume overload disease—leads to dilation with little hypertrophy. Whenever there is hypertrophy, afterload is high (the exception being infiltrative disease), and afterload is elevated with AR. The explanation for this is that the increased stroke volume of AR is ejected into the aorta causing a rise in systolic pressure, and thus an increase in LV afterload. In a sense, there is not enough room in the central circulation for the high stroke volume. With MR, the higher stroke volume (inevitable with any LV volume overload) is shared by the left atrium and aorta, so there is no increase in aortic systolic pressure.

Interestingly, the eccentric hypertrophy of AR is inadequate to normalize LV wall stress. Recall Laplace's law:

Wall stress or tension = pressure x radius of the chamber / 2 x wall thickness

Physiologists call the failure of the LV to thicken enough to normalize stress "afterload mismatch."
The enlarged LV accommodates the regurgitant volume with little increase in LV diastolic pressure, so there is no pulmonary congestion. This "chronic compensated" phase of AR may last for years. Eventually, the LV fails. There is a decline in contractility and a marked increase in LV end-systolic volume (so LVEF declines). LV diastolic pressure rises, leading to pulmonary congestion. Surgery early in this phase of decompensation may restore normal LV function, but there is also a chance that LV dysfunction will persist.

An important peripheral circulatory response to AR is vasodilation with low diastolic blood pressure. Pulse pressure is wide, and this is the best physical finding of significant AR. With chronic AR and a valve that is still somewhat competent, there is a considerable difference between LV and aortic diastolic pressure. If you think about it, LV diastolic pressure must be normal if there is no pulmonary congestion. Wide pulse pressure is responsible for a number of physical signs: Corrigans's pulse (sharp upstroke and rapid descent of the carotid pulse), DeMusset's sign (head bobbing), Quincke's pulse (pulsating color in the nail bed with pressure on the nail), Hill's sign (augmentation of the systolic pressure in the leg by more than 40 mmHg compared with the arm), and others. *If the pulse pressure is normal, AR probably is not hemodynamically significant.*

That is a simple and useful fact, yet it is common to see a patient in clinic because of "moderate-to-severe AR" on the echocardiogram, but with normal blood pressure, a soft or absent murmur, and normal LV dimensions. It is also common for the echo report to identify moderate-severe MR in a patient with no murmur, yet with normal LV and left atrial size. Most patients with chronic, advanced valve disease have typical murmurs.

Acute AR

The usual cause is endocarditis, most commonly with staphylococcal infection in a setting of drug abuse. Consider it when there is abrupt onset of heart failure in a young person. Look for peripheral signs of endocarditis (splinter or conjunctival hemorrhages, petechiae), and get blood cultures. A rash may indicate gonococcal sepsis.

The heart murmur may be soft or absent. Acute volume overload of the normal (not dilated) LV causes a marked rise in LV diastolic pressure and severe pulmonary congestion. The stiff pericardium helps to limit LV dilation. LV diastolic pressure may be similar to aortic diastolic pressure, and arterial pulse pressure is not wide. With a small diastolic gradient across the valve, the volume of diastolic regurgitation is minimal, reducing murmur intensity.

Diagnostic Procedures and Timing of Surgery for Chronic AR

LV end-systolic size, accurately obtained from the transthoracic echocardiogram, provides the best guide to timing of surgery, much as it does with MR. As long as the LV is able to contract down to a normal volume—or end-systolic diameter less than 4.0 cm—it is safe to continue observation. When the end-systolic dimension rises to 5.5 cm, it is time for surgery, even in the absence of symptoms. Between 4.0 and 5.5, any symptoms would indicate a need for surgery, and periodic echo surveillance is needed for the asymptomatic patient.

Box 3.1 Short Version of Surgical Timing

Both of the LV volume overload conditions—MR and AR—require surgical correction before the onset of symptoms. Waiting for symptoms can result in irreversible LV injury. The timing of surgery is based on LV size and function, so management is determined by serial echocardiograms. The opposite is the case with stenotic lesions (MS and AS).

The LV size that requires surgery is higher with AR (LV end-systolic dimension 5.5 cm) than with MR (4.5 cm). This probably is because of the higher afterload with AR; after surgery the LV is more likely to improve. Correction of AR is possible when there is LV dysfunction, but the outcome is better with early surgery. A large Mayo Clinic series divided patients into low (<35%), medium (35-50%) and normal (>50%) LVEF. Surgical mortality was 14%, 6.7%, and 3.7% in the three groups, and 10-year survival was 41%, 56%, and 70%.

An additional indication for surgery is increasing aortic root diameter, a common complication of Marfan's syndrome. When the root diameter exceeds 5.5-6.0 cm, the risk of aortic dissection is high, and prophylactic valve plus ascending aorta replacement is needed. Progressive dilatation of the proximal aorta and dissection are also possible with a bicuspid aortic valve.

Remember the rule of 55: fix AR when the LVEF falls below 55%, the end-systolic diameter reaches 55 mm, or the aortic root is larger than 55 mm.

The new guidelines have changed this rule for those with Marfan's syndrome or a bicuspid aortic valve; because of a higher risk of dissection surgery is recommended when the root diameter reaches 5.0 cm.

Medical Therapy

Afterload reduction therapy favors forward flow. Vasodilation with nifedipine has been shown to forestall the need for surgery in asymptomatic patients with good LV function by as much as 2-3 years. Angiotensin converting enzyme (ACE) inhibition has been shown effective in children, and probably works for adults, though it has not been studied. Afterload reduction therapy is the mainstay for symptomatic patients who will not or cannot have surgery, and the dihydropyradine calcium channel blockers and ACE inhibitors may be used. Congestion is treated with diuretics, and many improve with digoxin.

It is important to treat systolic hypertension, since high central aortic pressure favors regurgitant rather than forward flow. But this is one situation where beta blockade may be harmful. Regurgitation takes place during diastole, and at a slower heart rate, the total diastolic time is increased. Thus, drugs that cause bradycardia may aggravate the symptoms of AR (beta blockers, diltiazem, and verapamil).

Box 3.2 Marfan's Syndrome

Beta blockade has been shown to slow aortic dilatation and prevent dissection in patients with Marfan's syndrome; reducing LV contractility blunts the shear stress of the ejection wave. It must be used carefully when there is significant AR (regurgitation happens during diastole, and lowering heart rate increases the total diastolic time). Recent studies have cast doubt on the value of beta blockade in patients who do not have Marfan's syndrome.

Losartan, the angiotensin receptor blocker, was found to slow the progression of aortic root in an animal model, and in children with Marfan's syndrome. It blocks the action of transforming growth factor (TGF) beta, which modulates a step in the production of matrix metalloproteases (MMPs). MMPs break down collagen, and are at work when the aorta dilates. Sadly, randomized trials failed to demonstrate a benefit, but the science is tantalizing. (See Isselbacher's cogent description of how this story played out: J Am Col Cardiol 2018, 72: 1619-21)

TRICUSPID REGURGITATION

The most common cause of right heart failure is left heart failure. Left side failure is also the most common cause of tricuspid regurgitation (TR). Elevated LA and pulmonary venous pressure lead to high pulmonary artery (PA) pressure. High right ventricular (RV) pressure and RV dilation lead to TR. It is common for a patient having surgery for mitral valve disease to require tricuspid valve repair. Other causes of pulmonary hypertension, including cor pulmonale and primary pulmonary hypertension, may also cause TR.

Primary TR caused by structural damage to the valve is relatively uncommon. RV infarction, Ebstein's anomaly, endocarditis, and the carcinoid syndrome are illnesses you may encounter on board examinations. Levels of serotonin and its metabolites are higher in those with carcinoid plus TR than in others with a normal valve (drop that tidbit during morning rounds, and note the following discussion of appetite suppressant drugs). Clinically, the most common cause of isolated TR is endocarditis in drug users.

Presentation, Pathophysiology and Examination
The typical symptoms are those of right heart failure, including edema, ascites and fatigue. Hepatic congestion may lead to right upper quadrant pain, especially if the onset is rapid.

The apical impulse is not displaced unless there is LV disease. There is a parasternal lift (recall that the RV is the most anterior cardiac chamber, located just below the sternum and anterior to the LV). P_2 is loud when there is pulmonary hypertension, and this is one time you may hear both A_2 and P_2 at the right base (normally P_2 is soft and is heard only on the left side).

An RV gallop may be heard over the sternum, recognized as such by its increase with inspiration.

The murmur of TR is holosystolic and best heard along the right sternal border. It increases with inspiration. Negative intrathoracic pressure sucks blood into the chest, increasing RV filling and stroke volume, and increasing the TR volume. The murmur may not change with respiration if there is severe RV failure.

The jugular venous pressure is elevated, and it is important to examine the pulse wave. Normally, the dominant venous wave is the A wave, generated by atrial systole. But with TR there is no effective valve separating the RV from the jugular veins, so the pressure wave generated by RV contraction is dominant wave—the V wave. The key to examining the jugular pulse is to feel the brachial pulse. If the dominant venous pulsation is simultaneous with the arterial pulse, it is a V wave. If the visible venous pulse is just before the arterial pulse—presystolic—you are seeing an A wave. With TR, V>A (frankly, this is the only time I find assessment of the venous pulse wave helpful). The V wave may be reflected back through the great veins, leading to a pulsatile liver.

Treatment

The first step in the treatment of TR is treating the primary illness (left heart failure, mitral valve disease, pulmonary hypertension caused by lung disease, etc.). With or without left heart disease, therapy is aimed at relieving symptoms—edema—with diuretics. Isolated TR may be tolerated for years, and surgical repair may not be needed as long as edema is controlled.

TR often complicates mitral valve disease. The surgeon fixes the mitral valve, takes the patient off the pump and evaluates the tricuspid valve for persistent regurgitation. Traditionally this was done by sticking a finger through a hole in the right atrium and feeling the TR jet; transesophageal echo is now used for this purpose during surgery. If TR remains severe, the patient goes back on bypass and tricuspid annuloplasty is performed.

Box 3.3 The Serotonin Syndrome

Fenfluramine—a serotonin agonist—was used for appetite suppression in the early 1990s, and was found to cause valvular disease in 15-20% of those on chronic, high dose therapy (it is no longer on the market). Prolonged use of other serotonin analogues, methysergide and ergotamine, may also be complicated by valvular disease.

In vitro studies have shown that serotonin can stimulate the migration of fibroblasts to heart valve endocardium, promoting fibrosis. Although any heart valve can be affected, it is thought that AR is most common because the aortic valve is exposed to the highest flow rates and shear stress. Another cardiac complication of serotonin is pulmonary vasoconstriction leading to pulmonary hypertension and right heart failure.
Serotonin produced by carcinoid tumor can cause this illness. Eosinophils also produce serotonin, and Loeffler's endocarditis is a frequent complication of hypereosinophilic syndromes.

CARDIAC VALVE PROSTHESIS

None of them is perfect. My surgical colleague with special insight—and a sense of humor—used a slide in lectures that graded the different prosthetic valves with "units of disappointment." The major issues are durability and thromboembolic potential.

Tissue valves are the least thrombogenic, and there are a number of varieties (porcine aortic valves, bovine pericardial valves, etc.). Aspirin therapy is adequate long-term; warfarin is usually stopped at 3 months after surgery. The problem is that they begin to wear out after about 10 years and much earlier in young patients with active calcium metabolism.

Tissue valves are currently used when there is a contraindication to warfarin therapy or for the older patient where durability is less an issue. Deterioration of the valves tends to be gradual, and reoperation is rarely an emergency procedure. A patient who needs anticoagulation for chronic atrial fibrillation or prior embolism may as well have a mechanical valve.

The more durable mechanical valves have a thromboembolic rate of three to eight events per 100 valve-years, which is substantially reduced by warfarin therapy. Warfarin carries a risk of two hemorrhagic events per 100 valve-years, usually nonfatal gastrointestinal bleed. Most thromboembolic events are strokes. Thus, the evidence weighs in favor of warfarin therapy for all patients with mechanical valves. This is especially true for valves in the mitral position, where the embolic risk is higher than it is with aortic valve prostheses.

Anticoagulation

The target International Normalized Ration (INR) with a mechanical valve is 3-3.5. The addition of low-dose aspirin further lowers the risk of stroke, and may be considered for higher risk patients: those with atrial fibrillation, history of stroke or transient ischemic attack (e.g., a prior embolus), or a valve in the mitral position. To these recognized risk factors, many would add a greatly enlarged left atrium or a cardiomyopathic LV, especially if the echocardiogram shows evidence for stagnant flow ("smoke" in the LV).

The RE-ALIGN trial tested dabigatran (a novel oral anticoagulant, or NOAC) for stroke prophylaxis in patients with mechanical valves. It was not as effective as warfarin, and direct thrombin inhibitors are not approved for this indication.

Atrial fibrillation is common in patients with valvular heart disease. In such cases, an anticoagulant is given for AF, not the valve, and a NOAC is suitable. Many of these patients also have an indication for aspirin therapy; clopidogrel is a safer alternative in combination with the NOAC.

Another common issue is what to do with warfarin treatment when a patient with a mechanical valve needs a noncardiac surgical procedure. There are no clinical trials data to guide us. Prior to the late 1990s, many patients were admitted to the hospital for intravenous heparin as bridging therapy before surgery, and it was used postoperatively as well. This has been replaced by subcutaneous low molecular weight heparin that can be administered at home. Partly because it is easier to do, heparin bridging has become more commonly recommended. Risk factors for thromboembolism are history of stroke, valve prosthesis in the mitral position, atrial fibrillation, and low LVEF. With none of these risk factors, heparin bridging is unnecessary

INFECTIVE ENDOCARDITIS (IE)

As with most infections, IE requires a susceptible host and exposure to an infecting organism. The major component of susceptibility is a roughened valve or endovascular surface, usually the result of increased turbulence. Fibrin and platelets attach to the roughened surface, and circulating bacteria stick to this thrombus, becoming an independent site of infection able to seed the rest of the body. Valve lesions with a high degree of turbulence are more likely to promote colonization than large defects with high flow, but low turbulence (e.g., atrial septal defect).

Almost all bacteria may reach the circulation, but only those able to adhere to thrombus cause IE. For example, *Escherichia coli* and *Klebsiella pneumoniae* usually pass a roughened valve surface and do not stick, even though these are frequent causes of bacteremia in patients with cholangitis or pyelonephritis. On the other hand, *Staphylococcus aureus* is sticky, attaching to a roughened valve in the first circulatory pass and covering it within 24 hours.

Clinical Syndromes

Subacute IE

Fever and other constitutional symptoms such as weight loss, fatigue and weakness are common with subacute IE. Virtually every organ in the body may be a target of emboli from the vegetation. Stroke occurs in about one fourth of cases.

On physical examination there is usually a heart murmur. Classic skin lesions are found in just a small minority of patients, and include splinter hemorrhages, petechiae involving skin conjunctiva, or mucus membranes, painful subcutaneous nodules on fingers or toes (Osler's nodes), and painless hemorrhagic macules on the palms and soles (Janeway lesions). Clubbing of the fingers may occur with chronic endocarditis, but it is not specific (think of lung cancer as well). Roth spots are present in only 5% of cases, and can also be caused by leukemia, lupus, and profound anemia. Splenomegaly is found in as many as half the cases.

Acute IE

Rapid destruction of a valve is possible, most commonly with staphylococcal or gonococcal sepsis. Acute AR (or less commonly, MR) leads to severe pulmonary congestion or shock. As noted, the regurgitant murmur may be soft or absent.

Endocarditis is suggested by the abrupt onset of heart failure. Other clinical evidence of infection may include fever, the rash of gonococcal sepsis, and elevated white cell count. A history of intravenous drug use is common when the patient is young and has no prior history of heart disease. As with subacute IE, there may be evidence for peripheral embolus.

Associated Conditions

Right-heart (usually tricuspid valve) endocarditis is most common with intravenous drug use. Think of it, as well, for those with indwelling catheters. In urban centers a common cause is methicillin-resistant *S. aureus*, although enterococcus, viridans streptococci, and *Psuedomonas aeruginosa* can do it. These patients are also at risk for candida endocarditis, with associated endophthalmitis and left-side valvular infection.

More than half the patients with *Streptococcus bovis* endocarditis have lesions in the colon, including malignancies (a board question). Other malignancies may predispose to bacteremia and valve infection with unusual organisms such as *Clostridium septicum, Listeria monocytogenes,* and group B beta-hemolytic streptococci.

Laboratory Studies

One of the first three blood cultures is positive in more than 95% of cases. When there has been antibiotic treatment in the previous 2 weeks, the yield falls to 65%. For the initial evaluation of the untreated patient, three sets of cultures are adequate. A patient who has had antibiotic therapy should have blood cultures 2 and 10 days after treatment ends.

Constitutional symptoms are usually accompanied by elevated sedimentation rate or positive rheumatoid factor, but negative studies do not exclude IE. In Peterdorf's classic study, the mean Westergren sedimentation rate was 57 mm/hr. Normocytic anemia is present in most cases, and it worsens with time. The white cell count is elevated only occasionally.

The echocardiogram demonstrates valvular vegetations and is now included in diagnostic criteria for IE. Small vegetations may be detected with transesophageal study. But the echo may have either false-positive or false-negative results. The test is more sensitive than specific. Vegetations may persist for 2 years or longer after successful treatment, so a vegetation seen on echo does not prove active infection. Other imaging studies usually do not help (e.g., gallium scanning, although it is often ordered).

Treatment

A century ago, viridans streptococcal endocarditis was the usual illness; now it accounts for less than one-fourth of cases. The causes of IE we encounter more frequently are less susceptible to antibiotics and are trickier to manage. Few cardiologists are up to it, and we rely on infectious disease colleagues for the treatment of the infection.

An acutely ill patient may require empiric therapy, pending the culture results. Start a combination of nafcillin or vancomycin plus an aminoglycoside.

An issue for the cardiology consultant is the timing of surgery. The classic indications for valve replacement are heart failure, thromboembolism, or persistent bacteremia. In recent years there has been a trend toward earlier replacement of infected valves. For example, a patient with an increasing diuretic requirement may benefit from surgery. Difficult to treat organisms are relative indications for early surgery, including *P. aeruginosa* or fungi, especially when fever does not resolve with antibiotic therapy. Many believe that staphylococcal endocarditis requires early surgery, arguing that it is better to operate before perivalvular abscesses develop.

Prosthetic valve infection usually requires surgery. An exception is endocarditis more than 2 months after valve surgery with an especially susceptible organism such as strep viridans. Any dysfunction of the prosthetic valve, especially perivalvular leak, indicates a need for surgery. A key part of the physical exam is listening carefully for the murmur of AR. A mechanical valve leaflet that is blocked or frozen by vegetation or thrombus requires replacement.

When there is an indication for surgery it should not be delayed.
With time there is more opportunity for the organism to burrow
into the myocardium, cause abscesses (heart block is a potential
consequence of aortic valve endocarditis—watch the PR
interval), and generate emboli. Infection of a replacement valve
is infrequent, even when it is placed into tissue that may not be
sterile.

The new valve may not sit as securely into the valve ring
because of weakened tissue. Perivalvular leak complicates about
15% of the operations for IE. Antibiotic therapy after surgery is
a complex issue requiring infectious disease consultation (and
management).

Prevention of IE

Guidelines for antibiotic prophylaxis were revised in 2008, and
it is no longer indicated for the following cardiac conditions:
mitral valve prolapse, rheumatic heart disease, bicuspid aortic
valve, calcific aortic stenosis, atrial or ventricular septal defect,
and HOCM.

Prophylaxis is recommended for those with a prosthetic heart
valve, prior history of IE, cyanotic or otherwise complex
congenital heart disease, or heart transplant with valvulopathy.

Invasive dental, gastrointestinal, genitourinary and upper
respiratory tract procedures are indications for antibiotic
prophylaxis. On the other hand, restorative dentistry (filling
teeth), simple tooth extraction, endotracheal intubation,
esophageal endoscopy and vaginal delivery are not. Antibiotic
prophylaxis regimens are updated periodically by the American
Heart Association and are found in most standard texts (the
dentist usually has the information on his bulletin board).

Chapter 4: Lipid Disorders and Atherosclerosis

Abbreviations
ACE, angiotensin converting enzyme
ACEI, ACE inhibitor
ACC, American College of Cardiology
AHA, American Heart Association
ARB, angiotensin receptor blocker
ASCVD, atherosclerotic cardiovascular disease
CAC, coronary artery calcium
CAD, coronary artery disease
CRP, C-reactive protein
HDL, high density lipoprotein cholesterol
IDL, intermediate density lipoprotein cholesterol
HRT, hormone replacement therapy
LDL, low density lipoprotein cholesterol
MI, myocardial infarction
RCT, randomized clinical trial
VLDL, very low density lipoprotein cholesterol

Atherosclerotic cardiovascular disease (ASCVD) is the most
common cause of death in the United States, with almost one
million dying each year. Coronary artery disease (CAD) causes
a majority of these deaths. About 150,000 with no prior history
of ASCVD die suddenly.

Women are not immune; ASCVD is their leading cause of
death. They tend to develop it about a decade later than men.
The chance of a woman dying with heart disease is 10-times
greater than it is with breast cancer.

ASCVD is a disease of middle and older age; about 55% of
myocardial infarction (MI) occurs in people older than 65 years.
That has been true throughout history; prior to the 20th century
those who managed to survive into old age usually died from

heart disease. On the other hand, almost 40% of men and 30% of women who die of CAD are younger than 55.

RISK FACTORS FOR ASCVD

Sixty years ago, population studies established the concept of risk factors for premature ASCVD. It is still clinically useful. A recent trial calculated the risk of coronary events over 10 years of follow-up. In descending order of importance, the risk was influenced by age, LDL cholesterol, smoking, HDL cholesterol, systolic blood pressure, family history, diabetes mellitus, and triglycerides. Table 4.1 reviews known risk factors for ASCVD, plus a few of the more than 200 that have been suggested

---

Table 4.1. Risk Factors for Atherosclerotic Cardiovascular Disease (ASCVD)

Dyslipidemia: Lowering total cholesterol by 1% reduces the incidence of CAD by 2%.

Hypertension: $\geq$140/90, or on therapy. SHEP showed that control of systolic pressure lowers the risk of 1) fatal and nonfatal stroke, 2) nonfatal MI and coronary death, 3) combined ASCVD outcomes. A meta-analysis showed that lowering blood pressure 6 mm Hg reduces the CAD event rate 14%.

Diabetes mellitus: With diabetes there is also a worse prognosis

Abdominal obesity: The central element of the metabolic syndrome (see text), and an independent risk factor for ASCVD in the Framingham study.

Cigarette smoking: There is a dose-response curve, with the number of cigarettes smoked each day proportional to MI, stroke, and death.

Family history: Definite MI or sudden death in first-degree relative < 55 years old (for males), or < 65 (females). After stratifying for other risk factors, a positive family history increases risk 2-4 fold.

Male sex: Women develop ASCVD about 10 years later than men, and it is the most common cause of death in both women and men.

Age: > 45 yrs for men, 55 yrs for women. About 80% of fatal MI occur over age 65.

Left ventricular hypertrophy: An independent predictor of CAD and sudden cardiac death.

Physical activity: In the MRFIT study those who exercised had a 27% lower CAD mortality rate.

Systemic inflammation, high sensitivity CRP: Higher risk for developing CAD, plus a risk factor for becoming unstable (see text).

ASCVD, atherosclerotic cardiovascular disease; CAD, coronary artery disease; MI, myocardial infarction; CRP, C-reactive protein.

Epidemiologists emphasize that risk factors are useful for predicting who will get disease, but do not prove causality. This requires showing that treatment modifying the risk factor prevents disease (*primary prevention*) or halts progression of established disease (*secondary prevention*). Randomized clinical trials have shown that treatment of hypertension or dyslipidemia meets this level of proof. Our acceptance of other risk factors as causative is based on population studies, which, of course, are not randomized. For example, the Nurses Health Study found that women who maintain ideal body weight, exercise regularly, use alcohol in moderation and do not smoke lower their risk of ASCVD by 84% (but randomized study of such interventions is not possible).

Smoking

Half of all smokers die of smoking related causes, and they lose at least 10 years of life. ASCVD accounts for one-third of those deaths. For every 10 cigarettes smoked per day, cardiovascular mortality increases by 18% in men, and 31% in women. Continued smoking after MI halves life expectancy. Low tar cigarettes do not lower the risk of ASCVD.

Smoking has multiple actions that promote atherosclerosis. It lowers HDL cholesterol, adversely affects endothelial function, promotes vasospasm, raises fibrinogen levels, enhances platelet aggregation, is proinflammatory, and increases insulin resistance. In addition, there is an acute effect. The carbon monoxide from burning cigarettes raises carboxyhemoglobin levels, reducing the oxygen-carrying capacity of blood, and thus reduces the level of exercise that provokes ischemia (the angina threshold). Mention this to patients as an immediate benefit from stopping tobacco use. Smoking no longer counts as a risk factor for ASCVD 10-12 years after stopping.

There are a few drug therapies for nicotine addiction, beginning with nicotine replacement. Smoking has a mild antidepressant effect, and treating this with bupropion helps. Varenicline (Chantix) is a partial nicotine agonist that provides some nicotine effect to ease withdrawal symptoms. As a nicotine receptor blocker it inhibits the effect of nicotine from cigarettes if the patient resumes smoking. It was better than bupropion in comparison trials, and the combination of the two drugs has not been tested.

Many smokers go through multiple quit-attempts before they are successful, so never give up. The clinician's role is critical. Repeated mention of smoking by the practitioner has been shown to double the chance of a patient quitting, and it is recommended that smoking status as a vital sign is recorded at each clinic visit.

Vaping, or e-cigarettes, is not without cardiovascular risk. Compared with nonusers there is an increase in risk of MI, stroke and thromboembolic disease.

Obesity, Diabetes and the Metabolic Syndrome

Almost a third of American adults are obese, and another third are overweight. Most of them have hypertension. Obesity is the initiating element of the metabolic syndrome, thought to affect a quarter of American men and postmenopausal women. The consequence of this is an epidemic of diabetes, with an increase in diabetes related mortality.

Diagnostic criteria for the metabolic syndrome are summarized in Table 4.2. It begins with abdominal obesity, which causes insulin resistance. That is to say, for a given level of glucose, the insulin level is elevated. Not all obese people with insulin resistance develop diabetes, but those with a family history of beta cell dysfunction eventually do. These obese offspring of diabetic parents have high insulin levels for more than a decade before their beta cells wear out, serum glucose rises, and they are diagnosed with type 2 diabetes.

Table 4.2. The Metabolic Syndrome

Diagnostic criteria (those with three or more have the metabolic syndrome)

1. Abdominal obesity (Waist circumference >40 inches for men, or >35 inches, women)
2. Plasma triglycerides $\geq$ 150 mg/dL
3. HDL cholesterol <40 mg/dL (men), or <50 mg/dL (women)
4. Blood pressure $\geq$ 130/85 mmHg

5.   Fasting glucose $\geq$110 mg/dL (or A1c > 6)

Other conditions observed with the metabolic syndrome that may contribute to premature vascular disease
1.   Prothrombotic state (increased fibrinogen and platelet activator inhibitor-1)
2.   Abnormal endothelial and smooth muscle function
3.   Elevated C-reactive protein (ultra-sensitive CRP

Most obese people, and all of those with type 2 diabetes, thus have elevated insulin levels. Hyperinsulinemia is toxic, and is a risk factor for early vascular disease in those who are not diabetic. It causes endothelial dysfunction, possibly by increasing oxidative stress. Most patients with elevated insulin levels are hypertensive; whether this is from associated obesity or a pressor effect of insulin is uncertain. The hypertension contributes to endothelial dysfunction. Interaction with other risk factors has been described. Smoking aggravates insulin resistance, another potential mechanism of premature ASCVD.

Patients with abdominal obesity frequently have elevated C-reactive protein (CRP). Abdominal adipose is a source of proinflammatory cytokines, and the metabolic syndrome is an inflammatory condition.

Clinical Course and Treatment

Most obese people meet diagnostic criteria, even without diabetes. They may be assumed to have insulin resistance and hyperinsulinemia, and most of them have high triglycerides and low HDL cholesterol.

Premature vascular disease is such a common consequence type 2 diabetes that it is considered a surrogate for established CAD. Studies of treatment have shown that asymptomatic diabetic patients benefit from a secondary—rather than primary—prevention strategy.

Weight loss can cure the metabolic syndrome, and I point this out to patients. With bariatric surgery and substantial weight loss, diabetes resolves and with it, the risk of vascular complications. Grand obesity (an archaic description) has become a surgical illness.

Short of surgery, we now have an effective pharmacologic approach with the combination of phentermine and topiramate. Clinical trials show that it is effective, and patients who are taking it tell me they just are not hungry. Both drugs are given at low dose, and toxicity is uncommon. One question is how long to remain on therapy. Some experts are suggesting long-term treatment, since obesity is a chronic illness, like hypertension. You would not stop antihypertensives once blood pressure is controlled, and they suggest that appetite suppressive therapy is no different. That said, there has been no clinical trial of extended therapy.

Tighter control of blood sugar helps prevent the microvascular complications of type 2 diabetes, neuropathy, nephropathy, and retinopathy. Two large clinical trials tested whether tighter control, to a target HbA1c below 6.5%, could prevent macrovascular complications, MI and stroke. Neither ACCORD (10,251 patients in the US) nor ADVANCE (11,140 patients in the UK) found any benefit. A small increase in all-cause mortality in ACCORD led to premature discontinuation of the trial.

The modulation of insulin resistance with thiazolidinediones—rosiglitazone or pioglitazone—initially seemed promising, but clinical trials raised questions. Both drugs cause fluid retention and should not be used by patients with Class III-IV heart failure. Rosiglitazone may increase risk of MI (in Europe it is contraindicated for those with established vascular disease). Pioglitazone may lower the risk. There has been no head-to-head comparison study of the two.

The newest pharmacologic approach is SGLT2 inhibitors (empagliflozin and dapagliflozin).   These drugs inhibit glucose reabsorption in the proximal tubule, so there is increase secretion of glucose. This has been shown to lower insulin resistance and lower A1c, blood pressure, and body weight. Multiple trials have shown lower incidence of cardiovascular events, and recall that a survival benefit has been documented with HFrEF, even in nondiabetic patients (Chapter 1).

DYSLIPIDEMIA

Lipoprotein Metabolism

Oil and water do not mix. Cholesterol and triglycerides are hydrophobic, like other oils, and do not go into solution into aqueous media, such as blood. To get fats to dissolve in water requires a chemical that works like a detergent: a molecule that binds to fat on one side and to water on the other.

Lipoprotein particles have a core of fat packaged with a specialized protein that works like a detergent. This protein molecule, called an apoprotein, has regions that are nonpolar (hydrophobic) that bind with lipids, and other regions that are polar (hydrophilic) that face the surrounding aqueous phase and form hydrogen bonds with water. The lipid-apoprotein package is thus water-soluble.

Another useful property of apoproteins is binding sites that regulate steps in lipid metabolism. For example, the apoB-100 protein on the surface of the LDL cholesterol particle is recognized by the liver's LDL receptor, allowing hepatic uptake of LDL. Other apoproteins are cofactors for enzymes that interact with lipoproteins, such as lipoprotein lipase.

The core of fat in the lipoprotein particle includes fatty acids, cholesterol esters, phospholipids and triglycerides. Lipoproteins vary in density, and the first measurement techniques and classification schemes used ultracentrifugation. Larger, less dense particles contain more triglyceride and do not migrate as far in the centrifuge.

Very-low-density lipoprotein (VLDL) has 55% triglyceride, 19% cholesterol, and only 8% protein by weight—this fluffy particle migrates the least. The highest density lipoprotein (HDL) has just 5% triglyceride and a higher proportion of protein (40%) and cholesterol (22%), and it migrates the farthest in the centrifuge. Between the two is the LDL particle, which has the largest percentage of cholesterol (50%), 6% triglyceride, and 22% protein.

Antibody techniques allow measurement of surface apoproteins. ApoA is found on HDL, and apoB-100 primarily on LDL. Thus, a patient with a high apoB level will also have high LDL cholesterol.

It helps to know just what your clinical laboratory is measuring. Most common is the centrifugation technique that isolates the entire lipoprotein molecule (fat core plus the apoprotein envelope), then measures just the lipid component. Thus, when the laboratory reports the LDL cholesterol level, it is understood that the LDL component has been isolated from other lipoproteins by centrifugation, the apoprotein envelope separated from the lipid core, and the cholesterol contained in the lipid core measured and reported as mg cholesterol/dL. This is what you usually get from the clinical laboratory, although you will encounter research studies that refer to apoprotein levels.

Metabolic Pathways

The plasma lipoproteins are constantly being remodeled. Influenced by several enzymes, core lipids and apoprotein can be transferred from or among particles, altering their density (and therefore the lipoprotein class). Some particle alteration occurs in the liver, but much of it takes place in circulating plasma or in peripheral tissue. There are parallel systems that transport lipids: *exogenous transport* involves movement of lipid from the intestinal lumen, which uses a transport system distinct from *endogenous transport*, which processes either stored or synthesized fat.

The two systems have a lot in common (and here is the big picture). Both begin by packaging lipid, predominantly triglyceride but some cholesterol as well, into large, fluffy particles. The large particles circulate and are subjected to a series of lipolytic reactions, with hydrolysis of triglyceride to fatty acids that melt away from the particle and are used as fuel. The remodeled particle is smaller and denser, contains less triglyceride, and therefore has proportionately more cholesterol. Small particles are cleared from the circulation by the liver through the action of specialized receptors on the hepatic cell membrane.

Genetic defects may affect any of these metabolic steps, accounting for the familial nature of CAD.

Exogenous Fat Transport

Dietary fats are absorbed by the intestinal epithelial cell. In the cell, it is esterified into long-chain fatty acids. Apoprotein is added, and the particle is secreted as a chylomicron. Most of the fat in the chylomicron is triglyceride. *Lipoprotein lipase* located in vascular endothelial cells—especially in muscle and adipose tissue capillary beds—hydrolyzes the triglyceride to free fatty acid, either for storage or as a source of energy. What is left is the chylomicron remnant, which is cleared by liver cells. This process is rapid with most chylomicrons cleared from the circulation a couple hours after eating. The lipid profile measured after 12 hours of fasting does not reflect exogenous fat transport.

Endogenous Fat Transport

A 70-kg person has about 10 kg of triglyceride stored in adipose tissue. Lipases, inhibited by insulin and stimulated by epinephrine, hydrolyze stored triglyceride and release free fatty acid from adipose tissue into the circulation. It is bound to albumin and then cleared from the circulation by the liver.

Some of the free fatty acid is burned as fuel. The remainder is converted to triglyceride, which is packaged by the liver into lipoprotein particles of very low density (VLDL). Again, note the parallel between exogenous and endogenous pathways: the bulk of lipid at the origin of the cascade is triglyceride, and the lipoprotein particle carrying it is large and has low density.

The triglyceride in VLDL, like that in chylomicrons, is hydrolyzed by lipoprotein lipase to free fatty acids that melt away from the particle. In both the endogenous and exogenous pathways, apoC-II acts as a cofactor for lipoprotein lipase. The resulting particle is smaller, has less triglyceride, and proportionately more cholesterol, and it is called intermediate-density lipoprotein (IDL). This can be cleared by the liver, which has receptors for the apoE surface protein of IDL. Those IDL particles that are not removed undergo further hydrolysis to become LDL.

LDL has almost no triglyceride, and its lipid core is composed predominantly of cholesterol esters. The surface protein molecule is apoB-100. Transport of oxidized LDL into the endothelium is the beginning of the atherosclerotic process.

Regulation of LDL levels depends on the balance between production (via the lipolytic cascade described) and clearance. Clearance of LDL is governed by the number of hepatocyte LDL receptors. ApoB-100 on the LDL particle surface binds to the LDL receptor, and the LDL particle is then absorbed by the hepatocyte.

An excess of free cholesterol within the liver cell blocks production of LDL receptors, so that less LDL cholesterol is cleared from the circulation. A deficiency of intracellular cholesterol provokes a compensatory *increase in the number of LDL receptors* ("upregulation of receptors"). More receptors are able to react with LDL particles, increasing clearance of LDL from the circulation.

The final common pathway for treatment to reduce LDL cholesterol is the upregulation of hepatocyte LDL receptors. For example, decreasing cholesterol availability by dietary restriction or by blocking an enzyme in the cholesterol synthetic pathway (HMG-CoA reductase), causes a "deficiency" of intracellular cholesterol. The hepatocyte compensates by upregulating LDL receptors, and there is increased clearance of LDL particles from the circulation. This is a desirable effect, because it is *circulating* LDL cholesterol that is atherogenic.

The liver processes a large amount of cholesterol for a variety of purposes. The greatest proportion is used to manufacture bile. Some of the bile is recycled, and blocking its enterohepatic circulation with resins that bind bile salts in the gut creates a relative "deficiency" of hepatocyte cholesterol. The result: generation of more LDL receptors and further lowering of circulating LDL cholesterol.

HDL and Reverse Cholesterol Transport

Cholesterol that is not metabolized by peripheral tissue is excreted by the liver in bile. The reverse cholesterol transport system is responsible for moving excess cholesterol from the periphery, and eventually to the liver. HDL is the transport vehicle.

Production of HDL begins with secretion of apoA-I by both the liver and intestine. Apo A-I complexes with phospholipids, forming a disc-like structure called nascent HDL. This particle attracts free cholesterol from the cell membranes of peripheral tissue or from other lipoprotein particles, becoming a mature, spherical HDL particle. Free cholesterol contained in early atherosclerotic plaque may be absorbed by the developing HDL particle.

The liver does not have an HDL receptor. Instead, cholesterol is transferred from HDL to LDL. Cholesterol ester transfer protein (CETP) promotes this transfer. Thus, inhibiting CETP raises HDL and decreases LDL cholesterol levels. There was hope that CETP inhibitors would favorably affect atherosclerosis, but a clinical trial of the first of these agents found an increased risk of cardiovascular events. It is uncertain whether CV toxicity was from CETP inhibition itself or from some other action of the drug.

The level of HDL, expressed as mg/dL cholesterol by your clinical laboratory, is much lower than the level of LDL cholesterol. This gives the impression that the cholesterol removal system is comparatively small. But the HDL particle is composed of just 22% cholesterol, and remember that the laboratory measures just the cholesterol component of HDL. Furthermore, the HDL particle is small, weighing about one tenth of the LDL particle. In reality, the number of HDL particles (the molar concentration) exceeds that of LDL. The total surface area of HDL particles is greater than that of all other lipoproteins. The cholesterol removal system is thus quite large.

Treatment of Hyperlipidemia

In November 2013 the ACC-AHA Task Force on Practice Guidelines updated the guidelines for treatment of dyslipidemia, the first update since the NCEP recommendations of 2002. Since 2013 the ACC-AHA has updated the guidelines. Previously, therapy was targeted to an LDL cholesterol goal, depending on the level of risk. Thus, for secondary prevention of disease in those with a history of CV disease (MI, stroke, PVD), or diabetes, the goal was to lower the LDL to a target of 70 mg/deciliter. With the update, emphasis has shifted from LDL lowering (by any means), to the drugs which have been found to be efficacious, principally statins. The reason for this subtle change is that statins have beneficial effects in addition to LDL lowering (for example, their vascular anti-inflammatory action).

Since then, randomized trials have used fixed dose statin therapy, not titrated to an LDL goal. The new guidelines recommended fixed dose therapy for those with elevated CV risk, and they specify the use of either atorvastatin or rosuvastatin.

Risk is assessed using a "vascular risk calculator" based on data from large cohort studies; it can be loaded to your smart-phone as an app. The entry points are gender, age, total cholesterol, HDL cholesterol, hypertension, diabetes, and smoking. Family history and weight (or BMI) are not included. The program computes the 10-year risk of ASCVD, and if it is greater than 7.5%, statin therapy is indicated. Note that the calculator is used to decide whether a primary prevention strategy is needed. Patients with a history of ASCVD are automatically in the highest risk category, and receive high intensity statin therapy. Table 4.3 is a summary of the guidelines.

Table 4.3. 2013 Guidelines for Statin Therapy in Patients at Increased CV Risk

Patients > 21 years old without heart failure (NYHA class 2-4) or on hemodialysis: screen for risk factors, and measure LDL cholesterol.

1. Clinical ASCVD → high intensity statin Rx
2. LDL cholesterol > 190 mg/dl → high intensity statin Rx

3. <u>Diabetes (type 1 or 2)</u>, LDL 70-189; calculate 10-year ASCVD risk*. For risk < 7.5%, moderate-intensity statin Rx; ≥ 7.5% high-intensity Rx.
4. <u>No diabetes</u>, and LDL 70-189 mg/dl, calculate 10-year ASCVD risk*. For risk >7.5%, moderate to high-intensity statin Rx

<u>High intensity statin Rx</u> = atorvastatin 40-80 mg/day, or rosuvatatin 20-40 gm/day (lowering LDL cholesterol by about 50%)

<u>Moderate intensity statin Rx</u> = atorvastatin 10-20 mg, rosuvastatin 5-10 mg, simvastatin 20-40 mg, pravastatin 40-80 mg, lovastatin 40 mg (lowers LDL cholesterol 30-50%)

* Using the risk calculator

The new guidelines do not suggest statin therapy for some patients we previously treated, but for whom there are no data supporting treatment:
1. Patients > 75 years old, unless there is a prior history of ASCVD or the patient is already on a statin
2. Patients on hemodialysis
3. Patients with congestive heart failure

The guidelines simplify management:
1. There is no need to add additional treatment to raise HDL. Recent trials have studied the addition of fibrates, niacin and cholesterol ester transferase inhibitors, and have found no benefit, undermining the "HDL hypothesis" (see the editorial by Lloyd-Jones, N Engl J Med 2014;371:271-4).
2. In borderline cases, the guidelines indicate that tests with the greatest incremental risk prediction are CRP, coronary calcium scoring, and ankle/brachial index

(Morris, JACC 2014;64:190-206—she also reviews and compares the large number of conflicting guidelines). I would also consider family history.

Using the new guidelines, it would seem that we might miss treating some patients who need it. However, the opposite is the case. It doesn't take much for the risk calculator to indicate a 10-year risk above 7.5%, and the guidelines have increased statin use.

Raising HDL and Lowering Triglycerides

The first step for lowering triglycerides and raising HDL is weight loss. Triglyceride is the lipid fraction most sensitive to weight; an obese person who loses just 10-20 pounds may have a significant reduction. When triglycerides fall, the HDL rises.

Exercise has an effect on HDL that may be independent of its weight control benefit. The moderate use of alcohol, about two ounces of spirits a day, also increases HDL. Excessive drinking, on the other hand, raises triglycerides and lowers HDL.

Drugs

Statins

In addition to lowering LDL cholesterol, it is now well accepted that statin therapy stabilizes plaque. Cholesterol lowering accounts for some of this, as the cholesterol content of plaque is reduced and cholesterol-rich plaque is more prone to rupture. However, the major plaque stabilizing action is the vascular anti-inflammatory action of statins. C-reactive protein falls, and the near term risk of MI is reduced. This early benefit has made statins one of the therapies indicated for acute coronary syndrome (ACS).

One reason for the success of statin therapy is a relative absence of side effects when compared with other agents. After one year of treatment, more than 95% of patients on statins remain on therapy, compared with less than half of those on niacin, gemfibrozil or resins. That may surprise you, as there is such concern about liver toxicity and myositis with statins. Liver dysfunction is dose-related. Serial liver function testing is more important at high dose therapy, although a 3-fold rise in liver enzymes is still rare, developing in less than 1% of patients. Serial liver function testing is generally not recommended for those on low dose treatment.

Myositis also occurs at higher doses. It may develop out of the blue; serial testing of muscle enzymes is not useful. Statins are metabolized by the liver's CYP (a.k.a. cytochrome) enzyme system. Other drugs that share this metabolic route may inhibit degradation of the statin, leading to increased concentrations and adverse effects. These include gemfibrozil, amiodarone, cyclosporine, erythromycin (and other antibiotics), HIV protease inhibitors and large quantities (>1 quart/day) of grapefruit juice. Another important drug interaction is warfarin—the INR rises with statin therapy because protein bound warfarin is displaced by the statin.

Fibrates

The indication is hypertriglyceridemia and prevention of pancreatitis. In addition to lowering triglycerides, there is a modest (5-15%) increase in HDL. Fibrates increase the oxidation of free fatty acids in the liver, blocking synthesis of VLDL triglyceride.

Fenofibrate (Tricor) is a third-generation fibrate that is slightly more potent than gemfibrozil. The risk of myositis is lower with it than with gemfibrozil. It may be safer than gemfibrozil when used with statins. The combination of gemfibrozil with more than 20 mg simvastatin/day is discouraged.

Like other drugs that bind to protein, fibrates may displace warfarin from protein, requiring about a 30% reduction in the warfarin dose.

Niacin

In many ways it seems the ideal drug, substantially raising HDL while lowering LDL cholesterol. It is prescribed when there is statin intolerance. Niacin works by preventing mobilization of free fatty acids from the periphery (adipose), which leads to reduced hepatic production of triglycerides and secretion of VLDL. In addition, it inhibits conversion of VLDL to LDL.

At high doses, it can raise HDL concentrations by 30%, more than can be achieved with gemfibrozil. We tend to limit therapy to 1.5-2 gm of nicotinic acid per day, and this raises HDL slightly, while lowering triglycerides substantially.

Ezetimibe (Zetia)

It blocks both dietary and biliary cholesterol absorption. With less delivery of cholesterol to the liver, LDL receptor density increases, increasing LDL uptake from the circulation. The usual dose, 10 mg/day, reduces dietary absorption of cholesterol by 50%. It may be used in combination with statins to achieve the LDL target. There are no unfavorable interactions with statins or gemfibrozil; it is not metabolized by the CYP enzyme system. Consider adding it if LDL remains high despite maximum tolerated stating therapy.

PCSK-9 Inhibitors

Proprotein convertase subtilisin/kexin type-9 resides in the hepatocyte and is a participant the natural degradation of LDL receptors. PCSK-9 inhibitors are autoantibodies that block its action; this increases the number of LDL receptors, allowing hepatocytes to pull more LDL from the circulation. This therapy lowers LDL when nothing else works, and that is the indication

for its use. In general, we begin therapy when statins plus
ezetimibe fail to bring the LDL to the treatment target. The
response to the monthly intravenous autoantibody infusion is
dramatic with a >50% decline in LDL and a comparable
reduction in cardiovascular events.

Fish Oil

The polyunsaturated fatty acids (PUFAs) found in fish oil are
known to raise HDL and lower LDL cholesterol and
triglycerides. Fish oil supplements are especially helpful for
hypertriglyceridemia. Endothelial function improves, and there
is a reduction in inflammation. Multiple studies have
documented a reduction in ASCVD clinical endpoints.

An unexpected benefit has been a lower risk of sudden cardiac
death (SCD). An increase in dietary PUFA content has been
found to increase the PUFA level in the myocardial cell
membrane. This alters the action potential and may have an
antiarrhythmic effect. Reducing the vulnerability to ventricular
fibrillation may be more important than the effect on
atherosclerosis. The current AHA recommendation is that
everyone should have two servings of an oily fish meal per week
(such as salmon), and others have suggested additional
supplements for those at high risk for SCD. Supplements may be
safer given the level of mercury and other toxins in both farmed
and wild fish.

Hormone Replacement Therapy (HRT)

This is an odd story that underscores the importance of the
modern clinical trial. A series of observational studies,
beginning in the 1960s, suggested that HRT could lower the risk
of ASCVD by as much as 50% in postmenopausal women.
Some actions of estrogen make a protective plausible. It raises
HDL, while lowering LDL, Lp(a) and fibrinogen. It also inhibits
oxidation of LDL and improves endothelial function. On the

other hand, it raises triglycerides and C-reactive protein and promotes thrombosis. Adding progestin blocks the HDL benefit.

Most were surprised by a negative result from the first randomized trial of HRT, the Heart and Estrogen Replacement Study (HERS). There was no long-term benefit, and there was an unexpected increase in ASCVD risk during the first year after starting HRT. Since then, other randomized trials have confirmed the HERS result, finding no clinical or anatomic benefit from HRT for those with established CAD, and confirming increased risk emerging shortly after starting HRT.

More recently, *primary prevention* trials have indicated potential harm with HRT. The estrogen plus progestin arm of the Women's Health Initiative (WHI) was stopped early because of adverse effects. This study of healthy, normal women found that HRT caused a 29% increase in MI, a 41% increase in stroke, a 2-fold increase in venous thromboembolic disease, and a 26% increase in breast cancer.

One explanation for the discrepancy between the observational studies and clinical trials is the tendency for CV endpoints to appear soon after starting HRT. Observational studies are weighted with subjects who have been on treatment for some time. Those with early complications, especially if they are fatal, have "dropped out" before the observational study is done. Reexamination of the observational data, focusing on patients on HRT for less than one year, eliminated previously described benefits.

Possible explanations for the higher risk of vascular events soon after starting HRT include the prothrombotic and pro-inflammatory effects of estrogen. It is also possible that a subgroup of women genetically predisposed to adverse effects of HRT develop them promptly after starting treatment. The early clustering of adverse effects provided a rationale for the recommendation that a woman who is not on HRT should not start it, but that another who has been on it for some time need not stop it. This recommendation, however, does not appear in clinical guidelines, and HRT is not indicated for the primary or secondary prevention of ASCVD.

At present, HRT is indicated for the control of menopausal symptoms, including sleeplessness and hot flashes. The safest approach is the lowest dose for the shortest period of time. HRT is also approved for prevention of osteoporosis for those with early disease or declining bone density. The issue of ASCVD prevention is not entirely settled; different hormone combinations may be safer.

Diet Therapy

We are not good at it. The most successful diet approaches are impossible to sustain (try a vegan diet), or are complicated by side effects (i.e. the Atkins diet and stone formation). The Mediterranean diet remains the standard recommendation of organized cardiovascular medicine.

Surgical treatment of obesity has improved with laparoscopic techniques. It is difficult to subject it to randomized clinical trials, although the small CROSSROADS trial (< 50 patients), found that surgery resulted in greater weight loss and remission of type 2 diabetes when compared with intensive lifestyle modification. Larger studies would be needed to document a cardiovascular benefit.

Prospective although observational data have indicated both resolution of diabetes and dyslipidemia after gastric bypass. Weight loss commonly exceeds 100 lbs., and I am recommending gastric bypass for those who have been unable to diet successfully.

Diet supplements are commonly discussed. Flavonoids found in red wine and dark beer and spirits may be responsible for the

French paradox, a lower incidence of ASCVD despite a high fat diet. The mechanism of benefit may be improved endothelial function. Of particular interest, flavonoids block the endothelial dysfunction that follows consumption of a high fat meal.

Alcohol, used moderately, is another "dietary supplement" associated with a lower incidence of ASCVD in observational studies. It is known to raise HDL, reduce platelet aggregation and promote fibrinolysis. Up to 2 ounces of spirits a day may prove beneficial, but the evidence is not compelling enough to recommend that nondrinkers take it up. Heavier consumption raises triglycerides, and can depress left ventricular function or provoke atrial fibrillation. In addition, even modest alcohol use can make hypertension treatment-resistant.

Atherosclerosis

Here is the general picture: at high circulating levels LDL traverses the endothelial barrier and is oxidized in the intima. The oxidized particles in turn provoke formation of adhesion molecules on the endothelial surface. A number of risk factors trigger endothelial cell expression of adhesion molecules; ACE inhibitors and statins inhibit their production.

Adhesion molecules attract monocytes and facilitate their transport to the intima. Monocytes become macrophages when activated by oxidized LDL in the intima. These cells scavenge LDL, become foam cells, and form the fatty streak observed on the arterial endothelium. Activated macrophages produce cytotoxic substances that promote endothelial injury, and growth factors that stimulate proliferation and migration of smooth muscle cells into the early plaque. In turn, smooth muscle cells are transformed to fibroblasts, and as the plaque matures, a fibroproliferative process dominates. Mature, stable plaque has a small lipid core that is acellular (few white cells), and the lipid core is insulated from the arterial lumen by a thick fibrous cap.

Inflammation and Unstable Plaque

Conversely, unstable plaque has a thin, fragile cap and large lipid core, rich in macrophages and T cell lymphocytes. The thin cap is vulnerable to rupture. When this happens the exposed lipid core and raw connective tissue activate platelets, and the result is thrombosis and the acute coronary syndrome (ACS).

Inflammation is probably responsible for thinning of the cap and destabilizing plaque. Macrophages in the lipid core produce matrix metaloproteases (MMPs), which remodel the collagen in the plaque cap, thinning it.

What provokes the inflammatory process is not clear. It is not a localized process. Intravascular ultrasound studies of ACS have found that plaque throughout the coronary circulation appears unstable (thin cap, large lipid core), not just the plaque of the culprit lesion. Autopsy studies have found this unstable plaque morphology in the carotid arteries of those who died after MI.

One cause of panvascular inflammation is <u>systemic inflammation</u>. Population studies have found an association between a wide spectrum of inflammatory conditions and ACS, including MI. These include influenza and other pulmonary infections, urinary tract infection, periodontal disease, asthma, rheumatoid arthritis (RA) and other autoimmune conditions with unremitting inflammation. The intensity of inflammation counts; MI in patients with RA is related more to sedimentation rate than to usual risk factors for ASCVD. The risk of MI with RA is increased by about 50%; but with systemic lupus the risk is increased 4-5 fold.

The mechanism linking systemic and vascular inflammation is uncertain, but appears related to activated T lymphocytes ("killer T cells"). T cell memory may be long-lasting, since childhood infectious illnesses predict higher ASCVD risk decades later. As an example, there are interesting data relating the MI epidemic of the 1950-1980's to the Spanish influenza pandemic of 1918, which commonly affected young adults. We might encounter an MI epidemic decades in the future among those who had Covid-19 infection; it is admittedly speculative, but many of you will be in practice and may witness it. In any event, the data identifying systemic inflammation as a risk factor for ACS are comparable in quantity and quality to the observational data that originally identified hypertension, smoking, diabetes and family history as risk factors for ASCVD.

C-reactive protein (CRP) is a marker of inflammation that has been found to predict myocardial infarction, sudden cardiac death, stroke and peripheral arterial disease. It is independent of other risk factors for ASCVD. A level of 1-3 mg/L corresponds to moderate risk, and >3 mg/dl, to high risk. Note that these are low levels; with bacterial infection the CRP may approach 100 mg/dl. A highly sensitive CRP assay is required for accurate measurement of these low levels. When the CRP is above 10 mg/L the test should be repeated and other processes excluded (low grade infection, malignancy).

The metabolic syndrome is now considered an inflammatory condition; abdominal adipose produces inflammatory cytokines. CRP levels correlate with the level of insulin resistance, endothelial dysfunction and impaired fibrinolysis, features of the metabolic syndrome that are not easily measured. Thus, CRP helps differentiate high from low risk patients with the metabolic syndrome.

The CRP level tends to be stable in an individual, without circadian variation. Eating does not influence it; fasting blood sampling is unnecessary. It is not age or sex dependent, but it is higher during hormone replacement therapy. The molecule has a long half-life, and is stable during storage; this has made it possible to return to earlier clinical trials and measure CRP using stored serum. There are other biomarkers of inflammation that predict ASCVD events (interleukin-6, cytokines, cellular adhesion molecules, CD40 ligand and others), but they are no more sensitive or specific than CRP and are more difficult to measure. The erythrocyte sedimentation rate and white blood cell count have not proven useful.

Suppression of inflammation may help. Among men in the Physicians' Health Study, aspirin for primary prevention was most effective in those with high CRP. Statins are vascular anti-inflammatory agents, suppressing the CRP levels. This action is independent of the lipid lowering effect of statins. The anti-inflammatory effect is prompt, leading to a reduction in ischemic event rates within a week of beginning statin therapy.

The inflammation hypothesis is being tested. CANTOS showed a lower CV event rate with a monoclonal antibody targeting interleukin. Another trial with low dose methotrexate did not. Stay tuned…

Treatment of Atherosclerosis

Subsequent chapters will review the management of CAD in detail. But let us reemphasize the three treatments that are indicated for all who have ASCVD, the guidelines directed medical therapy or GDMT.

Aspirin
Statin (or if necessary, a PCSK-9 inhibitor)
ACE inhibitor (or ARB)

The indication for treatment is any atherosclerotic disorder, including CAD, cerebrovascular and peripheral arterial disease, *plus diabetes*. Since each of these medicines has been shown to improve survival, you should document a reason for not using one of them.

Chapter 5: The Evaluation of Chest Pain and Management of Chronic Coronary Artery Disease (CAD)

Abbreviations

ACS, acute coronary syndrome
AHA, American Heart Association
ASCVD, atherosclerotic cardiovascular disease
AV, atrio-ventricular
CABS, coronary artery bypass surgery
CAD, coronary artery disease
CHF, congestive heart failure
CK, creatine kinase
COX, cyclooxygenase
CPUE, chest pain of uncertain etiology
CRP, C-reactive protein
ECG, electrocardiogram
ED, erectile dysfunction
ER, emergency room
H2, histamine-2
LAD, left anterior descending (coronary artery)
LDL, low density lipoprotein (cholesterol)
LV, left ventricle (ventricular)
LVEF, LV ejection fraction
MET, metabolic unit
MI, myocardial infarction
MVO_2, myocardial oxygen demand
NCEP, National Cholesterol Education Program
NSTEMI, non-ST elevation MI
USAP, unstable angina pectoris

Scientific medicine in the 20th century evolved in a series of steps. The first was the recognition of the pathology and physiology of a disease. Next was the development of mechanical solutions (when possible), followed by their replacement with pharmacologic therapy. Take the case of

peptic ulcer disease: the recognition of gastric acid as a cause
was followed by surgical procedures to resect the ulcer and
block acid secretion. The Billroth procedure was the general
surgeon's bread-and-butter when I was a medical student in the
1960s. Then development of H2 blocker and proton pump
inhibitors eliminated the need for surgery.

We are watching a similar story unfold with the treatment of
coronary artery disease (CAD). My early years in practice
witnessed the evolution of mechanical treatment. Coronary
artery bypass surgery (CABS) was new when I trained, and had
its golden era in the 1980-90s. Its turf has been steadily eroded
by percutaneous coronary intervention (PCI) over the last 20
years.

But the hot news of the last decade has been the rapid
development of pharmacologic therapy. While there may be a
bias to "fix the blockage," often among patients and those who
do the fixing, the reality is that stable CAD can be a medical
illness.

EVALUATING CHEST PAIN OF UNCERTAIN ETIOLOGY (CPUE)

There is no diagnostic code for chest pain of uncertain etiology
(CPUE), but I think of it as a clinical entity because its
evaluation is such a common clinical exercise. I am not referring
to the evaluation of a patient with known CAD and typical
angina pectoris. Instead, CPUE refers to the patient in the
emergency room (ER) or clinic with somewhat vague,
"atypical" pain and no electrocardiographic (ECG) changes that
indicate acute ischemia.

It may or may not be cardiac. After a careful history and
physical exam, I know that my best guess about etiology of a
person's chest pain can be wrong. We are used to being fooled
and understand that our job is often about managing uncertainty.

Nevertheless, because chest pain is so common (3 million emergency room visits a year), most who practice general medicine become adept with the differential diagnosis (Table 5.1). The first goal is recognition of cardiac pain and dissection of the aorta as they may be fatal while most other causes of chest pain are not.

Table 5.1 Differential Diagnosis of Chest Pain (Associated Conditions, History and Physical Exam, Laboratory Exam)

Angina pectoris: Typical chest pain is seldom misleading. There usually are risk factors for CAD. The exam is usually normal but an S4 gallop or soft systolic murmur (papillary muscle dysfunction) are possible during pain. ST segment depression during pain. Positive stress test.

Ascending aortic dissection: Marfan's syndrome in young patients, hypertension/ASCVD in older patients. Abrupt onset of pain (see text), unequal pulses, AR murmur if proximal. Wide mediastinum on chest x-ray is common; make the diagnosis with transesophageal echo or CT scan.

Pulmonary embolus: Clinical setting may suggest the diagnosis, venous disease (although acute phlebitis seldom causes PE). Pain may or may not be pleuritic, and often there is no pain. New atrial flutter (right heart strain), low PaO2, elevated d-dimer. Diagnosis with CT angiography.

Gastroesophageal reflux or esophageal spasm: Distinctive history, normal exam. GI evaluation may not confirm the diagnosis.

Esophageal rupture: Follows severe vomiting. Subcutaneous emphysema.

Pancreatitis: History of alcoholism or gallbladder disease. Epigastric tenderness. Elevated amylase, lipase, white blood cell count.

Chest wall pain: Often a history of arthritis. History and physical exam make the diagnosis.

Herpes zoster: Old age, immunocompromised, history of shingles. Pain may precede rash by a couple days. Usually a clinical diagnosis.

Pericarditis: Young patient, may follow a flu-like illness. Pleuritic pain or pain with swallowing (a clinical pearl). Friction rub common. ST elevation on the ECG, elevated sedimentation rate, usually normal white count, small pericardial effusion on echo in some cases.

Table 5.1 describes a number of noncardiac causes of chest pain. The most common are gastroesophageal reflux and chest wall syndromes. In these cases, the history, alone, may allow a diagnosis. A patient with pain at night when recumbent that is relieved by sitting up, is associated with a sour taste, and is provoked by a late meal has reflux. Esophageal diagnostic studies are seldom helpful. If you suspect gastroesophageal reflux, try a therapeutic trial of antacids (a proton pump inhibitor in the morning and an H2 blocker at night are effective), elevation of the head of the bed, avoidance of late meals, and so forth. If the symptoms do not resolve, then consider GI evaluation. If you decide on a therapeutic trial, there should be a follow-up visit.

Musculoskeletal chest pain is aggravated by movement: deep breathing, reaching, twisting, or use of the arms. It may be positional, worse lying on the wrong side. The diagnosis of chest wall pain—usually costochondritis—is confirmed when there is chest wall tenderness, and reproduction of symptoms with light pressure on the chest wall. There may be point tenderness, often over a costochondral joint. When the bedside evaluation indicates one of these conditions, and the ECG is normal, additional cardiac work-up may be unnecessary.

Aortic dissection is a rare cause of chronic chest pain. The pain of acute aortic dissection is abrupt in onset and at its maximum when it begins; angina is mild at the onset and builds up slowly. Multiple studies have identified this difference in the onset of pain as the best way to distinguish the two conditions. Radiation of pain to the back occurs in just a minority of patients with dissection.

On physical examination, there are two physical findings that may occur during pain that indicate ischemia. Ischemia causes diastolic dysfunction, since muscle relaxation is an energy requiring process, and with an increase in stiffness, an S4 gallop can appear. It goes away with resolution of angina. The second transient finding is the systolic murmur of papillary muscle dysfunction. If you are at the bedside of a patient having angina, listen for these objective signs of ischemia. (Plus, it gives you something to do while someone fetches the ECG machine.)

Laboratory Evaluation of Chest Pain

The need for blood work varies. Most benefit from a complete blood count. Anemia alone does not cause angina, but it lowers the angina threshold in the presence of CAD. Inflammatory conditions that with CV effects may not raise the white blood count. A normal erythrocyte sedimentation rate excludes pericarditis. A more sensitive marker of inflammation, the C-reactive protein (CRP), can be elevated in chronic CAD, but more so with acute coronary syndromes (ACS).

None of the chest pain syndromes alters electrolytes, but it is always worth checking serum potassium and magnesium in a patient who is on diuretics. I do not order the chem-20 unless there is a specific reason (e.g., a new patient, one who is being admitted to the hospital, other medical problems that should be monitored, suspicion of gallbladder disease). If the differential diagnosis includes angina, a lipid panel will be useful, although it is not a part of the ER evaluation.

Cardiac enzymes, troponin or creatine kinase, are frequently measured as part of the ER evaluation of chest pain. The indication for drawing enzymes is to rule out myocardial infarction (MI). *If there is no clinical suspicion of MI, there is little need to measure them.* Cardiac enzymes are drawn frequently when they are not indicated, and elevated levels that are false positives lead to unnecessary further work-up. Chapter 6 discusses cardiac enzymes in some detail.

The resting *ECG* is essential when evaluating a patient with chest pain. It is cheap, safe, easy to do and universally available. If there are ST segment or T wave changes that could be from ischemia, and that are not known to be chronic, the patient should be admitted to hospital for more evaluation.

On the other hand, the ECG may be normal between episodes of angina. During angina—e.g., active ischemia—there usually is ST segment depression, and an absence of ECG changes during pain is suggestive evidence against ischemia. Unfortunately, it is not absolute proof, since there are some myocardial regions that can be electrocardiographically "silent." In particular, ischemia involving the lateral wall of the LV supplied by the circumflex artery may not cause ST segment alteration. For this reason, a normal or unchanged ECG does not support discharge from the ER when the history is suggestive.

The chest x-ray is a crude screen for thoracic aneurysm; mediastinal widening is present in 80% who have aortic dissection. A normal study does not exclude dissection, and the work-up for aortic dissection requires a transesophageal echocardiogram or CT angiogram.

Deciding to Admit or Not Admit

Unstable angina is the usual criterion for admission (Table 5.2).
An initial diagnosis of unstable angina could be wrong, and the
patient may be having noncardiac chest pain. Nevertheless, a
clinical impression of unstable angina justifies admission. A
minority of patients with unstable angina is at low risk for MI in
the near future, and they may be safely evaluated as outpatients
(vide infra). But when in doubt, admit.

Table 5.2 Classification of Angina Pectoris
Chronic Stable Angina:

Clinical syndrome:
1. Angina at a predictable level of exertion (the angina
threshold).
2. Relief with rest or nitroglycerin.
3. No change in the angina pattern for ≥ 2 months.
4. The ECG may be normal.

Prognosis: Annual mortality $< 3\%$ with normal LV function.
Low short-term MI risk.
Coronary artery lesion: Flow-restricting stenosis (>70 reduction
in lumen diameter), but smooth plaque surface, a thick fibrous
cap, and a small, acellular lipid core.

Unstable Angina:
Clinical syndrome: Angina with any of the following:
1. New onset (< 2 months)
2. Accelerating pattern (more frequent, with less exertion)
3. Angina at rest
4. Nocturnal angina
5. Long episodes of pain
6. New ST-T changes on the ECG

Prognosis: 10-20% chance of MI or death within 3-4 months.

<u>Coronary artery lesion:</u> The stenosis may not be tight. The lipid core is large and packed with white blood cells (active inflammation), covered by a thin fibrous cap that is prone to rupture. This exposes collagen and lipid which incites thrombus formation. Angiography may show ragged or ulcerated plaque surface.

Chest pain centers have used a couple protocols to exclude a cardiac etiology of pain for the patient who is not believed to have unstable angina. With one of them, a repeat ECG and troponin are done six hours after admission to the ER, and if all are negative, a stress perfusion scan is performed before discharge. A normal study indicates that the near term risk of MI is low, and hospital admission is unnecessary.

A more useful alternative is cardiac CT angiography (CCTA). Called the triple rule-out study, it can exclude (or diagnose) aortic dissection, pulmonary embolus and proximal coronary artery plaque. It can be done in minutes, soon after ER admission (no need to wait hours), is less expensive, and exposes the patient to less radiation than stress perfusion imaging. For the patient with no ischemic ECG changes and negative troponin, the strong negative predictive value of CCTA allows a shorter ER stay.

STABLE ANGINA PECTORIS

The clinical definition of chronic stable angina is *exercise-induced discomfort that is relieved in minutes by rest or nitroglycerin, with symptoms that have been stable for more than two months (e.g., no change in the frequency or severity of angina,* Table 5.2). In the absence of left main coronary artery stenosis, the mortality rate is under 3% per year. The number of angina episodes per week is not related to prognosis, as long as the spells are exercise-induced and brief.

Pathophysiology

Myocardial ischemia occurs when oxygen supply falls below myocardial oxygen demand (MVO_2). The typical coronary stenosis causing stable, effort angina is fairly tight, reducing the vessel diameter by $\geq 70\%$. The lesion tends to be calcified, concentric, and has a smooth plaque surface. It has an hour-glass appearance on the angiogram. The lesion is not a "dynamic;" that is to say, the percent stenosis changes little, and there is no thrombus at the site of the lesion.

The hydraulics of coronary blood flow with stable angina is similar to fuel line hydraulics in any machine (this is a good way to describe it to patients). A car with a fuel line "stenosis" runs normally when idling. Opening the throttle increases the workload of the engine, but fuel flow is limited and the engine misses. Because of the fixed nature of the fuel line stenosis, you would expect the engine to begin missing at the same workload—speed—every time. That workload might be considered the "angina threshold." Back off the throttle, and the engine stops missing.

The same holds true for stable, exercise-induced angina. Myocardial oxygen demand (MVO_2) is proportional to heart rate and systolic blood pressure. The heart rate-blood pressure product is proportional to cardiac work, and the HR-BP product at which angina occurs defines the *angina threshold*. Serial exercise testing in patients with stable angina shows that the angina threshold is consistent from day to day. Patients usually identify the level of physical work that provokes angina, and try to avoid it.

A change in the angina threshold usually means a change in the plaque. Developing angina at a lower workload–a worsening of the angina pattern–is one of the clinical definitions of unstable angina, and it signifies a higher risk of MI.

Variable Threshold Angina: A Qualification of the Fixed Plaque Model

The supply-demand model with a fixed lesion is a generally reliable explanation for angina. But some patients with exertional angina have variation in the angina threshold. For example, they may describe good days, with no angina despite much exercise, or bad days when angina develops with little exertion. Another common example of this is the warm-up phenomenon: angina with minimal exertion early in the day, with improvement later and no angina despite vigorous activity.

A possible explanation is variability of the coronary artery lumen at the site of plaque. Although uncommon, this may occur when the plaque is eccentric, and does not cover the entire circumference of the arterial wall. The uninvolved arterial segment may relax or contract, and thus change luminal diameter and flow.

More common is a change in vascular resistance distal to the stenosis (Figure 5.1). Coronary blood flow is limited by resistance in the entire vascular bed, not just at the site of stenosis. Lowering downstream resistance can improve overall blood flow, raising the angina threshold.

Blood flow in distal coronary artery branches is auto-regulated, controlled largely by local factors. Vasodilatation occurs with increased tissue CO_2 tension and endothelial nitric oxide. The major vasoconstrictor influence is alpha adrenergic stimulation. When there is a tight proximal stenosis that limits flow and creates persistent, low-level ischemia, auto-regulation of the distal vessel is maxed out. There is no "vasodilator reserve" to counter an alpha adrenergic, vasoconstrictor stimulus.

Figure 5.1 Variable Threshold Angina

$$\text{Flow} = \frac{\text{Pressure}}{\text{Resistance}}$$

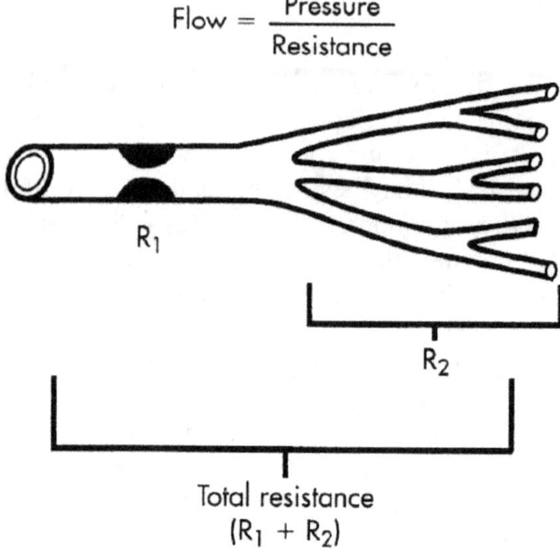

Figure 5.1 Blood flow is proportional to perfusion pressure and inversely proportional to vascular resistance. We are used to thinking that resistance to flow is from the fixed coronary stenosis in the patient with effort angina (R_1). However, the total resistance to flow comes from the combined resistances at the stenosis (R_1) and downstream (R_2). R_1 probably does not change with vasodilator therapy, but R_2 may (this has been shown with calcium channel blockade). In addition, the angina threshold may fall when R_2 is high, explaining why a patient with "fixed" coronary stenosis can have variation in symptoms (e.g. good vs. bad days, the warm-up phenomenon).

This was initially demonstrated in cardiac catheterization laboratory experiments using the cold pressor test, which provokes alpha-adrenergic discharge. Placing the patient's hand in ice water lowered coronary blood flow by causing peripheral vasoconstriction. A change in alpha tone affecting distal coronary resistance may be the link between angina and emotional stress, the warm-up phenomenon or walking into a cold wind. Calcium channel blockers appear to contribute to distal coronary vasodilator reserve; nifedipine blocked the changes seen during the cold pressor test.

Calcium channel blocker therapy is especially effective for the patient whose history suggests variable angina threshold.

Evaluation of the Patient with Angina

Stable angina tends to be stable, and a patient who has had it for years does not require frequent cardiac reevaluation. Lipid lowering therapy (as well as other medical therapy) should be monitored, and an updated ECG in the record is useful for comparison if symptoms change. Repeated stress testing with or without imaging is of little use unless there is a change in the angina pattern. The stress test should be positive, since the patient does, after all, have angina. Most importantly, it does not help to predict the future; a yearly stress test does not predict when the patient will become unstable or have an MI.

This is worth emphasizing, since it is common for a patient with CAD to ask for a test to determine "how I am doing" despite stable or no symptoms. This requires some time to explain, and in that process, it is worth noting that annual survival with stable CAD plus GDMT is in the 97% range.

On the other hand, a patient who first presents with angina needs evaluation to exclude a risk for early MI or death, even if it is "chronic stable angina" with consistent symptoms for more than two months. Clinical features indicating worse prognosis weigh in favor of angiography (Table 5.3).

Table 5.3 Predictors of Poor Prognosis with Coronary Artery Disease

1. More extensive coronary artery disease: Natural history studies in the 1970s, before modern medical therapy, found annual mortality rates of 2-3% with single-vessel CAD, 4-6%

with two-vessel CAD, and 7-10% with three-vessel disease. The mortality risk is much lower with current medical therapy (vide infra). Tight (≥70%) left main coronary artery stenosis is especially dangerous with an annual mortality >50%. Infarction of this vessel means the simultaneous loss of 2 of the 3 vascular regions, the anterior and lateral walls. Early evaluation thus screens for high risk coronary anatomy, either left main and/or multivessel CAD.

2. Exercise intolerance during treadmill testing: Effort intolerance—poor functional class—is as bad with CAD as with CHF. Patients who have to stop the exercise test before completing stage 2 in the Bruce protocol (less than 6 minutes of exercise) have 6-10% annual mortality risk, compared with 1% for those who reach stage 4 (9+ minutes). Thus, a patient with poor exercise tolerance plus ischemia during an exercise test would be a candidate for angiography, while good exercise tolerance would make us more comfortable with a trial of medical therapy. An ability to exercise more than 7 minutes indicates a good prognosis, independent of ECG changes; e.g., those with a positive test still have a good prognosis if exercise tolerance is good.

3. Poor left ventricular (LV) function: This is true for most adults with heart disease, and especially with CAD. Defining LV function is an important part of the initial evaluation. LV dysfunction is suggested by a history of MI, Q waves on the ECG, or symptoms of congestive heart failure, including easy fatigue. Poor LV function identified by noninvasive testing weighs in favor of angiography, even when the angina pattern is stable.

4. Comorbidities: Elevated creatinine and diabetes suggest a worse prognosis. And it makes sense that another debilitating illness adversely affects survival.

5. ECG changes: ST-T wave changes, LV hypertrophy, ST segment changes during angina, new bundle branch block, and long QT interval are associated with worse prognosis.

6. Stress test indicators: >2 mm ST segment depression with exercise, ST depression in exercise stage I, ST depression in multiple leads, ST depression persisting for >5 minutes during recovery, symptoms and ST depression at heart rate <120 (off beta blockers), angina during exercise, a drop in systolic blood pressure >10 mmHg with exercise (may indicate left main CAD), exercise-induced PVCs or ventricular tachycardia (PVCs at baseline that improve with higher heart rate do not indicate poor prognosis), delayed recovery of heart rate (it should fall >12 beats/min in the first minute of recovery).

7. Perfusion scan abnormalities: Defects in multiple vascular distributions (indicates multivessel CAD), anterior plus lateral defects (possible left main CAD), an anterior perfusion defect (left anterior descending CAD) suggest a worse prognosis. There are markers of ischemia-induced LV dysfunction that indicate extensive ischemia and poor prognosis, including post-exercise LV dilation and increased lung uptake of the isotope. On the other hand, increased lung uptake without other indicators of ischemia is not associated with poor prognosis and is not considered a positive test.

8. LV function imaging during stress: Low LVEF at rest is the most prominent indicator of poor prognosis with CAD. Poor prognosis is also associated with a fall in LVEF during exercise ($\geq$10 percentage points), LV dilation with exercise, and exercise induced wall motion abnormalities involving multiple vascular regions.

9. Coronary and LV Angiography: the following are markers of poor prognosis and also are indications for revascularization.
Left main CAD*
Three-vessel CAD

Proximal left anterior descending CAD (when present, it upgrades the risk, moving two-vessel disease into a higher risk category)

Ragged plaque surface and associate filling defects (thrombus)—indicators of unstable plaque,

Depressed LV function—when present it increases the need for revascularization for those with active ischemia. It is a graded effect: the worse the LV, the greater the need for revascularization

MI, myocardial infarction; LVEF, left ventricular ejection fraction; CAD, coronary artery disease; METS, metabolic unit (1 MET is the energy used sitting at rest, 4 METS is the equivalent of walking up stairs or doing housework); PVC, premature ventricular contraction; CABS, coronary artery bypass surgery.

*"Stenosis" and "disease" indicate luminal diameter reduced $\geq 70\%$.

Noninvasive Screening for CAD

Stress Testing

The resting ECG tends to be normal, but during angina, there is ST segment depression. As noted, an absence of ST segment changes weighs against angina. If you are on the wards and are able to get an ECG during chest pain, be sure to note—on the tracing and in a progress note—that the ECG was obtained during pain. If you do not, you will have difficulty identifying the chest-pain ECG later.

The coronary arteries are on the epicardial surface of the heart, and they send perforating branches into the myocardium (Figure 5.2).

Figure 5.2 Coronary Artery Anatomy

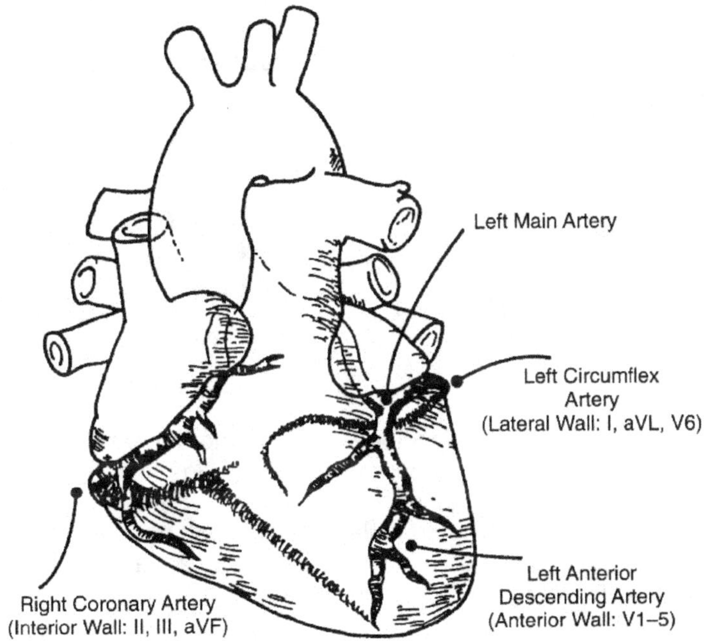

Figure 5.2 The figure also identifies the ECG leads that reflect changes in each vascular distribution. The left main artery divides into two major branches, the left anterior descending (LAD), and left circumflex (LCX) arteries. The LAD is positioned over the interventricular septum, giving rise to septal perforating branches and diagonal branches to the anterior wall of the LV. The LCX and right coronary arteries (RCA) encircle the heart in the atrioventricular groove. Branches of the LCX leave the groove to supply the lateral wall of the LV. Proximal branches of the RCA supply the right ventricle, and the most distal branch, the posterior descending artery (PDA), is positioned over the inferior part of the interventricular septum (opposite the LAD), and also sends septal perforating branches up from the inferior wall. The PDA supplies the inferior wall of the LV.

Exercise-induced ischemia first affects the muscle farthest from the epicardial source, the subendocardium (the layer of muscle adjacent to the ventricular cavity). Thus, angina usually produces the ECG pattern of subendocardial ischemia, ST segment depression (Figure 5.3).

Figure 5.3 Positive Stress ECG, Ischemic ST Segment Depression

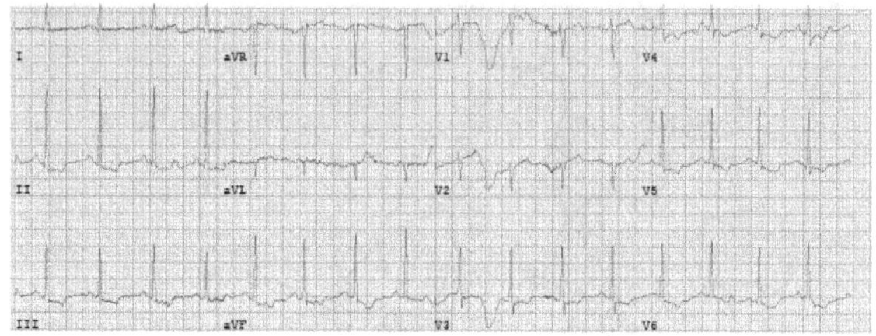

Figure 5.3 The patient developed angina and down sloping ST segment depression in inferior and lateral leads after 3 minutes of exercise. The changes persisted for 5 minutes into recovery. This would be considered a high risk positive because 1) angina, 2) positive at low workload, Bruce stage 1, and 3) the changes did not resolve promptly with rest.

The treadmill ECG (a.k.a. stress test, graded exercise test) is straightforward. The goal is to provoke ischemia in a controlled setting so that both symptoms and the ECG may be evaluated. The test is positive when the coronary stenosis is tight enough to limit flow, when the luminal diameter is reduced $\geq$70%. That is usually the case with exercise-induced angina, and stress testing has good sensitivity in chronic stable angina.

Table 5.4 Bruce Exercise Test Protocol
(The patient walks in each stage for 3 minutes)

Stage 1: 1.7 mph, 10% grade, 5 MEts*. The average peak cost of most activities of daily living (walking up stairs, sex with a spouse).
Stage 2: 1.5 mph, 12% grade, 7 METs
Stage 3: 3.4 mph, 14% grade, 9.5 METs. An ability to walk 7 minutes indicates good prognosis, even when the stress ECG has ischemic ST segment depression.
Stage 4: 4.2 mph, 16% grade, 13 METs. The average exercise capacity for a moderately active young man.

*1 MET (metabolic equivalent) is the energy used sitting quietly at rest; at this baseline the average oxygen consumption is 3.5 ml/kg/min (thus, 5 METs indicates that oxygen consumption is 17.5 ml/kg/min). Achieving 5 METs assumes completion of stage I, or at least being able to exercise comfortably at that level. Walking slowly on level ground requires about 3 METS.

While it is a useful screening study the stress ECG has limits. It does not identify the artery responsible for ischemia. For example, inferior wall ischemia does not cause changes in just the inferior ECG leads. Most positive stress tests have ST segment depression in lead V_5, regardless of the location of the culprit lesion.

ST segment depression in multiple leads, and a failure of the ST segments to return to baseline with 6 minutes of recovery indicate worse prognosis. A drop in blood pressure during exercise suggests left main coronary stenosis; there usually is ST depression as well. Blood pressure normally increases with exercise, even during ischemia involving smaller coronary branches, but left main ischemia affects a large portion of the LV, causing transient pump failure and hypotension.

The stress ECG is less sensitive in unstable angina, because the lesion may be changeable, and may not be tight. The person with a normal stress test who has an MI the next day or week probably had unstable angina and a 30-50% stenosis, not tight enough to cause ischemia during exercise. But such "non-critical" lesions can have an unstable plaque surface, leading to thrombosis, the usual mechanism of acute coronary syndrome (ACS). Clot may reduce luminal diameter and cause angina at rest, or it may occlude the artery and cause MI. For this reason, I usually tell patients that a normal stress test indicates low risk for MI, "but not zero risk."

Despite this limitation, the stress ECG is still an effective tool for evaluating chest pain of uncertain etiology, particularly when the pain is exertional. False positives happen in 10-15%, and are more common in women, in patients taking digoxin, and when there are baseline ST-T wave changes. A patient with stress induced ST depression, but good exercise tolerance and no angina, usually has a false positive study. Repeating the stress study with imaging can prove this.

With CAD and a number of other cardiac conditions, exercise tolerance—or functional class—is the best predictor of longevity. It is no surprise that the time on the treadmill documents this. Patients who can walk for more than 7 minutes in the Bruce protocol, and certainly for 9 minutes or more, tend to do well.

Stress ECG without Imaging

Believe us, the old-fashioned treadmill stress test is reliable, and current practice guidelines recommend it as the initial test for the patient who can exercise, including women, especially when the resting ECG is normal. Insensitivity of the stress ECG is generally overstated. When the stress ECG is normal, and the patient has walked for 9 minutes on the treadmill, an imaging study adds nothing (in fact, if there is a perfusion abnormality it usually is an artifact). A stress ECG costs less than a third of a stress imaging study. Despite all this, many young physicians assume that all stress testing should include imaging, but that is not the standard of care. If it becomes your standard practice, you will be identified as a high-cost operator.

Perfusion Imaging

Most of the isotope is extracted by muscle with the first pass, and myocardial accumulation is proportional to myocardial blood flow. A normal scan shows homogenous uptake by all LV segments. With ischemia there is a "cold spot" on the scan, less uptake in the vascular distribution of the stenosed or occluded coronary artery.

An anterior defect indicates left anterior descending artery stenosis, a lateral defect usually indicates circumflex artery disease, and inferior defect, right coronary disease (Figure 5.2). Defects involving more than one region may indicate multivessel CAD and a worse prognosis. Large defects affecting more than 10-15% of the LV myocardium suggest high-risk coronary anatomy, and prognosis is better with small lesions.

To differentiate scar from ischemia, two scans are obtained. Ischemic but viable muscle does not accumulate isotope with the stress images, but it looks normal on the resting scan. A perfusion defect on both the stress scan and the resting scan indicates scar.

Stress perfusion imaging is not as reliable for those with unstable angina. As with the stress ECG, the coronary artery must be narrowed by > 70% to restrict flow enough to produce an abnormal stress study, with or without imaging. That may not be the case with unstable angina, where unstable, variable plaque may not be that tight at the time of the stress study. It seems that everyone knows someone who had a normal nuclear stress study, and soon thereafter had an MI. The explanation is that the patient had unstable angina. Stress testing with or without imaging can be misleading in that case.

Pharmacologic Stress Test

Exercise testing should be done when possible. It allows assessment of exercise tolerance, which is related to prognosis. An ability to complete an exercise stress test is another predictor of better outcome when the perfusion scan is normal. However, many of our patients cannot walk on the treadmill.

There are two approaches to pharmacologic "stress." The first really is a stress test. Dobutamine is infused at progressively higher doses to raise heart rate and blood pressure in an attempt to provoke ischemia. The perfusion scan is first done at rest and then during maximum dobutamine infusion.

The second non-exercise approach is the coronary vasodilator scan, using adenosine or dipyridamole (which blocks the uptake and removal of adenosine). Adenosine is a powerful coronary vasodilator, at least doubling coronary blood flow. It does not cause an increase in cardiac work, so it does not provoke ischemia. Instead, there is "differential dilatation," with a normal coronary artery dilating more than a stenosed vessel. Flow thus increases to the normal area, but much less in the stenosed region. This heterogeneous flow pattern creates the illusion of ischemia and a positive scan—or you may argue that there is "relative" ischemia. But most patients do not have chest pain with ST segment depression.

Some patients have chest pain but no objective evidence for ischemia (ST changes or a perfusion abnormality). The probable mechanism is that adenosine is the neurotransmitter at cardiac sensory nerve endings, and stimulation of pain receptors may be the mechanism (note the discussion of silent ischemia and Syndrome X near the end of this chapter).

Adenosine (and dipyridamole) can provoke bronchospasm or
AV nodal block and bradyarrhythmias. Both effects are
promptly reversed by intravenous theophylline, and this is kept
on hand in the stress testing lab.

Coronary Steal Syndrome

About 10% do have angina and ST changes during a vasodilator
study; this usually indicates an occluded artery supplied by
collaterals. Adenosine dilates the vessel that is the source of the
collaterals, thus increasing antegrade flow. This reduces flow
through the collaterals—the coronary steal.

Stress Echocardiogram

Like perfusion imaging, LV function and wall motion studies
raise the sensitivity and specificity of stress testing, and they are
able to identify the ischemic region. There is prompt cessation
of contractility when muscle becomes ischemic. The stress test
report will describe a new "wall motion abnormality" or region
of akinesis. A large ischemic region indicates a worse prognosis.
Anterior wall ischemia tends to be more dangerous than inferior
or lateral wall disease, since the left anterior descending artery
(LAD) supplies a larger amount of myocardium. Likewise, a
substantial fall in LV ejection fraction during exercise and
ischemia indicates higher risk (LVEF normally increases during
exercise).

Choosing a Noninvasive Imaging Technique

The sensitivity and specificity of stress perfusion imaging and
stress echo are similar. Studies of these tests are from centers
with medical and technical personnel who work full time on
either nuclear imaging or echocardiography. Although self-
evident, this is worth mentioning, since both techniques are
operator-dependent. The average cardiologist reading
echocardiograms—me for example—is not qualified to interpret
a stress echo. That requires further training, then a relatively
high practice volume to maintain skill. The same holds true for

nuclear stress testing. If your scans are being read by a radiologist who has no cardiac training and minimal experience, you will see a lot of false positives. Day in and day out, use the technique favored by your center.

Left bundle branch block (LBBB) affects wall motion. The septum contracts late, and this reduces stroke volume (note the discussion of resynchronization therapy in Chapter 1). Vasodilator perfusion imaging is the most accurate noninvasive technique with LBBB. This special case has made it to the internal medicine board exam.

Cost may influence choice. In our hospital, the retail cost of a stress perfusion scan is more than twice that of stress echo. Isotopes are expensive.

Radiation exposure is an issue with perfusion imaging. Sestamibi is the commonly used isotope, and the radiation dose is the equivalent of 200 chest x-ray. Thallium, which is used less frequently, delivers the equivalent of 600 chest x-rays. Repetitive nuclear imaging should be avoided; but we occasionally encounter an asymptomatic patient who has had serial nuclear stress studies "to be sure everything is ok." At the least, patients should be informed about radiation exposure.

CT Angiography

Contrast is injected in a peripheral vein, and the images of the proximal coronary arteries are quite good. Radiation exposure and cost are lower than nuclear studies. The study also provides a calcium score. It is a good test for evaluating chest pain of uncertain cause, especially when the clinical impression is that it is a non-cardiac symptom. When assessing the cause of pain with known coronary disease, stress testing can be more helpful.

Coronary Angiography

The indication for cardiac catheterization is suspicion of high risk based on the history and results of noninvasive studies (Table 5.3). Remember that myocardial injury is cumulative, and the chance of a patient with MI dying is much higher when there is a history of prior MI. Thus, a history of MI and known depression of LV function are both clinical indicators of high risk CAD. The most frequent indication for angiography in a patient who has had chronic stable angina is a change in the frequency or severity of the angina. When this happens, the patient has essentially developed unstable angina. "Unstable angina" is probably the most common diagnostic code used as an indication for catheterization.

Angiography is considered a low risk, though invasive procedure. The chance of a major complication—death, MI, stroke or another embolic event, bleeding, loss of a limb—is about 1 in 700. The risk is higher for those with peripheral artery disease or diabetes, yet it is remarkable how well critically ill patients with advanced disease tolerate the procedure.

The radial artery approach is preferred for those with normal sized arteries. With correct patient selection it has proved as safe as the femoral artery approach. Hematoma is less common but can occur. A firm knot at the puncture site can persist, but the scar disappears over a few months. If the knot is pulsitile, there may be concern about pseudo-anerysm (the arterial puncture wound has not closed and is in communication with the adjacent scar). This can be diagnosed with ultrasound.

Box 5.1 Contrast Nephropathy

Most studies define it as a rise in creatinine ≥ 0.3 mg/dL over baseline. It usually occurs in those with elevated creatinine or diabetes. For those with near normal renal function, spontaneous recovery during the week after angiography is the rule. However, with advanced renal disease, contrast exposure may be the final insult leading to dialysis. When on the fence about the need for angiography, severe renal dysfunction weighs against it.

A variety of mechanisms have been identified with related prophylaxis regimens. Presently, our approach is extra hydration pre-procedure.

Treatment of Stable Angina

It is useful to think about what you will accomplish with any therapy. In particular, you should distinguish treatments that prolong life from others that just relieve symptoms. Both goals are important, but highest on the list would be the life-prolonging therapies. In general, these appear in practice guidelines and are referred to as "guidelines directed medical therapy," GDMT. If your patient is not receiving GDMT, you would be wise to document the reasons in the medical record (previous side effects, low blood pressure or heart rate, etc.)

GDMT for ASCVD: survival with CAD is better with statin therapy, aspirin, and angiotensin converting enzyme (ACE) inhibitors or receptor blockers (ARBs). Trials have shown that patients with diabetes should also receive this GDMT. For those with a history of MI, add beta blocker therapy to the list.

LDL Lowering Drugs

Statins have a vascular anti-inflammatory effect that stabilizes arterial plaque. Therapy should be started soon after establishing the diagnosis of any vascular disease, since there is a survival benefit within the first weeks of treatment (Chapter 4). In addition, LDL lowering has been shown to stabilize plaque, although the angiographic appearance of the stable lesion is probably less important than plaque stabilization.

Antiplatelet therapy

Aspirin prevents MI and lowers the risk of death in patients with established ASCVD—including CAD—as well as those with multiple risk factors for ASCVD. Clopidogrel (or other thienopyridine class antiplatelet drugs) is a good substitute for those who do not tolerate aspirin. The CAPRI trial compared aspirin 325 mg/day with clopidogrel 75 mg/day in about 19,000 patients with stable vascular disease. The risk of MI, stroke or vascular death was 8.7% lower in the clopidogrel group (5.3% vs. 5.8%). While statistically significant, the difference is not great enough to justify its use for all patients, especially considering the low cost of aspirin. Perhaps more important, CAPRI documented the safety of clopidogrel.

Because of recent observations, patients may tell you that aspirin doesn't work. They are referring to a trial showing no aspirin benefit in low risk middle-aged or older people with no history of or risk factors for ASCVD. But higher risk patients definitely benefit.

Nonsteroidal Anti-inflammatory Drugs (NSAIDS), and COX-2 Inhibitors

Cyclooxygenase (COX) plays a role in the production of both thromboxane A_2, which activates platelets, and prostacyclin which both blocks inflammation and inhibits platelets. Aspirin, a nonselective COX inhibitor, blocks the generation of thromboxane A_2, and is thus antithrombotic. Selective COX-2 inhibitors affect the inflammatory, prostacyclin pathway. There has been concern that this leaves prothrombotic pathway unopposed, increasing the risk of atherothrombosis (including MI and stroke).

This "imbalance hypothesis" has not been confirmed in animal models of athero-thrombosis. Most of the clinical evidence came from population data-base studies showing an association of Cox-2 inhibitor therapy and MI. However, they were unable to control for systemic inflammation, a known cause of vascular inflammation MI. Arthritis is the usual indication for NSAID therapy, and it is an inflammatory condition. So what was the cause of MI in these retrospective studies, systemic inflammation or the medicine?

More recently, the issue has been resolved with a large, prospective trial specifically addressed the CV safety of Cox-2 inhibitors. It compared celecoxib with naproxen or ibuprofen nonselective COX inhibitors—and celecoxib was as safe (the PRECISION trial, NEJM, Dec 29, 2016), so there is no reason to avoid effective treatment for arthritis. I find myself commonly prescribing meloxicam or celecoxib in cardiology clinic, because primary care providers are unnecessarily concerned about risk.

Angiotensin Converting Enzyme (ACE) Inhibitors

ACE inhibition has direct vascular effects. It is interesting how this understanding developed. Early studies of hypertension demonstrated a renoprotective effect of ACE inhibition in patients who also had diabetes. Assuming this was a vascular effect, the next step was to test benefits in patients without diabetes.

The HOPE trial proved vascular protection using ramapril, and a smaller clinical trial of enalapril supports it. It is believed to be a class effect, one shared by angiotensin receptor blockers (ARBs). ACE inhibitor or ARB therapy is thus recommended for all with ASCVD, with or without diabetes.

Box 5.3 The HOPE Trial

This was a study of 9297 patients <55 years old with a history of CAD, stroke, peripheral vascular disease or diabetes, plus one additional risk factor for ASCVD. It compared treatment with ramipril 10 mg/day to placebo. During 5 years follow-up, ramipril lowered death from MI 20%, death from stroke 32%, and death from any cause 16%. Before treatment, 37% of the patients had diabetes, and in this group ramipril reduced "diabetic complications" (a composite of nephropathy, need for dialysis or need for laser treatment for retinopathy). Most interesting, ramipril also prevented the development of new diabetes; the explanation for this is uncertain. The benefit of ramipril was considered a direct vascular effect, independent of the small reduction of blood pressure noted in the study.

Beta Blockade

A survival benefit has been demonstrated with beta blocker therapy after MI. The treatment of stable angina has not been well studied, but most clinicians extrapolate the post-MI data to the treatment of chronic CAD. Thus, the AHA practice guidelines recommend beta blockers as the initial therapy to control angina symptoms, citing the "consensus opinion of experts." On the other hand, GDMT does not include beta blockers for the treatment of stable, asymptomatic CAD.

The efficacy of available beta blockers is comparable. Bronchospasm is a relative contraindication, and would be an indication for a cardioselective, beta-1 agent, metoprolol or atenolol. At low doses, they do not provoke bronchospasm in those with mild-moderate reactive airway disease. At higher doses, all beta blockers tend to lose their selective effects; when treating a patient with lung disease, start with a low dose and slowly uptitrate it (as we do with beta blockers for congestive heart failure).

Vasospasm is a potential problem with beta blockade that is often overlooked. Beta adrenergic stimulation causes both coronary and peripheral artery dilatation. Blocking this leaves alpha vasoconstriction unopposed. An increase in claudication is fairly common after starting beta blockers. Unopposed alpha activity is a concern in cocaine users as well. Cocaine blocks the reuptake of epinephrine, and coronary spasm is the probable mechanism of sudden cardiac death with cocaine use. It is theoretically safer to treat cocaine users with labetolol, which has a combined alpha and beta blocking effect (we occasionally choose carvedilol for this reason as well).

Consider vasospasm in the rare patient with worsening angina after beta blockade. The first patient I encountered with Prinzmetal's angina developed it after starting metoprolol for hypertension.

We usually avoid beta blocker therapy when there is bradycardia. However, pindolol (Visken) and acebutalol (Sectral) have "intrinsic sympathomimetic activity," and may be considered. They have little effect on resting heart rate, but limit the rise in heart rate with activity.

Nitrates

Nitroglycerin relaxes vascular smooth muscle, predominantly in the venous system. With vasodilatation, there is less blood return to the heart. Lower preload reduces ventricular size, lowering wall tension and MVO_2 (the Laplace relationship, Table 1.4). Because its effect depends on pooling of blood in the lower body, nitroglycerin is less effective when the patient is recumbent. Conversely, the Trendelenberg position reverses any hypotensive effect. Advise your patients to sit, but not to lie down when they have angina and take nitroglycerin.

Both beta blockade and nitroglycerin reduce the heart's mechanical activity. The patient is able to perform more work before reaching the angina threshold. The time on the treadmill is longer, but the heart rate-blood pressure product that causes angina is not changed. This is another way of saying that nitrates and beta blockers to not increase coronary blood flow, but instead reduce oxygen demand.

At the cellular level, nitroglycerin does not work on the endothelium, but goes directly into the smooth muscle cell where it is converted to nitric oxide (NO). Nitroglycerin is thus an "NO donor." The endothelium is a separate source of NO, but nitroglycerin remains active when the endothelium is not intact.

Continuous therapy leads to *nitrate tolerance.* This may occur with all of the long acting nitrate preparations, with evidence of tolerance apparent after 24 hours of a constant blood level of the drug. A brief, nitrate free interval restores responsiveness. Limiting nitrate exposure to 12-14 hours/day prevents tolerance. That requires the patient remembering to take a nitroglycerin patch off before retiring. Most patients would prefer taking a pill to the use of patches, and patch therapy has fallen from favor. The sustained release form of isosorbide mononitrate (Imdur) works for 12 hours, so it is just right when given once a day (30-240 mg). The timing of the single dose is tailored to the patient's needs; nocturnal symptoms may be controlled by an evening dose. We occasionally find a patient taking it bid, and that is an error.

An occasional patient is reluctant to use sublingual nitroglycerin because it is a "pain pill." Explain that it works to change blood flow and has no central or addictive effect. Also, recommend taking it as soon as angina begins. The duration of action is about 20 minutes, and thus may prevent angina if taken just before angina-provoking activity.

Headache is the most common side effect of nitrate therapy. It may improve with dose reduction and with time. But I am struck by how often I see patients who have been kept on long acting nitrates despite headache. Nitrates do not prolong survival or prevent MI, and there are good alternatives, so there is no reason to continue therapy when there are side effects.

Calcium Channel Blockers

Because there is no survival benefit, calcium blockers tend to be used infrequently for control of angina. Consider them for symptom relief, since they are effective and well tolerated, especially by elderly patients. Serial treadmill testing has shown an increase in the angina threshold with calcium blockers. Thus, unlike beta blockers and nitrates, they appear to improve coronary blood flow. They do not dilate the coronary artery at the site of stenosis, but instead dilate the downstream vessel, lowering overall resistance in the system and improving flow (Figure 5.1). A fall in peripheral vascular resistance (LV afterload), and mild depression of contractility with some agents adds to the antianginal effect by lowering cardiac work.

Diltiazem is a reasonable substitute for beta blockers in the patient with severe bronchospasm, since it lowers heart rate. Verapamil has a greater effect on heart rate, but is a relatively weak vasodilator; it has the greatest negative inotropic effect and should be avoided when LV function is depressed. Although it does not affect LV function as much as verapamil, diltiazem should not be used when LV ejection fraction is below 40%. The dihydropyridines are pure vasodilators, and reflex tachycardia may be an issue. This could be beneficial when there is bradycardia, or when beta blockade is needed (e.g., a patient with depressed LV function). Patients with poor LV function can use them safely.

Ranolazine

This unique anti-angina drug inhibits fatty acid oxidation, shifting ATP production to the more efficient carbohydrate oxidation pathway (in a sense, making the heart a more effective anaerobe).

Like nitrates and calcium blockers, it has no survival benefit. It has been shown to provide additional relief of symptoms when added to either beta or calcium channel blockers. There is supposed to be no effect on heart rate or blood pressure, so it can be added when other meds can be pushed no further. That said, a small number of patients on beta blockers have a fall in blood pressure when ranolazine is added, and the beta blocker dose may need to be lowered.

Ranolazine prolongs the QT interval, and that should be monitored while on therapy. QT prolongation is a contraindication, and ranolazine should be used with caution

with other meds that affect the QT.   There are reports of it
causing high-degree AV block.

It is the last drug I add to control angina because of its expense.
There is no reason for using it before trying calcium channel
blockers.

Table 5.5 Summary: An Approach to Medical Therapy for Chronic Stable Angina

1. Correct associated problems that may aggravate angina
(anemia, hyperthyroidism, uncontrolled hypertension, valvular
heart disease).

2. Modify risk factors.

3. Treat all patients with a statin, aspirin (or clopidogrel), and an
ACE inhibitor, the medicines that prevent MI and prolong
survival.

4. Initiate symptom control using beta blockers and sublingual
nitroglycerin.

5. If symptoms are not controlled, add either a calcium blocker
or a long-acting nitrate.

6. When heart rate and/or blood pressure place limits on the use
of other medicines, add ranolazine.

Revascularization

The COURAGE trial confirmed that prognosis with stable CAD
is as good with medical therapy as it is with revascularization.
(It is worth reading the study: 2287 patients were randomized to
optimal medical therapy alone, or medical therapy plus stenting,
and follow-up was 5 years.) It confirmed that revascularization

does not prevent MI or death for those with stable or no angina. Other studies have supported the result.

Generally, there are two indications for angiography and revascularization for patients with chronic stable angina:

1. There is high risk for MI or cardiac death based on clinical and noninvasive evaluation (Table 5.3, and note that COURAGE excluded patients with low LVEF, heart failure, a markedly positive stress study, or left main coronary disease).

2. Medical therapy fails to control symptoms—symptoms are intolerable.

Accepted anatomic indications for revascularization include left main coronary disease, 3-vessel CAD, and multivessel CAD with poor LV function.

Intolerable angina despite medical therapy is a common indication for revascularization. "Intolerable" for some may be an inability to play competitive sports. On the other hand, elderly or sedentary patients may prefer to live with exertional angina, adjusting activities to avoid symptoms (and invasive therapy). Angina at low workloads, after just a couple minutes on the treadmill, is a relative indication for angiography, since it indicates poor prognosis. In practice, the indications for revascularization often overlap.

Percutaneous Coronary Intervention (PCI)

This is the mode of revascularization for most patients

Be aware that restenosis of the stented artery may occur within a year. Think of it as hyperactive scarring at the site of vascular injury—and PCI involves controlled injury of the arterial wall. Drug eluting stents (DES) have dramatically lowered the risk of restenosis, below 5% in many trials. The polymer coating of the stent contains an anitproliferative drug that leeches out over about 30 days and inhibits scarring.

On the other hand, since the antiproliferative drug inhibits growth of endothelium over the stent, there is an increased risk of late thrombosis. Presently, clopidogrel, ticagrelor, or another P2Y12 receptor addition to aspirin—dual antiplatelet therapy, or DAPT—is recommended after placement of a drug-eluting stent. The duration of therapy is a moving target, with more recent studies suggesting that months-long therapy may be unnecessary. The interventional cardiologist will prescribe therapy based on the stent that was placed.

Follow-up after PCI is straightforward. The patient still has coronary artery disease and should be on the medicines that promote survival: statin, antiplatelet and ACE inhibitor therapy. Those who have had MI should be on a beta blocker.

Practice guidelines allow noninvasive screening for restenosis, but do not require it. I do not feel that routine screening is the "standard of care," and few of my colleagues have patients return for expensive follow-up studies. Most patients with restenosis have a recurrence of angina. An exception may be the patient who initially presented with silent ischemia or an angina equivalent such as dyspnea on exertion or exercise induced, episodic fatigue. In such cases, consider a follow-up perfusion scan or stress echo, not another angiogram. If you are going to screen for restenosis, wait until the restenosis period has expired: 6 months with the BMS, 12 months with a DES. A screening study done earlier does not exclude the possibility of restenosis.

Coronary Artery Bypass Graft Surgery (CABG)

It is common to see an elderly patient with new angina who had CABG many years earlier. When dealing with these often-difficult cases, it helps to remember that CABG was probably responsible for the patient reaching old age—it was a therapeutic triumph. I often mention that to patients and families to maintain perspective.

A number of technical advances have improved outcomes with CABG. These include the routine use of the left internal mammary artery for grafting the anterior descending artery, better myocardial protection and monitoring during surgery, and minimally invasive, off-bypass surgical techniques. Endoscopic surgical techniques are being developed that will allow some patients to avoid thoracotomy.

Perhaps the major determinant of the risk of surgery is patient selection. There is increased risk with advanced age, depressed cardiac function and poor general health ("How brightly does the fire of life burn?"). It is noteworthy that the average age of patients having CABG has steadily risen, since younger patients with less extensive CAD have PCI. A 78 year old woman with low LV ejection fraction undergoing a second bypass operation would have a mortality risk as much as 15 times that of an otherwise healthy 55 year old man having a first, elective operation (not that you could find a surgeon who would take her case). The quality of the artery distal to the obstructive lesion is another determinant of patient selection. With diffuse distal disease—a poor target for the graft—surgery is usually not offered.

Box 5.4 Ejection Fraction Does Not Tell the Entire Story

Patients with depressed LVEF but good exercise tolerance and no history of heart failure tend to do well with CABG. When there has been clinical heart failure, and the patient is functional class III or worse, the risk is much higher. Viability studies are commonly requested, but I've found that a scan showing viable but stunned muscle rarely generates enthusiasm for the operation. This widely held clinical impression has been supported by the STITCH trail, which randomized patients with multivessel CAD and low LVEF to medical therapy or CABG. There was a survival benefit for those with good exercise tolerance, but not for those without. Results from viability study did not predict outcome.

Other comorbidities that increase the risk of surgery include recent MI, CABG in emergency circumstances, ventricular arrhythmias, diabetes, cerebral vascular disease, obstructive lung disease and elevated creatinine. The potentially fatal complications of CABG include stroke, deep wound infection, MI, and renal or pulmonary failure.

Follow-Up After CABS

Though "fixed," the patient still has CAD and should be on the usual life-prolonging therapy (statin, aspirin, ACE inhibitor and a beta blocker when there has been MI). During the first couple months after surgery, most have easy fatigability and poor exercise tolerance. They may be alarmed because they have been told they will be ready to return to work after six weeks. In reality, it is a small minority that is able to return to normal activity this quickly. Those who do physical work require more time. Older patients commonly take six months to recover. Cardiac rehabilitation speeds the recovery process, and helps with risk factor modification.

With better coronary blood flow, the cardiac risk of exercise is lower after surgery than it was before. There are few activities that must be avoided, and walking and other aerobic exercise are key elements in the recovery process. Chest wall soreness will limit upper body exertion, and symptoms are a reasonable guide. The chest wall is stable after surgery, and nothing will fall apart if the patient over-exerts and is sore. Most who are walking regularly can resume driving 3-4 weeks after surgery while avoiding prolonged sitting and long trips at first. There is no reason to delay resumption of sexual activity; the usual recommendation is "if you can walk up the stairs to the bedroom, you can have sex."

Complications After CABG

Patients are now being discharged just a few days after uncomplicated CABG. There are a few complications of CABG you may encounter in a primary care practice:

Atrial fibrillation **(AF)**—AF occurs in 15%-20% during the week after CABG. It is not related to the severity of heart disease, does not injure the heart, and is not an indicator of a poor surgical outcome. Reassure your patient that while AF is aggravating, it has few serious consequences (stroke may occur but it is rare). The usual treatment principles apply (Chapter 7). Cardioversion with ibutelide or countershock is effective and safe. If it persists for longer than 48 hours, anticoagualation is indicated. Late recurrence is rare, and anticoagulants can be stopped a couple months after cardioversion.

Note that low magnesium or potassium is a common cause AF after any operation, and electrolyte replacement may correct the arrhythmia. Small studies have suggested that prophylactic beta blockade and/or aggressive magnesium replacement may prevent perioperative AF. Do not stop beta blocker therapy preoperatively for those already on it. It is common to see patients on amiodarone after CABG—AF is the usual reason it was started, and there is no reason to continue it long term (stop it after a month).

Potspericardiotomy syndrome—This is another complication of heart surgery that brings patients to their family doctor. It is an autoimmune illness with fever and pleuropericarditis that develops 1-6 weeks after surgery. Any mechanical manipulation of the pericardium can cause it, including cardiac trauma or perforation of the heart by a pacemaker wire. The serositis is like that of Dressler's syndrome. The incidence is about 10% with heart surgery, with mild cases unrecognized.

It is easy to diagnose when you are aware of it. The usual clinical picture is fever, cough and pleuritic chest discomfort, plus flu-like symptoms. The patient usually feels poorly out of proportion to physical findings. Patchy pneumonitis is common, and often is mistaken for pneumonia. There may be a pericardial friction rub, and ECG and echocardiography may suggest pericarditis. Granulocytosis is uncommon, but there may be mild lymphocytosis. All patients have a *high sedimentation rate*, above 60 mm/hr. That is the key test for making or excluding the diagnosis.

Mild cases respond to non-steroidal anti-inflammatory drugs. A short course of steroids (e.g., a Medrol dose-pack) is frequently needed. Most patients have a single episode, but some have intermittent recurrence, with episodes as late as one year after surgery. Recurrence is easily identified by symptoms and re-elevation of the sedimentation rate. Postcardiotomy tends to burn out with flare-ups becoming farther apart and less severe with time. While rare, pericardial fibrosis and constriction are possible. We reassure patients that the inflammatory process does not hurt the heart and that they may expect to do well long term.

Neurocognitive dysfunction—It is a long suspected but recently described complication of CABG, and the results of the small studies are controversial. It may appear to be transient, with some improvement in the months after surgery, but this can be followed by later decline. Predictors of late, persistent cognitive dysfunction after surgery are advanced age, cognitive dysfunction before or early after surgery and low educational level. The severity of the heart disease and the duration of cardiopulmonary bypass have not been identified as risk factors for cognitive dysfunction. On the other hand, many suspect that the heart-lung bypass machine plays a role, and suggest that cognitive decline may be avoided with off pump surgery. Provoking dementia is another argument for PCI as palliation in elderly patients.

Choosing Between Coronary Stenting and CABG

About 60% of the patients with multivessel CAD treated with CABG or PCI could have been treated with either procedure. After reading the above descriptions, you can see that arguments can be made for or against either procedure. Comparison studies have shown that survival is similar with each approach.

There is a trade-off. With PCI, the patient avoids major surgery, but has chance of restenosis leading to repeat angiography, re-stenting and rarely, CABG. With CABG, the patient is less likely to need a subsequent revascularization procedure. In practice, most are willing to go through a lot to avoid a major operation, and choose PCI. A rare patient wants to know he is "fixed for good" and chooses CABG. As an initial revascularization strategy, PCI costs less.

Diabetes and multivessel CAD is a unique circumstance; long-term survival is better with CABG. That said, with improving technology and operator experience, the indications for PCI have broadened to include higher-risk patients, including those with left main coronary artery disease.

OTHER CLINICAL SYNDROMES, AND SPECIAL ISSUES

Prinzmetal's Variant Angina

This "variant" of angina pectoris occurs at rest and is not provoked by exercise. During pain there is ST segment elevation—not depression—and angiography confirms coronary artery spasm as the cause. Spasm may occur at the site of atherosclerotic plaque, as with Dr. Prinzmetal's initial cases, but also may occur in normal-appearing arteries. It may coexist with other vaspospastic disorders, including Raynaud's phenomenon or migraine headache.

There is no apparent etiology for most patients. The most common identifiable cause is cocaine. It blocks the presynaptic uptake of norepinephrine and dopamine, increasing alpha-adrenergic tone. Similarly, beta-adrenergic blockers may aggravate coronary spasm by leaving alpha stimulation unopposed. An occasional patient develops Prinzmetal's angina after starting beta blocker therapy for hypertension. There are also reports of coronary spasm after treatment with 5-fluorouracil or cyclophosphamide.

The attack frequency may wax or wane, with occasional symptom-free intervals. The quality of angina discomfort is typical. Pain usually occurs at rest, and it tends to occur at the same time every day, commonly at night. Continuous ST segment monitoring has shown that many ischemic episodes are painless, especially when they are brief. Exercise tolerance is usually normal. Another presentation is syncope. Ischemia may be severe enough to provoke ventricular tachycardia. Heart block may occur with right coronary spasm and AV nodal ischemia.

Laboratory Evaluation

The diagnosis of coronary spasm is confirmed when an ECG during chest pain shows ST segment elevation. A patient with no ST changes during typical pain probably does not have spasm and would not benefit from angiography. Exercise stress testing may be considered to screen for fixed coronary stenosis but is of no use for the diagnosis of spasm.

Angina at rest is, by definition, unstable angina, so many of these patients have coronary angiography. It is justified when there is ST segment elevation with pain, and when there is uncertainty about the diagnosis. In addition to identifying spasm, an angiogram determines the extent of atherosclerotic CAD.

Provocative testing with ergonovine maleate during angiography is the standard test for spasm. After identifying normal appearing coronary arteries, the patient is given increasing doses of ergonovine. With spasm, a repeat angiogram shows occlusion or near-occlusion of a segment of coronary artery, with ST elevation plus typical anginal pain. Spasm is focal. An overall reduction in the caliber of the vessel is a normal response to ergonovine, and does not cause pain or ST elevation.

In the past provocative testing was frequently done to exclude spasm in the catheterization laboratory in patients with chest pain and normal coronary arteries. However, the yield was low. Patients with atypical chest pain syndromes seldom have coronary spasm. The ergonovine stress is now reserved for those with normal arteries and typical angina at rest. The test is both sensitive and specific for coronary artery spasm.

Ergonovine testing is considered safe. Angina and ST segment elevation are usually relieved by sublingual nitroglycerin, but some require intracoronary nitroglycerin. For this reason, provocative testing has been a cath lab procedure. There are reports of using ergonovine stress with noninvasive imaging, but this approach has not been validated by large studies.

Therapy

Calcium channel blockade is the mainstay of therapy. These agents are so effective that I think of coronary spasm and Raynaud's phenomenon as illnesses of the calcium channel (realizing that the basic mechanism has not been identified with certainty). All of the long-acting preparations work, and may need to be given at high dose. An occasional patient who does not respond to one of them will respond to another. A rare patient needs treatment with two different calcium blockers, from different drug classes.

There may be rebound of symptoms when calcium blockers are stopped, such as perioperatively. Intravenous diltiazem may be used if symptoms have been frequent.

Angina attacks are relieved by nitroglycerin, and long-acting nitrates may be used with calcium blockers. Since the mechanism of action is different with the two drug classes, combination therapy makes sense. One reason it is important to recognize spasm as the mechanism of angina is that two of the standard therapies for CAD and angina may cause worsening of symptoms. *Beta blockers* leave alpha adrenergic stimuli unopposed. Consider coronary spasm if your patient with hypertension develops angina after starting a beta blocker. *Aspirin* inhibits synthesis of prostacyclin, a coronary vasodilator, and may thus aggravate spasm. Avoiding aspirin may help the patient with variant angina with no underlying ASCVD. With coronary artery plaque plus spasm, benefits of aspirin probably exceed risks—but monitor symptoms.

Hypomagnesemia may cause spasm. Serum magnesium often falls after major surgery, and spasm is a rare complication. It responds to magnesium replacement.

Pure vasospasm with no underlying atherosclerosis is a medical condition, not a surgical one. A failure to recognize that a stenosis is from spasm rather than plaque may lead to a surgical/interventional disaster. Spastic arteries are touchy, and often develop spasm at the site of manipulation or graft insertion. Postoperative ST segment elevation, arrhythmias and infarction may follow. (Remember magnesium replacement!) On the other hand, when spasm develops at the site of a tight plaque, stenting or CABS is effective.

Natural History

As noted, symptoms may wax and wane. Many patients are better 4-6 months after initial presentation. When symptoms resolve, it is reasonable to slowly taper therapy, and possibly to stop it. If symptoms recur, they respond to the same medicines.

The risk of MI and death is highest for those with spasm and underlying atherosclerosis. Those with angiographically normal coronary arteries have a good prognosis, with 5-year survival about 95% and MI risk less than 10%. If cocaine use is the cause of spasm, continued use confers higher risk.

Silent Ischemia

A reported 20%-60% of heart attacks are unrecognized by the patient (my experience favors the lower end of this range). About half of these are truly painless. There are some patients who have a defective angina warning system, and are at risk for MI and death. Others have angina with longer episodes of ischemia, but also have shorter, asymptomatic spells. Ischemia is bad, regardless of the presence or absence of symptoms. Exercise-induced ST segment depression without angina indicates a 4-5x increase in cardiac mortality.

Pathophysiology

Pain-sensing nerves, the C fibers, accompany cardiac sympathetic afferents. They follow the path of the coronary arteries, originating at the base of the heart and moving to the apex, and are primarily subepicardial. The sensory nerves pass through ganglia in the heart, mediastinum and thorax, then to the nucleus of the solitary tract, and finally with other visceral and somatic afferents in the spinothalamic tract. After passing through the hypothalamus and thalamus they are projected bilaterally to the frontal cortex.

At the myocardial end, adenosine is the neurotransmitter. Chest pain without ischemia (e.g., there is no ST segment change or perfusion abnormality) is common during adenosine or dipyridamole stress testing; it is a neurotransmitter effect.

Silent ischemia may result from peripheral neuropathy. This is
the probable cause with diabetes, where asymptomatic ischemia
is common. It is more common when there is autonomic
neuropathy.   Nociceptive dysfunction has also been described
after reperfusion therapy for acute MI; the prolonged ischemia
before reperfusion apparently damages cardiac nerves, and
subsequent infarct-zone ischemia is more likely to be silent (the
patient is left with "stunned nerves and live muscle").

Box 5.5 Testing Autonomic Function at the Bedside

Autonomic dysfunction is common in diabetic patients, and is
another manifestation of peripheral neuropathy. Peripheral
neuropathy affects long nerves first, like the vagus nerve. An
easy way to test for it at the bedside is to monitor the heart rate
response to the Valsalva maneuver (monitoring the radial pulse).
With strain heart rate slows, and with release, there is transient
tachycardia. Try it on yourself. A diabetic patient whose heart
rate does not vary during or after Valsalva has autonomic—
vagal nerve—dysfunction, and is more likely to have silent
myocardial ischemia.

Asymptomatic ischemia may also be a central phenomenon.
Study of hypertensive patients with silent ischemia
demonstrated a generally higher pain threshold (to tooth pulp
stimulation, of all things). They may have higher endorphin
levels. PET scans in others with painless, dobutamine-induced
ischemia showed activation of the thalamus, but a failure of the
impulse to project to the left frontal cortex.

The duration of ischemia often determines symptoms.
Ambulatory ECG monitoring shows that a majority of patients
with stable angina also have brief periods of ST segment
depression without pain. They develop pain only when ischemia
is present for 2-5 minutes.

Management

Observational studies have found that prognosis with CAD is related to the extent of disease and LV function, and not to the presence or absence of symptoms. It has been argued both ways: 1) with a defective warning system, the patient must have a higher risk, or 2) the absence of symptoms may mean less severe ischemia and therefore, lower risk. However, available data show that silent ischemia indicates neither lower nor higher risk.

Silent ischemia is usually discovered with stress testing or following an asymptomatic MI. The size of the ischemic defect on the stress perfusion study is a fair indicator of prognosis. A low-risk scan—a small defect—is not an indication for coronary angiography, especially if exercise tolerance is stable.

Since diabetes carries an increased risk of CAD, autonomic dysfunction, and therefore, silent ischemia, there has been question about preemptive screening. However, clinical trials have found no benefit using stress testing with imaging. The American Diabetes Association has suggested coronary calcium scoring if there is a desire for testing. On the other hand, there is not much in it for the patient, since those with diabetes should already be on GDMT for CAD (diabetes being a surrogate for CAD).

Syndrome X: Microvascular CAD

This syndrome has been defined as angina or angina-like chest pain with normal appearing epicardial coronary arteries. It is a mixed bag, and most are having noncardiac pain.

Some truly have microcirculatory disease and ischemia. The stress test is abnormal and there may be patchy thallium perfusion defects. Increased myocardial lactate production during induced angina has been demonstrated in such cases. Microvascular constriction, or inadequate vasodilator reserve are possible mechanisms, since coronary blood flow does not increase with exercise or dipyridamole infusion.

In other cases, there is abnormal cardiac pain perception. I think of this as the flip side to silent ischemia—the heart is hypersensitive. In such cases, low dose adenosine infusion may cause severe pain without objective evidence for ischemia. Some of these patients with sensitive hearts have heightened visceral pain sensitivity elsewhere (e.g. an abnormal pain response to esophageal stimulation).

The rare patient with Syndrome X who has objective evidence for ischemia will respond to antianginal therapy. However, treating those with chest pain, normal coronary arteries and no objective evidence for ischemia with antianginal drugs rarely helps. It is important to reassure the patient. Most have spontaneous resolution of symptoms with time. The risk of MI and death is low, even for those with ischemia on the stress ECG or perfusion scan.

Erectile Dysfunction and Phosphodiesterase 5 Inhibitors (PDE5i)

Erectile dysfunction (ED) affects almost 30 million men in the United States. Risk factors for ED parallel those of ASCVD. A survey of men in their late fifties with diabetes, hypertension or both found ED in 62%, 46% and 67% of the three groups. The evaluation of a patient with heart disease before sildenafil therapy is a common cardiology consultation.

As part of your initial evaluation, be aware that many of the cardiovascular drugs may cause ED (diuretics, beta blockers, statins, fibrates and digoxin to name a few). Impotence is among the intolerable complications of medical therapy, and there are few cases where I feel compelled to continue therapy (perhaps an exception is beta blockade that has had a dramatic effect on survival and LVEF in a patient with heart failure).

PDE5i's are safe for men with CAD. A study of hemodynamic changes after 100 mg sildenafil in men with flow-restricting coronary artery stenosis found a trivial drop in arterial and pulmonary artery pressure, no change in cardiac output or pulmonary wedge pressure, and no change in coronary blood flow in the stenosed artery measured using intracoronary Doppler. Clinical trials in men with stable CAD, congestive heart failure or with hypertension have shown no increase in cardiac risk with PDE5i treatment. While there are reports of death or MI during sex with Viagra, an FDA survey found that the number of cases is below what would be expected considering the large number of men who have received prescription. The usual workload associated with sex with a spouse is 4-6 METS. If there is uncertainty about exercise tolerance based on history, a treadmill test may be appropriate.

Mechanism of Action and the Interaction of Viagra and Nitroglycerin

This is worth reviewing since nitrates contraindicate the use of Viagra. Relaxation of arterial smooth muscle is promoted by c-guanylate monophospate (cGMP), which through a series of steps affects an ion channel, reducing intracellular calcium. (Calcium ion in the cell stimulates muscle contraction.) Phospodiesterase (PDE) leads to the degradation of c-GMP; PDE *inhibitors* thus lead to higher levels of cGMP, and to vasodilatation. Nitric oxide, produced by the endothelium or from a nitrate donor like nitroglycerin, stimulates the production of cGMP.

The net effect of increasing cGMP production (nitroglycerin), and impeding its breakdown (PDE inhibitor) is maximal vasodilatation. This combination can lead to severe hypotension. This does not require simultaneous administration of the two drugs, but may be delayed. Recent guidelines suggest a 24-hour interval between administration of sildenafil and nitrates. In practice I do not prescribe Viagra when the patient is on any nitroglycerin preparation.

There are some cardiologists who feel that any patient with CAD should carry nitroglycerin, even an asymptomatic person after revascularization. But remember that nitro does not prevent MI or sudden cardiac death; it is used just for relief of symptoms. If an asymptomatic man with stable CAD and fair exercise tolerance wants to use Viagra, there is no contraindication to stopping nitro.

Palliative Care for End Stage Coronary Artery Disease

Everyone with CAD reaches a point where another revascularization procedure is not feasible. This can be distressing news for the patient and family. It is even more distressing when the doctor tells the patient, "There is nothing more we can do for you."

It is not a useful phrase. Not only is it emotionally devastating, it is factually incorrect. Medical therapy is remarkably effective, and even patients with advanced CAD may expect to have symptoms and survival improve. It is better to tell the patient that "in your case medical therapy is superior to revascularization," and then to emphasize what we know to be true: the medicines we use to control symptoms also prolong life, including aspirin, clopidogrel, beta blockers, and ACE inhibitors.

At the same time, we must be truthful about prognosis. I tell the patient with end-stage disease that the condition may be fatal. But the timing of death is uncertain. With metastatic lung cancer, we know that most are dead in six months. With advanced CAD, some will be dead in six months, but it is possible to live much longer.

How about this? "If I hear that you have died three months from now, I will be surprised, although I realize that is a possibility. On the other hand, if we are still visiting in clinic three or five years from now, I will not be surprised, because I know that is possible." This is an honest yet hopeful message. When you have had the experience of following patients for years, you will realize that many with "end-stage heart disease" stabilize and do quite well. In addition to usual therapy for angina, consider these treatments for the end-stage patient.

A common finding is occlusion of all native vessels, and loss of all bypass grafts except for the left internal mammary artery (LIMA) grafted to the left anterior descending artery. The LIMA supplies everything through collateral vessels to other vascular distributions. Flow through the collaterals is not good enough to prevent angina and MI. Experience has shown that this anatomy is remarkably stable, and patients can live for some time with good medical therapy. Calcium channel blockers may be especially useful.

Calcium channel blockers are often overlooked when treating chronic CAD, since they are not on the list of medicines that prevent death or MI. But they are quite effective in controlling symptoms and are well tolerated by sick and/or elderly patients. They are easy to use in combination with other antianginal drugs. Dihydropyridines do not slow heart rate, so may be used when there is bradycardia. Diltiazem does slow the rate, and is the choice for the patient with tachycardia. It may depress the myocardium, so must be used with caution when there is heart failure or low LVEF. All calcium blockers may lower blood pressure.

Adding *clopidogrel* to aspirin often helps. Patients with end-stage CAD usually have some rest angina, and thus have "unstable angina." This justifies more aggressive antiplatelet therapy, and it may control symptoms.

Ranolazine–discussed above–is the next drug to add.

Morphine is commonly used to treat end stage heart-failure, but it also palliates angina when all else has failed. In addition to its analgesic effect, it is a venodilator, reducing blood return to the heart and therefore, cardiac work—a nitroglycerin-like action, but without the problem of nitrate tolerance.

Hospice care is appropriate by the time a patient with angina needs morphine. While hospice is not required when prescribing opioids, I usually recommend it. Some consider morphine an unconventional treatment for CAD, and hospice involvement obviates any medical-legal question. More important, hospice nurses are good at monitoring opioid therapy. Patients with heart disease frequently improve with the attention of a skilled hospice nurse. After a few months many are ready for discharge from hospice.

Home oxygen has not been tested in clinical studies, but an occasional patient has less angina with it. Some of this may be a placebo effect, a well-documented and important component of all therapies for angina. Oxygen is easier to justify for those with low arterial oxygen saturation on room air.

Correcting mild anemia has been shown to relieve symptoms. A patient with advanced illness often has the anemia of chronic disease, and boosting the hematocrit from 30% to 33-35% changes the angina threshold.

Smoking cessation is worth pursuing, even for the end-stage patient. There is an immediate effect on arterial oxygen carrying capacity. Smoke contains carbon monoxide, and active smokers have elevated arterial carboxyhemoglobin levels. There is an acute effect: treadmill testing found that time on the treadmill declined shortly after smoking a couple cigarettes (as carboxyhemaglobin level increased). A person with advanced symptoms may note an improvement within days of reduced smoking.

Spinal cord stimulation has been tested using electrodes implanted in the epidural space, and with transcutaneous stimulation (TENS). Randomized small studies have found improved exercise tolerance and decreasing frequency of angina episodes. By reducing the number of hospital admissions, this may be cost effective.

Chelation therapy. Originally, the rationale for chelation was the removal of calcium from plaque using EDTA infusion, debulking it. A more recent clam is that EDTA plus vitamins have an antioxidant effect that improves endothelial function. A recent clinic trial (TACT) suggested a clinical benefit that was limited to diabetic patients, and another trial, TACT-2, is in progress. Chelation clinics continue to peddle this expensive technique, and there are stories of miraculous cures. The placebo effect of any treatment for CAD can be remarkable.

Rest therapy often is the final step in palliation. One of my mentors, Dr. Julian Beckwith (1910-1982), taught me that a sensible treatment option for uncontrolled symptoms is reduced activity, a "bed-to-chair" lifestyle. This was a common approach before the1960s, and at times is still appropriate. There is no doubt about the efficacy of aerobic activity for patients with heart disease, both CAD and heart failure. But there comes a time when it no longer works, and reduced activity offers palliation.

Chapter 6: ACUTE CORONARY SYNDROMES (ACS)

Abbreviations

ACS, acute coronary syndrome
CABG, coronary artery bypass surgery
CAD, coronary artery disease
CCU, coronary care unit
CHF, congestive heart failure
CRP, C-reactive protein
CV, cardiovascular
ECG, electrocardiogram
ER, emergency room
GDMT, guidelines directed medical therapy
LAD, left anterior descending (coronary artery)
LV, left ventricle (ventricular)
LVEF, LV ejection fraction
MI, myocardial infarction
NSTEMI, non-ST segment elevation MI
PCI, percutaneous coronary intervention (e.g. stenting)
STEMI, ST segment elevation MI
UA, unstable angina

Pathophysiology

The acute coronary syndromes include unstable angina pectoris
(UA), non-ST elevation MI (NSTEMI), and ST segment
elevation MI (STEMI). They are a continuum of the same
process. In some cases, distinguishing between them is an
exercise in semantics. For example, some studies of USAP
include patients with elevation of troponin. You would be
correct claiming that any patient with elevated troponin has had
an MI—that is to say, muscle damage.

STEMI is often considered separately from the other ACS
syndromes because total occlusion of the infarct artery with
STEMI requires a different approach to treatment, and the

consequences of the larger infarction can be different. The therapy of USAP and NSTEMI share the same "ACS protocol." In this chapter we will consider USAP and NSTEMI as acute coronary syndrome and approach STEMI in the next.

The initiating event in stable angina is exercise leading to an increase in myocardial oxygen demand. The reverse is true with ACS. This was discovered by studies using ambulatory 12-lead ECG and blood pressure monitoring. With exercise induced angina, a rise in heart rate and blood pressure, e.g. increased cardiac work, precedes ST depression and chest pain: *demand exceeds supply.*

But with rest angina, *what comes first is a drop in supply.* On the ambulatory monitors, ST segment changes and chest pain occurred before any change in heart rate or blood pressure (which often rose after pain developed). That is to say, ischemia preceded pain, and without any increase in cardiac work. By some mechanism the lesion of unstable angina becomes tighter and causes ischemia, unrelated to a change in cardiac work. That mechanism is thrombosis.

Of interest, another finding of the ambulatory monitoring studies was a delay in onset of pain. Often 3-5 minutes of ischemia (ST segment depression) was needed before chest pain developed, and that was true with both exertional and rest angina. Those with angina at rest commonly had multiple, brief episodes of silent ischemia during the day and while asleep.

Atherosclerotic plaque morphology is different with stable and unstable coronary disease. Paradoxically, those with stable angina often have tighter stenosis. At least a 70% reduction in vessel diameter is needed to cause effort angina (or a positive stress test). This is the oxygen-demand-outweighing-supply, physiology of stable angina, with exercise the usual cause of increased demand. The stable plaque even looks stable. Its fibrous cap is thick, and the lipid core is small with few inflammatory cells (Figure 6.1).

Figure 6.1 Plaque Morphology

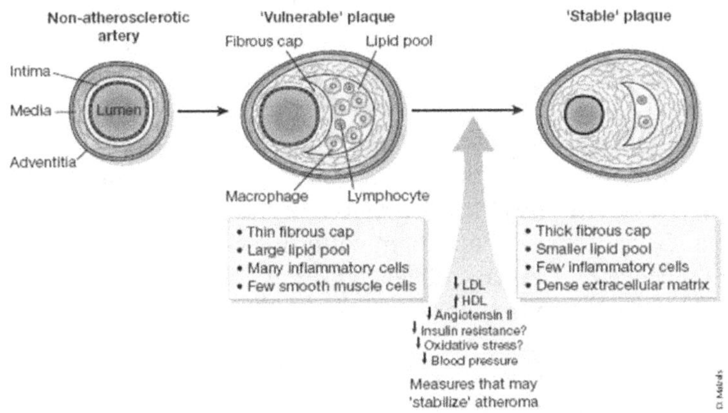

Figure 6.1 The stable lesion, far right, has a thick, dense cap of fibrin separating the lipid core from the arterial lumen. We could add vascular anti-inflammatory agents to the measures that promote plaque stability, including statins and ACE inhibitors. A deficiency of this cartoon is that the plaque of stable angina tends to be concentric, with the lumen in the middle of the artery; on the angiogram the stenosis has an hourglass appearance, and looks the same from different projections.

In contrast, the culprit lesion of ACS often is not stenotic enough to cause effort angina. Instead, something happens to disrupt the less stenotic but "vulnerable" plaque, leading to plaque rupture, platelet activation, thrombosis and ischemia. The vulnerable plaque has a thin fibrous cap, ragged plaque surface, and a large lipid core containing macrophages and lymphocytes. Rupture of the plaque usually occurs at its shoulder, where it meets normal arterial wall, a site that is susceptible to shear forces. When rupture occurs, the lipid core is exposed to

207

circulating blood and platelets are activated. If the resulting thrombus occludes the vessel, there is STEMI. If it does not occlude, but instead creates tight stenosis with continued antegrade blood flow, the result is UA or NSTEMI

Multiple lines of evidence implicate inflammation in plaque instability and rupture. Postmortem examination indicates a concentration of inflammatory cells, mostly macrophages, in ruptured plaque. Macrophages release matrix metalloprotease (MMP) that can weaken the thin fibrous cap, leading to rupture, and MMP levels are high in ACS. The degree of instability with ACS is proportional to the degree of elevation of C-reactive protein (the biomarker of inflammation), and most patients with MI preceded by UA have elevated CRP. Conversely, angiography commonly reveals no evidence for unstable plaque in the patient with a diagnosis of ACS who has a normal CRP. Intracoronary angioscopy and ultrasound indicate that ACS plaque morphology—thin cap, big lipid core—involves plaque at multiple sites in the coronary tree, in addition to the culprit lesion, suggesting a systemic process, or panvascular endothelial inflammation.

Thus, ACS involves the interaction among plaque anatomy, plaque inflammation, coagulation, and exogenous factors such as vasomotor tone, plaque location (there is more turbulence at branch points), and systemic inflammation (see below).

Once plaque rupture initiates thrombosis, several things can occur. If the thrombus completely occludes the artery, it causes STEMI. If thrombus occludes intermittently, or just forms tight stenosis, unstable angina or NSTEMI is the result. A balance between endogenous thrombolysis and the thrombosis mediates this process. With thrombus forming and breaking up, ischemia occurs at rest, and angina may come and go.

This is the treatment strategy for ACS: 1) interrupt thrombosis with antiplatelet therapy, 2) stabilize the coronary artery with either PCI or CABG. GDMT also includes suppressing vascular inflammation with a statin. Beta blocker therapy is also is a GDMT (vide infra).

Systemic Inflammation; a Risk Factor for CAD

In Figure 6.1, interventions that promote plaque stability are listed, and all have anti-inflammatory effects. Dentists claim they prevent MI, and they probably do. Periodontal disease is associated with increased risk of ACS. That is true of all infectious illnesses that have been studied. For example, when influenza is epidemic, there is a rise in the incidence of MI except in the vaccinated subset of the population. There is a higher risk of MI with connective tissue diseases including systemic lupus and rheumatoid arthritis. Essentially any condition that causes enough inflammation to raise CRP has an association with MI. Systemic inflammation may provoke plaque inflammation by activating T cell lymphocytes (killer T cells).

Throughout history, the most common cause of death in old people has been coronary artery disease. Steadily rising longevity in the developed world is often attributed to improved diet. But a reduced lifetime burden of inflammation may be more important; consider vaccination, improved sanitation, fluorination, dental care, and effective treatment of infectious disease.

The Clinical Syndrome

The term *unstable* is more than descriptive. UA is a well-defined clinical syndrome associated with a 10%-40% increased risk of death or myocardial infarction within 4 months.

The clinical definition of unstable angina includes angina at rest, prolonged episodes of pain, worsening of the angina pattern, or recent onset of symptoms (within 2 months).

The prognosis varies with the severity of symptoms, and risk stratification is largely based upon the history. Findings that indicate the *highest risk* for MI or early death are prolonged and on-going chest pain, angina within the last day, new ST segment or T wave changes on the resting ECG, angina with heart failure or hypotension, angina with a new or worsening mitral regurgitation murmur, and elevation of cardiac enzymes. A common presentation is the patient with prolonged pain and new T wave inversion—changes that look like those of non-Q wave MI—but no rise in cardiac enzymes.

Conversely, another patient may have minimal or no ECG changes, but a small rise in troponin, which by definition is NSTEMI. Both patients fall in the high-risk category and should be admitted to hospital for early angiography.

Figure 6.2 ECG Changes with NSTEMI

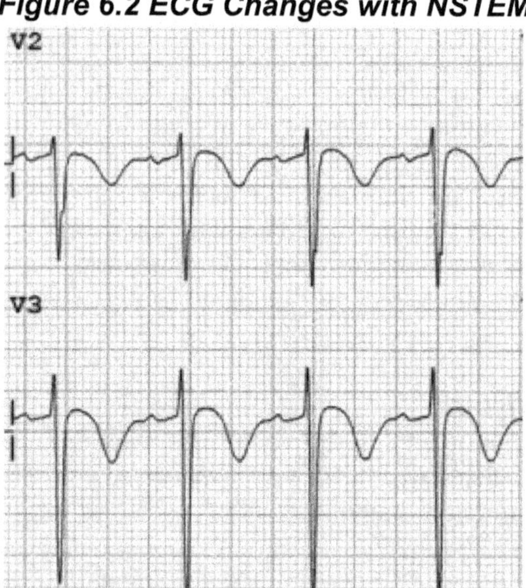

Figure 6.2 Deep, symmetrical T wave inversion in anterior leads—Wellens T waves—indicates proximal LAD stenosis. In addition to T inversion, there may be QT interval prolongation.

The patient usually has an elevated troponin. On the other hand, ST-T wave changes may not be as specific; they may look like the changes seen with LV hypertrophy or transient ischemia, but when accompanied by troponin rise and chest discomfort, make the diagnosis of NSTEMI.

There are *lower risk patients* who meet UA diagnostic criteria. This group is comprised of patients with exertional angina, but with onset of *symptoms < 2 months* before, without angina in the two days before evaluation, and no new ST or T wave changes on the resting ECG. In a sense, the patient has stable effort angina that is not yet chronic. If the history indicates that angina is probable, coronary angiography is the next step. However, since the patient is relatively stable, immediate hospitalization is not required, and the test can be performed within the next few days.

What about stress testing? Remember that ACS often occurs with non-stenosing, but unstable plaque. If the stress study is performed when obstructive thrombus is not present, it could be negative. That is why a convincing history of UA is an indication for angiography. (Patients will often tell you about an acquaintance who had a negative nuclear stress test, and had MI the next week.) On the other hand, we commonly evaluate those with chest pain that is not typically anginal, and stress testing helps sort this out. That is the usual indication for stress testing: is CAD the cause of the patient's chest pain?

Medical Therapy of Unstable Angina and Non ST Elevation MI

Antithrombotic Therapy

Unstable angina and non ST-elevation MI is about platelets and thrombosis (period). Treatment with aspirin reduces subsequent MI by 50%, and aspirin should be started if there is any suspicion the patient may have CAD and/or ACS. Heparin provides an additional benefit and should be added if ACS is *likely*. Comparative trials have found enoxaparin superior to unfractionated heparin, and practice guidelines indicate that it is the preferred agent, especially if troponin is elevated. On the other hand, a benefit of intravenous, unfractionated heparin is reversibility with protamine. For that reason our interventional team prefers intravenous heparin.

The addition of a $P2Y_{12}$ inhibitor such as clopidogrel to aspirin and heparin further reduces cardiac death or MI by 20%. A benefit with clopidogrel therapy was apparent within 24 hours and persisted during the next year. Clopidogrel is best started at least 6 hours before angiography and PCI, and a loading dose may be given.

Box 6.1 Choice of $P2Y_{12}$ Inhibitor

For convenience, this discussion cites clopidogrel as representative of drugs in this class. Other platelet ADP receptor blockers have similar benefit—in some cases an increased benefit. The PLATO trial compared clopidogrel and ticagrelor and found a 16% reduction in combined CV endpoints with ticagrelor. But the absolute benefit was small: the incidence of MI was 6.9% vs. 5.8%, and cardiac death was 5.1% vs. 4.0%. Another choice would be prasugrel. There are other considerations when choosing one of them, and the interventional cardiologist usually makes the choice.

A curious side effect of ticagrelor is worth remembering. As many as 20% on chronic therapy have dyspnea, usually at rest and with a normal chest exam. The symptom is usually mild, but bothersome. It can be transient, but there is no reason to continue the drug when there are good alternatives.

Clopidogrel given 5 days before CABG increases the risk of serious perioperative bleeding at least 50%. When it is likely that CABG will be needed, clopidogrel may be held until angiography. The drug strategy may relate to logistics, and the length of delay until study. If cath cannot be done for days (e.g.

a Friday afternoon admission with cath scheduled for Monday morning), clopidogrel makes the wait safer.

It seems like a lot: triple antithrombotic therapy—aspirin + clopidogrel + heparin. The trials that demonstrated benefit involved their use as adjunctive therapy before and during PCI. Since most patients with ACS need PCI, the GDMT includes this three-drug combination before cardiac cath.

Bleeding is the usual complication with this aggressive anticoagulation regimen. Patients at high risk for bleeding should have more urgent angiography. In such cases, use of a bare metal stent may be preferable because the recommended duration of clopidogrel post-stenting is just 6 weeks (and we occasionally shorten that to 4 weeks). In practice, fewer bare metal stents are being used.

What about the patient with unstable angina who has angiography but does not have CAD suitable for revascularization? Clinical trials showed that such patients on medical therapy also benefit from long-term clopidogrel + aspirin.

Statins

Their anti-inflammatory effect improves clinical outcome when started immediately, and they are now included as GDMT for ACS.

Beta Blockade

Meta-analysis of studies of UA found that beta blockers reduce the risk of MI by 13%. Many of the trials of beta blockade were done before we understood the role of thrombosis in ACS, and a number of them did not even include aspirin therapy. It is uncertain whether beta blockade would add benefit in patients on three-drug antithrombotic therapy. Nevertheless, it is included as GDMT. Various beta blockers have similar efficacy.

The dose should be titrated to bring the heart rate between 50 and 60 beats/minute.

Nitroglycerin

Intravenous nitroglycerin can be prescribed for on-going ischemic pain. It will relieve angina, but if you think about it, chest pain is seldom an issue for a patient with ACS who has been admitted to the hospital. Usually, the patient gives a history of chest pain that has resolved. The critical issue at that point is prevention of thrombosis that would lead to a return of pain. Nitroglycerin has no effect on thrombosis.

Furthermore, nitroglycerin in any form does not prevent MI or death in patients with CAD. Despite this, it is common to consult on a patient with ACS and find a messy gob of nitroglycerin ointment on the chest, making auscultation awkward. It just is not a component of the ACS protocol (and ordering it betrays a lack of understanding).

Revascularization

The benefit of angiography and revascularization patients with ACS is well established. Recall that revascularization does not prevent MI or death in patients with stable angina and preserved LV function (Chapter 5). The pre-cath diagnosis for most of our patients having coronary angiography is unstable angina. Remember that the definition of UA includes acceleration of symptoms as well as new-onset angina. Many of them turn out to not have unstable anatomy, and either do not or cannot have revascularization. As often, they may not have CAD, and the clinical diagnosis was incorrect. Still, UA is the usual indication for cath.

There may be concern about sending a patient to the catheterization laboratory with 3-drug antithrombotic therapy on board. While there is a risk of bleeding and hematoma, clinical trials have shown a better outcome with this aggressive treatment.

Outcomes have been slightly better with early angiography. There is no benefit from a cooling off period with medical therapy. On the other hand, angiography is not an emergency procedure (unlike STEMI). Rather, the patient with UA may be scheduled for "the next available" slot in the catheterization lab. Next day cath is best because it shortens the exposure to multi-drug antithrombotic therapy. I worry about the patient who is put on ice for a three-day weekend.

Thrombolytic Therapy

Early clinical trials comparing thrombolytic therapy with placebo included patients who had ACS with and without ST segment elevation. In the absence of ST segment elevation there was no benefit; because of this empirical observation, thrombolytic therapy is not used to treat UA or NSTEMI.

An absence of benefit makes sense when considering the pathophysiology. With STEMI, thrombus totally occludes the artery, and disrupting the clot is needed to restore antegrade flow. On the other hand, *without* ST elevation—UA or NSTEMI—angiography shows that the artery is not totally occluded. There is antegrade flow, even though the plaque is unstable. Effective anti-thrombosis (aspirin + heparin + clopidogrel) effectively preserves that flow, and adding a thrombolytic agent provides no additional benefit.

The role of fibrinolysis will be discussed in the next chapter.

Chapter 7: ST Segment Elevation Myocardial Infarction (STEMI)

Abbreviations

ACE, angiotensin converting enzyme
ACS, acute coronary syndromes
AICD, automatic implantable cardioverter-defibrillator
AIVR, accelerated idioventricular rhythm
CAD, coronary artery disease
CK, creatine kinase
CPR, cardiopulmonary resuscitation
EMS, emergency medical services
EP, electrophysiology
IABP, intra-aortic balloon pumb
ICD, implantable cardioverter/defibrillator
LAD, left anterior descending (coronary artery)
LV, left ventricle (ventricular)
LVEF, LV ejection fraction
LBBB, left bundle branch block
MI, myocardial infarction
MVO2, myocardia oxygen demand
NSTEMI, non-ST segment elevation MI
PCI, percutaneous coronary intervention (e.g., stenting)
PVC, premature ventricular contraction
RCA, right coronary artery
rt-PA, recombinant tissue plasminogen activator
RV, right ventricle (ventricular)
RBBB, right bundle branch block
SCD, sudden cardiac death
STEMI, ST-segment elevation MI
t-PA, tissue plasminogen activator
VF, ventricular fibrillation
VT, ventricular tachycardia

Over the last two decades, the incidence of myocardial infarction (MI) has declined, while that of unstable angina has increased. Patients are coming to the emergency room earlier with warning symptoms, rather than later with infarction. Nevertheless, more than one million Americans have an acute MI each year, and about one-third of them die. Many still die within an hour of the onset of symptoms, before reaching the hospital.

PATHOPHYSIOLOGY

When blood flow to the heart muscle is interrupted, contractile activity stops within a few heartbeats. Energy is then devoted to maintaining cellular viability. During the subsequent minutes to hours, cell death occurs. The cell membrane deteriorates, and cellular contents, including the contractile proteins, troponin (Tn) and creatine kinase (CK), leach out of the infarct zone and into the circulation. These muscle proteins are often referred to as "cardiac enzymes" or "biomarkers of injury."

The underlying illness is atherosclerosis. With stable angina, the atherosclerotic plaque that causes ischemia during exercise is tight, reducing the cross-sectional diameter of the coronary artery > 70%. The pathophysiology of acute coronary syndromes (ACS), including unstable angina and non-ST elevation MI (NSTEMI), was reviewed in Chapter 6. With these illnesses, the culprit lesion often is not flow-restricting. Instead, a "vulnerable plaque" with relatively large and white cell-filled lipid core covered by a thin fibrous cap ruptures, exposing the lipid core to the circulation. This activates platelets and the clotting cascade, and the abrupt accumulation of thrombus is responsible for rapid progression of symptoms, angina at rest, or ischemia that is severe enough to cause injury and a troponin (Tn) leak.

Acute MI with ST segment elevation is at the worst end of the ACS spectrum. The process of coronary thrombosis is the same, but the clot totally occludes the artery. The ECG pattern indicating occlusion and total interruption of blood flow is ST segment elevation (Figure 7.1).

Figure 7.1 Patterns of STEMI

A. Evolution of ST-T changes and Q waves

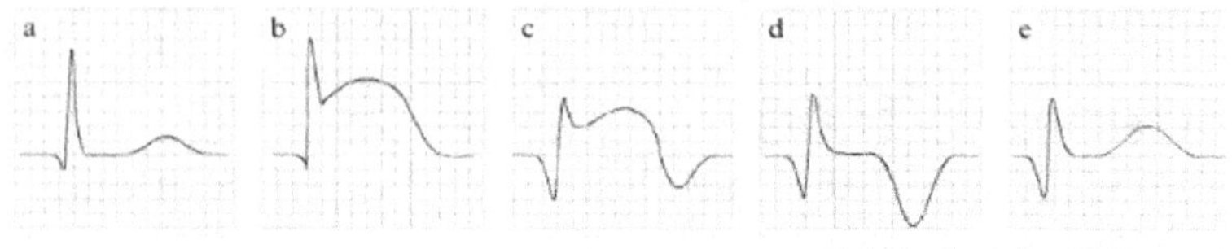

B. Anterior-Lateral infarction

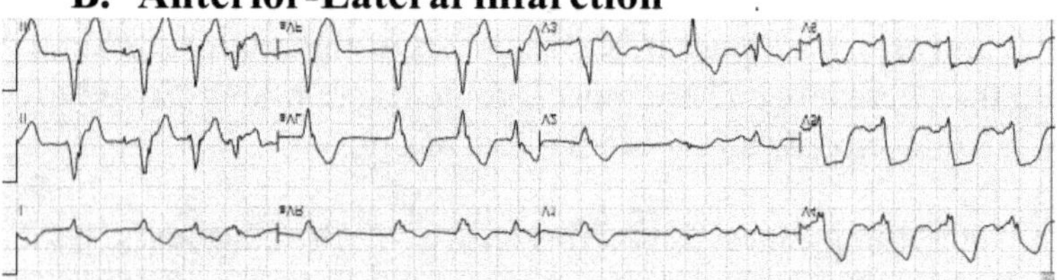

C. Inferior infarction

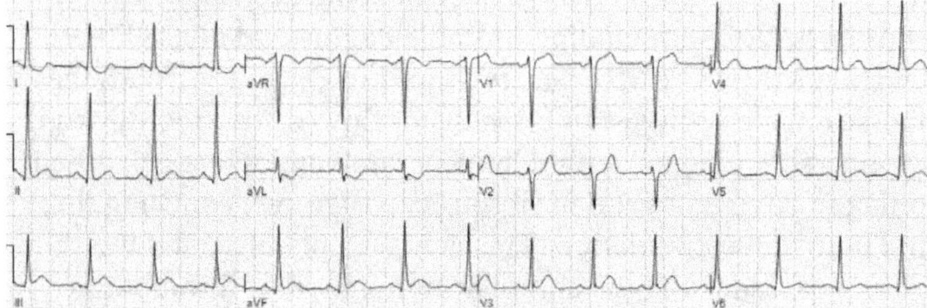

D. Lateral infarction

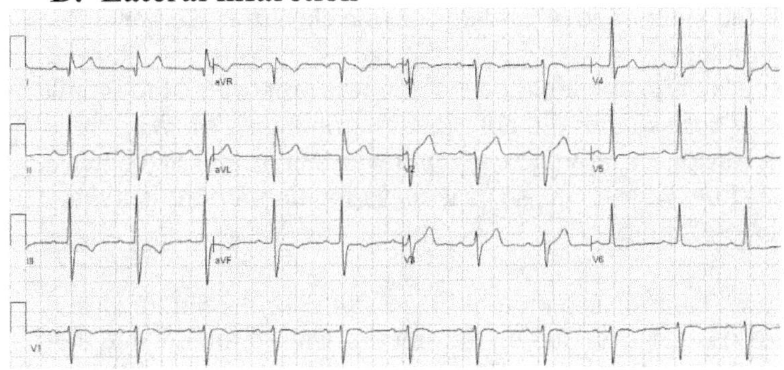

Figure 7.1 **A.** Evolution of the ECG pattern, beginning with the normal ECG. Immediately upon occlusion, there is ST-segment elevation. Over the next few hours, the T wave inverts and Q waves appear. ST segments then return toward baseline, and the T wave may become upright; a persistent Q wave is the chronic pattern. (From ECGpedia.org). **B.** Antero-lateral MI. Generally, the size of an anterior MI is proportional to the number of leads with ST elevation. This one is huge with ST elevation in 6 precordial leads plus I and aVL. **C.** Inferior MI. The ST elevation in II, III and aVF, though definite, is not that pronounced; the reciprocal ST depression in I and aVL confirms the diagnosis of acute ischemia. **D.** Lateral MI. There is persistent ST elevation in I and aVL, and Q waves have evolved. (For additional examples, and for practice, there are a number of online tutorials.)

Prognosis, Infarct Size and Cumulative Injury

The measurement most useful for predicting the prognosis of an adult with heart disease is left ventricular ejection fraction (LVEF). There are a few exceptions, but this is generally true, and it certainly is for those with coronary artery disease (CAD). EF is a simple measurement: LVEF = 50% simply means that the ventricle ejects 50% of its content with each heartbeat, and normal is $\geq$ 50-55%.

The size of the infarct is determined by the size of the artery that occludes, and it is roughly proportional to the loss of EF points and the magnitude of cardiac enzyme elevation. Earlier studies of uninterrupted MI—before the age of reperfusion—showed that peak creatine kinase elevation was proportional to infarct size. Those studies did not measure troponin (Tn). With reperfusion therapy there is rapid washout of muscle contents, including Tn and CK, so peak elevation does not reflect the degree of injury.

The vascular distribution of the left anterior descending artery (LAD) is large, including the anterior wall of the LV and the interventricular septum. Thus, uninterrupted anterior MI is usually the largest: peak creatinine kinase CK may be 3,500 IU, and LVEF after recovery is often <30%. Both the right and circumflex arteries supply smaller LV regions, and inferior or lateral infarction push the CK to the 1,000 IU range, with minimal effect on LVEF. On the other hand, there is considerable anatomic variation. An occasional patient has an especially large right coronary artery supplying a large portion of the lateral as well as the inferior walls of the LV; occlusion causes a large "inferolateral" MI.

Cardiac injury is cumulative. Following infarction, dead muscle cannot regenerate. I tell patients that losing heart muscle with an MI is like losing a toe; neither can grow back. Thus, a patient who loses 10 EF points with a first MI, and loses another 10 with a subsequent MI must then live with an LVEF in the 30% range. When a large anterior MI, or multiple smaller MIs, have pushed the LVEF below 30%, there may be a loss of exercise tolerance or heart failure. In fact, a Social Security Administration criterion for disability benefits with heart failure is LVEF <30%.

Since damage is cumulative, a major goal after MI is the prevention of future ischemic injury. The mortality risk with a second MI is much higher than that of the first. You may tell your patient with MI, "You have lost all the muscle you can afford to lose."

ST-Elevation Versus Non-ST-Elevation MI (STEMI vs. NSTEMI)

This is now the preferred nomenclature, replacing non-Q and Q-wave MI. As noted, ST elevation indicates total occlusion of the infarct artery, and ischemia that is transmural (e.g., it involves the full thickness of the LV ass in the affected region). The progression of ECG findings begins with ST elevation, then T inversion with or without persistent ST elevation, then formation of Q waves (the chronic post-MI pattern, Figure 7.1).

NSTEMI (Chapter 6), MI with ST depression or T wave inversion—also called non-Q or subendocardial MI —has ischemia largely confined to the subendocardial region (Figure 7.2).

Angiography during infarction has taught us a lot. With ST segment elevation, the infarct artery is totally occluded. When the artery is opened in the catheterization lab, the ST segment elevation resolves quickly, within seconds. Without reperfusion, the infarction runs its course, and Q waves develop the next day (Figure 7.1). It is useful to think of this as a *completed MI*. That is to say, there is completed injury of all of the muscle supplied by the infarct artery, and the infarct zone will become a scar.

But here is an interesting wrinkle. With reperfusion, Q waves usually develop abruptly, within minutes. The ECG evolutionary pattern, Figure 7.1, is compressed. In this case, Q waves do not reliably indicate full thickness scar, since there is viable muscle in the reperfused zone.

Figure 7.2 NSTEMI vs. STEMI

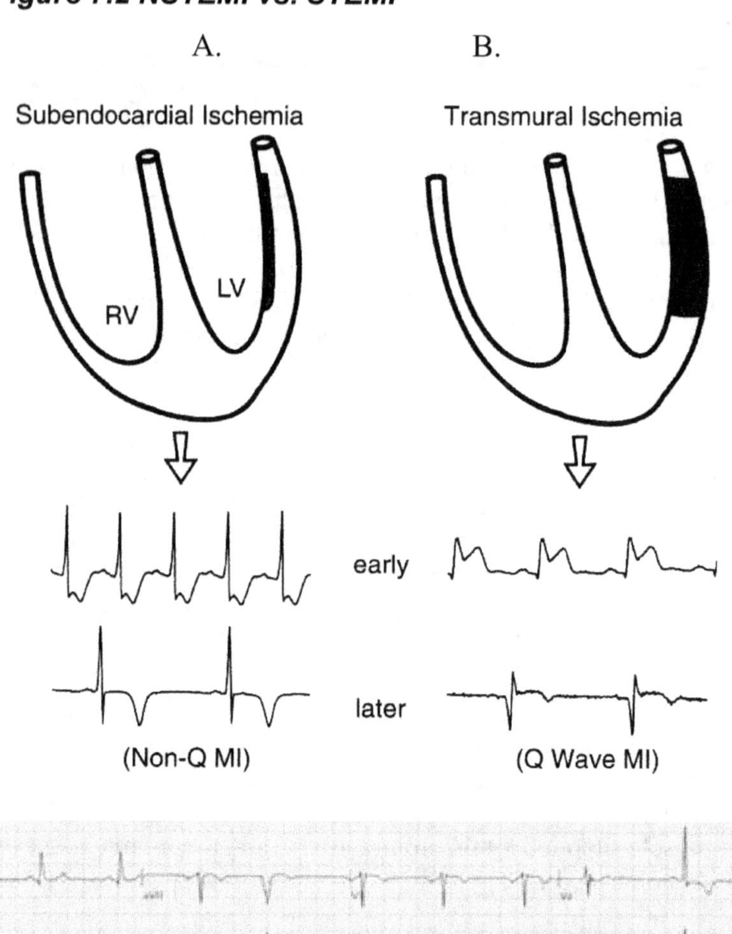

Figure 7.2 A: Patterns of myocardial infarction (MI). Tight stenosis of a coronary artery but with some antegrade flow causes subendocardial ischemia and ST segment depression. If ischemia persists long enough to cause necrosis, there may be T wave inversion the next day. This has been called non–Q MI, or at its outset, non–ST–segment elevation MI (NSTEMI). Total occlusion of the coronary artery affects the full thickness of the myocardium causing ST–segment elevation (STEMI). With necrosis, Q waves develop.

B: ECG from a patient who had 1 hour of chest pain the night before admission. The symmetrically inverted T waves in anterior leads are new. These are the "Wellons" waves of anterior NSTEMI, and indicate proxomal LAD disease.

A completed infarct—absent reperfusion—tends to be stable— scar tissue is not subject to further ischemic injury. We have always thought there is no need to open or bypass the totally occluded artery since it is not possible to turn scar back into muscle. Furthermore, totally occluded vessels have been considered more stable than tightly stenosed ones. But who knows what will happen to the patient with a tightly stenosed coronary artery when that vessel finally closes?

These long-accepted concepts about clinical stability with coronary occlusion—essentially our notions about completed infarction—have been questioned. Small studies have claimed better LV function and exercise tolerance after opening a persistently occluded artery a month after MI. The argument is that restoration of flow salvages stunned and non-functioning muscle that is still viable in the infarct and peri-infarct zones. The issue should have been settled by the only randomized study of late intervention, the Occluded Artery Trial (OAT). It found no benefit with late reperfusion, but the procedure is still being done despite incorporation of the OAT result in practice guidelines.

Box 7.1 The Occluded Artery Trial (OAT)

A study of PCI 1-30 days after STEMI, in which 2166 patients were randomized to PCI of the infarct artery + medical therapy, or medical therapy alone. Most had an occluded artery, and PCI was generally successful, including a high rate of patency at one year. Five-year follow-up showed no benefit with PCI. Although there was a measurable improvement in LV size (e.g. remodeling), the primary endpoint—death, MI or heart failure—was 17.2% with PCI compared with 15.6 with medical therapy alone (P = not significant). Individual endpoints of death or MI were slightly higher in the PCI group.

One of the surprises with early reperfusion therapy was the rapid appearance of Q waves with restoration of flow. It can happen within minutes of opening an infarct artery that has been occluded 3-6 hours. In such cases, the infarct zone may have viable muscle, and the infarction has not been "completed." This is another problem with the Q wave as the indicator of transmural injury or scar. During the course of acute MI (not treated with PCI), the artery may spontaneously open and close. If it is closed long enough, and then opens, a Q wave can develop.

A clinical entity seldom encountered since reperfusion therapy for MI is "infarct extension." Initially, the patient had ST elevation and a few hours of chest pain with evolution of Q waves. Several days later, there was recurrent pain and ST elevation, so called extension of the original infarct. The probable pathophysiology was spontaneous thrombolysis during the original infarct, with resolution of pain and evolution of Q waves. Because the infarct was interrupted before completion there was residual viable muscle in the infarct zone. With reocclusion—essentially reinfarction—the remaining viable muscle in the infarct zone was lost. Like a number of other complications of STEMI, it is prevented by stabilizing the infarct artery with PCI.

Angiography during an NSTEMI usually documents a stenosed vessel with antegrade flow. The surface of the stenotic plaque appears ragged and hazy, possibly with a filling defect in the contrast shadow, all characteristics of thrombus on the plaque surface. It does not have the concentric shape and smooth endothelial borders seen with stable angina. (We realized this description is redundant but feel it is justified, because the pathophysiology is a key concept.)

Persistent flow in the vessel means there is less injury. NSTEMI causes a smaller rise in cardiac enzymes and leaves the patient with a near-normal LVEF. On the other hand, the patient is left with an incomplete MI, and the unstable vessel may occlude causing ST-elevation infarction. Formerly, NSTEMIs were considered mild heart attacks, but follow-up studies found that the one-year mortality equalled that of STEMI. That is because reocclusion is common with NSTEMI; it is the most unstable of the acute coronary syndromes.

Clinical Presentation

The chest discomfort of MI is like that of angina pectoris, though it becomes more severe. With both, the discomfort is mild at first and then worsens with a crescendo pattern, "like a balloon blowing up in my chest." This is different than chest pain with dissection of the thoracic aorta where the pain has sudden onset and at maximum intensity. This may be the best clinical feature that distinguishes the two illnesses (and has figured into board questions).

The quality or location of pain does not point to the location of MI. Those with inferior infarction may have more vagal symptoms including nausea, but nausea is a common enough feature of anterior and lateral infarction as well. While severe, the pain of MI does not knock the patient down, leaving him writhing in agony. Usually, a person with MI sits quietly and appears anxious. There is a sense of "impending doom," even though the pain is not as severe as that of some other illnesses (i.e. pancreatitis, kidney stone, or migraine headache). But there is a connection between the heart and brain that tells the patient that something is profoundly wrong.

The peak incidence of MI is between 6 AM and noon, a pattern that coincides with an elevation of plasma catecholamines and cortisol, and an increase in platelet aggregability during the morning hours. Patients who are taking beta blockers or aspirin do not exhibit this circadian variation in the timing of MI.

There are a number of well-recognized triggers of MI: heavy physical work, particularly when fatigued or exposed to temperature extremes (heat and cold); stress (MI is more common on Monday mornings!), anger and upsetting life-events; hypoxemia from any cause, including anemia; and drugs that may provoke coronary spasm (cocaine, ergot preparations, beta blockers, and rarely, 5-fluorouricil or cyclophosphamide). Sexual activity can trigger the onset of MI, but this is uncommon, occurring in less than 1% of cases. MI is especially rare when sex is with a spouse or regular partner. On the other hand, a syndrome of "sudden motel death" has long been recognized.

At least a third of patients with acute MI describe a symptom during the days or weeks before admission that, in retrospect, was unstable angina. On the other hand, less than 10% of patients admitted with unstable angina develop MI. Actually, 10% is an old number, and with modern treatment including antithrombotic and revascularization, it would be unusual for a patient with UA to have acute MI in the hospital.

Painless, silent MI accounts for at least 10% of cases. It is more common in those with diabetes or hypertension, and in patients with no history of angina before MI. Silent MI is more commonly followed by silent ischemia, a positive stress ECG without angina. The prognosis of silent MI is similar to that of MI with symptoms.

Physical Examination

There is a sense of urgency when a patient with acute MI comes to the ER, but a methodical exam is still important. Take a careful stroke and bleeding history and look for signs of bleeding or trauma. The most common cardiac finding is an S4 gallop. A soft systolic murmur indicating papillary muscle dysfunction is more common with inferior or lateral MI. A loud friction rub suggests pericarditis as a cause of chest pain. Soft and transient friction rubs are common during the three days after transmural MI, but not NSTEMI. With transmural injury there is inflammation of the epicardial surface.

It is important to note the presence or absence of rales. The Killip classification relates the severity of heart failure during acute MI to the risk of death during hospitalization.

Box 7.2 Killip Class and Mortality

<table>
<tr><td>

Hospital mortality with MI and heart failure:

Killip Class I: no rales, mortality risk = 6%
Killip II: rales, 17%
Killip III: pulmonary edema, 38%
Killip IV: cardiogenic shock, 81%

(Data are from Dr. Killip's 1967 study. Survival is much better with modern therapy, but this gives you an idea. At that time overall mortality with MI was above 15%.)

</td></tr>
</table>

Sinus tachycardia during the week after MI is frequently overlooked. Resting tachycardia in a patient no longer having pain indicates a worse long-term prognosis than does successfully treated ventricular fibrillation (VF) during the acute phase of MI. That is because sinus tachycardia at rest is a marker of poor LV function. VF *during the early hours* of MI is an electrical event that may occur with a small MI, and does not indicate LV dysfunction. At any other time, complex ventricular ectopy *is* associated with low LVEF. (That is why low LVEF is the indictor for ICD therapy.)

LABORATORY EVALUATION

Electrocardiogram (ECG)

ST-segment depression is the pattern of subendocardial ischemia and is the earliest change with NSTEMI. This is followed by T wave inversion (Figure 6.1). Occluding a coronary artery with a balloon catheter causes ST segment elevation after a few heartbeats, and that is the pattern of transmural ischemia and STEMI (Figure 7.1).

If there is persistent occlusion of the coronary artery—in the absence of reperfusion therapy—the ST segments usually remain elevated for a day, and T wave inversion occurs. It is common to see T wave inversion while the ST segment is still elevated. (That combination excludes pericarditis, *vide infra*.) By the day after STEMI, ST elevation begins to resolve, and Q waves have developed. This process is accelerated with reperfusion.

Anterior MI

Anterior infarction follows occlusion of the left anterior descending (LAD) artery (Figure 5.2). It tends to be a large MI because of the size of the vessel, and a vascular distribution that includes both the free anterior wall and much of the interventricular septum. Occlusion of the proximal LAD is the worst, because there is loss of largest diagonal branches (supplying the antero-lateral wall of the LV) and septal branches. Most patients with heart failure after a first MI had proximal LAD occlusion. Occlusion distally is less devastating, because some of the diagonal and septal branches are spared.

Occlusion of the LAD causes ST segment elevation in the V leads (the so called precordial or anterior leads). It is possible to estimate the size of an anterior MI from the initial ECG: the number of leads with ST segment elevation is proportional to infarct size (Figure 7.1). ST elevation in leads V_{1-4} plus aVL usually means occlusion proximal to the first diagonal branch. ST elevation of just a couple V leads is more consistent with mid-LAD occlusion.

Septal Infarction, a Misnomer

The ECG computer often diagnoses "septal infarction" when there are Q waves in V_{1-2}. A review of previous and subsequent ECGs usually shows R waves in V_2 (e.g. an absence of Qs). This pattern is an artifact caused by changes in lead placement.

Furthermore, septal branches of the LAD are small vessels that penetrate the septum. Because they are intramural, they do not get atherosclerotic plaque. *Isolated* septal infarction is not a clinical entity. There is infarction of the interventricular septum with proximal LAD occlusion, but the infarction includes the anterior wall of the LV as well (it's a huge MI with ST elevation, then Q waves across most precordial leads).

We now have a clinical model of isolated septal infarction: alcohol septal ablation for hypertrophic obstructive cardiomyopathy—HOCM. The first septal perforating branch of the LAD is cannulated, and alcohol is infused which causes a "chemical infarct." Subsequent MRI with late enhancement shows a circumscribed scar in the proximal septum, reducing the volume of muscle and relieving outflow tract obstruction. The procedure does not cause Q wave formation in V_{1-2}. Rather, the usual ECG pattern after this localized, proximal septal infarct is right bundle branch block, occasionally with left anterior fascicular block. The right bundle branch traverses this region and is damaged.

Inferior MI

Most (85%) are caused by occlusion of the right coronary artery (RCA). The RCA is "dominant" and supplies the inferior wall. The remaining 15% have a left dominant circulation; the RCA is small, and the left circumflex coronary artery (LCx) is large and reaches the inferior wall. Both the RCA and LCx encircle the heart in the atrioventricular (AV) groove (Figure 5.2). The "dominant" vessel is the one that reaches the base of the heart and is the source of the large posterior descending (PDA) that extends toward the apex along the inferior wall. Loss of flow to the PDA causes inferior MI, regardless of whether it originates from the RCA or LCx.

RCA occlusion causes ST segment elevation in limb leads, II, III and aVF (the "inferior leads," Figures 7.1 and 5.2). It is also possible to estimate the size of inferior MI from the initial ECG, but in a manner different from that for anterior MI. Rather than the number of leads with ST elevation, the sum total of ST elevation in the inferior leads (II, III and aVF) is proportional to infarct size (Figure 7.3). Thus, a patient with 3-5 mm ST segment elevation in the inferior leads is having a much bigger infarct than another with 1-2 mm ST elevation. Another marker of large inferior MI is "reciprocal ST depression" in anterior (V_{1-4}) or lateral (I, aVL, V_{5-6}) leads.

Figure 7.3 Two Patients with Inferior MI

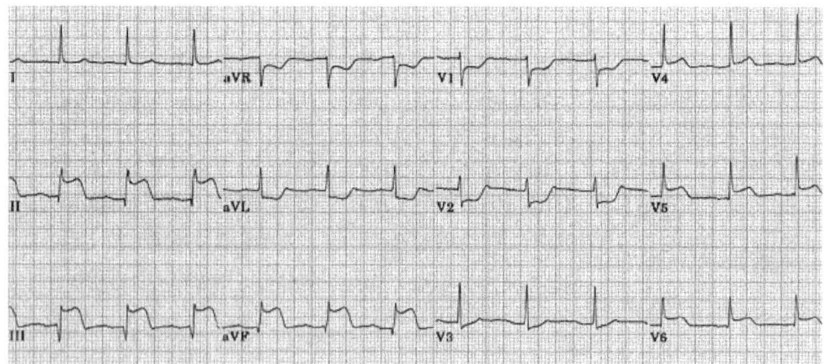

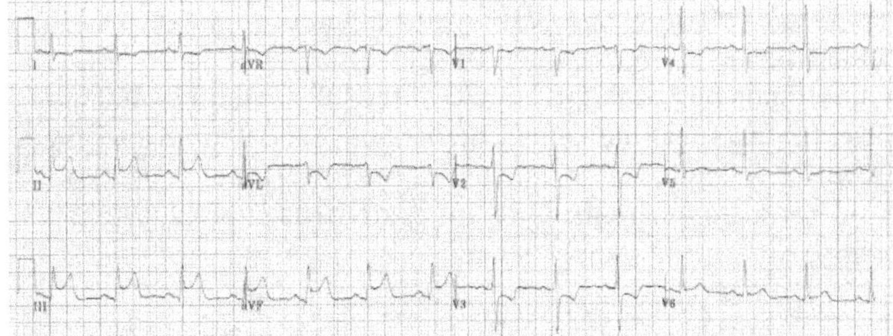

Figure 7.3 First patient: the sum of ST elevation in the 3 inferior leads is greater than it is in the second patient's ECG, so the infarct is larger. In addition, the first patient has ST elevation in V3-6 as well, indicating that the right coronary artery supplies a portion of the lateral wall, making this an inferolateral-MI, and a big one. Compare both with the inferior MI in Figure 7.1, where ST elevation is far less, indicating a smaller infarct. In all three cases there is reciprocal ST depression in anterior and lateral leads, further evidence of ischemia (differentiating it from pericarditis).

Bundle Branch Block

New bundle branch block occurs more commonly with anterior MI, because the LAD supplies most of the interventricular septum. Early placebo-controlled trials found improved survival with coronary thrombolysis for those with new right or left bundle branch block (RBBB, LBBB).

When anterior MI causes RBBB—indicating proximal septal injury—the infarct is quite large and prognosis is poor. Studies of ischemic cardiomyopathy and RBBB have documented a large amount of scar tissue on MRI.

LBBB usually is not caused by ischemic injury of the nerve, but is the result of stress in the proximal interventricular septum. MRI in patients with cardiomyopathy and LBBB usually finds little scar tissue. In a setting of acute MI, LBBB is an indicator of poor prognosis because in it occurs with depressed LV function. Furthermore, LBBB obscures the ECG diagnosis of acute MI; the RV is activated first, and the initial phase of LV activation is buried in the middle of the QRS complex. In a rare case, findings that indicate ischemia with LBBB are ST segment elevation in leads where the QRS is positive (usually V_{5-6}), or ST depression where the QRS is negative (usually the inferior leads).

The usual problem with bundle branch block is deciding whether it is old or new. With a prior ECG for comparison that shows LBBB, new ST segment elevation or depression may indicate acute ischemia in a patient with chest pain.

Lateral MI

The usual finding is ST elevation in the lateral leads (leads I, aVL or V_{5-6}, Fig 7.1). On the other hand, the posterolateral wall of the LV can be electrocardiographically "silent." Occlusion of a small circumflex artery branch may not cause ST segment elevation in lateral leads. There may be minimal ST depression or T wave inversion in V_{5-6}, a pattern more consistent with nontransmural ischemia. Subsequent angiography proves occlusion of the lateral wall branch, with akinesis of that region, and the CK rise is higher than usual for NSTEMI.

Because there is no ST elevation or Q wave development, this technically is a NSTEMI. But total occlusion of the LCx and akinesis of the afflicted LV region identify completed infarction.

An occasional patient with lateral MI presents with no ECG changes at all. In fact, patients who are having MI without ECG changes are usually having lateral infarction. This is the rationale for observing a patient in the hospital who has convincing chest pain but no ECG changes, at least until serial cardiac enzymes—or perhaps cardiac CT angiography— excludes MI.

Anterolateral and Inferolateral MI

Acute MI usually affects just one vascular distribution. It would be a remarkable coincidence for two different coronary branches to occlude simultaneously. When the distribution of infarction extends from the anterior or inferior walls into the lateral wall, based on ECG changes in lateral leads (Figure 5.2), it is not because a second artery has occluded. Instead, it indicates that the infarct artery—either the RCA or LAD—is unusually large, with branches to the lateral wall (Figure 7.1 and 7.3 for examples).

Pseudoinfarction

The ST segment elevation of *pericarditis* can mimic the changes of transmural ischemia. Usually they are diffuse, involving both anterior and inferior leads. With persistent inflammation, T wave inversion may develop. However, with pericarditis, the ST segment usually returns to baseline before the T waves flip. With ischemia, T inversion occurs while the ST segment is still elevated. ST depression is not seen with pericarditis and would support a diagnosis of ischemia.

An occasional patient with *myocarditis* has ST segment elevation, then T wave inversion and evolution of Q waves, a pattern indistinguishable from acute MI. There may be elevation of cardiac enzymes as well. Diffuse ST elevation involving multiple vascular distributions suggests myocarditis, but angiography may be needed to sort it out.

ST segment elevation may also occur with left bundle branch block, hyperkalemia, left ventricular hypertrophy and in the Brugada syndrome. Early repolarization is a normal variant; there is J point elevation in multiple leads but with a normally shaped ST segment. With these conditions the changes in ST segments are not associated with a chest pain syndrome and usually are present on previous ECGs.

The delta wave of Wolff-Parkinson-White syndrome may appear as Q waves, usually in inferior leads. A short PR leads to the correct diagnosis, and is supported by the history (no prior MI) and echocardiogram (no regional wall motion abnormality). Pseudo-Qs may also occur with hypertrophic cardiomyopathy or with an infiltrative cardiomyopathy such as amyloidosis.

Cardiac Enzymes

The diagnosis of acute MI has been based on a triad of chest pain, ECG changes, and a rise in cardiac enzymes. When drawn at least 4-6 hours after the onset of pain, a normal troponin would make the diagnosis of MI unlikely—the test is quite sensitive for myocardial necrosis. In fact, "cardiac biomarkers"—enzymes—are now so sensitive that a European Society of Cardiology/American College of Cardiology committee has suggested a universal definition MI that *requires* elevation of cardiac troponin, plus one of the following: 1) ischemic symptoms, 2) ECG changes (ST segment changes early, or evolution of Q waves or T inversion), 3) coronary angiography that documents CAD.

This definition of MI requires more than just an enzyme rise since it is important to distinguish between myocardial necrosis and infarction. The cardiac troponins are more sensitive and specific than CK-MB allowing detection of necrosis of < 1 gm of myocardium. Because of its sensitivity, Tn can be elevated with stressful noncardiac illnesses (Table 7. 1)

Table 7.1 Non-ischemic Causes of Troponin Elevation (Myocardial Injury or Demand Ischemia)

Cardiac trauma (contusion, pacing, ICD firing, cardioversion, biopsy, cardiac surgery)
Congestive heart failure
Hypertension
Hypotension/shock
Renal failure

Rapid atrial fibrillation (or other tachyarrhythmia)
Postoperative (noncardiac surgery)
Critical illness (especially in diabetic patients)
Drug toxicity (e.g. adriamycin, 5-fluorouracil, Herceptin)
Hypothyroidism, hyperthyroidism
Myocardial inflammation (myocarditis, sarcoidosis)
Sepsis
Pulmonary embolus
Burns (usually extensive)
Myocardial infiltrative disease (sarcoidosis, amyloidosis)
Acute neurological disease, including stroke
Rhabdomyolysis with cardiac injury
Transplant vasculopathy
And others…

These conditions with Tn elevation involve myocardial necrosis though without ischemia (they do not indicate ACS). On the other hand, an elevated Tn is not benign. It is associated with increased mortality with most illnesses, especially heart failure or chronic kidney disease. With acute illness it may reflect increased cardiac demand, enough so that there is myocardial necrosis.

Elevation of Tn in the absence of acute MI may be referred to as demand ischemia, or as a Type-2 MI. Without new ECG changes or chest pain to indicate active ischemia, it is not necessary to approach the Tn rise as an indicator of ACS, or a harbinger of acute MI. This is often a judgment call, and excessive testing after demand ischemia and small Tn elevation can lead to unnecessary procedures.
Troponin (molecular weight 33,000 D) tends to appear in the circulation a bit earlier than CK-MB (86,000 D) and usually is elevated 3 hours after the onset of pain. The persistent elevation of troponin 10-14 days after MI helps with a late diagnosis of infarction.

A marker of injury that is abnormal even sooner after the onset of MI would be useful for early diagnosis. Smaller molecules are able to leach out of the infarct zone faster. Myoglobin weighing 18,000 D may be elevated one hour after the onset of chest pain, but it is not specific for myocardium, and a reliable assay is not widely available. It is important to remember that none of the available biomarkers is elevated at the onset of MI. That is why a decision about reperfusion therapy is based on the history and ECG, not cardiac enzymes.

INITIAL TREATMENT OF NON—ST-SEGMENT ELEVATION MI (NSTEMI)

Angiography during the early phase of MI without ST segment elevation usually shows antegrade flow and a tight, ragged coronary artery lesion. The pathophysiology, presentation and treatment of acute coronary syndromes (ACS) are reviewed in Chapter 6. Thrombolytic therapy has been tested and found no better than anticoagulation, probably because there is antegrade coronary blood flow. Three drug antithrombotic therapy is indicated using aspirin, clopidogrel, and heparin. Beta blockade has been shown to prevent recurrent ischemia and progression of the MI. Diltiazem is a reasonable substitute when beta blockade is not possible.

By the time we see these patients in hospital, the chest discomfort has usually resolved. Ongoing pain despite medical therapy is an indication for immediate angiography. In most centers, urgent, next-day angiography is scheduled for the patient without pain who is stable on antithrombotic therapy. Same-day catheterization may be advantageous, but it may not be feasible, and it is not presently the standard of care.

INITIAL TREATMENT OF ST-SEGMENT-ELEVATION MI (STEMI)

Reperfusion Therapy—PCI

Reperfusion therapy is now the standard of care of STEMI and for MI with new bundle branch block. Cell death begins within 15 minutes of coronary occlusion and is progressive beyond that point. With each quarter hour that passes more heart muscle is lost. Early reperfusion saves more lives than later reperfusion. A patient in the ER does not have time to wait for a cardiologist to arrive a make a diagnosis and decision. The first doctor to see the patient in the ER should initiate treatment.

It is now apparent that the best reperfusion technique is PCI, usually coronary artery stenting. Randomized trials showed that balloon angioplasty is superior to thrombolytic therapy. Later trials found that stenting is better than POBA (plain old balloon angioplasty).

An issue is what to do in a hospital without a cardiac cath lab. Early studies showed that patients transferred from a community hospital to a tertiary referral center for PCI did better than those who were treated on site with thrombolytic therapy. But that was true only when the time from presentation to stenting was under 2 hours.

The time of transfer is a problem. The trials that found transfer for PCI superior to thrombolysis had angioplasty delayed by 43 minutes on average (compared with on-site thrombolysis); 95% were treated within two hours of the initial presentation. That is remarkably slick. Minimizing "door to balloon time" was obviously a goal of these studies, which were as much about logistics as about the therapies. More realistic—and reflecting real world experience—are data from a large U.S. registry that showed a door-to-stent time averaging 185 minutes for those requiring transfer. Just 3% in the registry were treated within 90 minutes.

The survival advantage of PCI over lytic therapy disappears when fibrinolytic therapy can be started $\geq$ 60 minutes before angioplasty. The data suggest that if the delay caused by transfer is going to be $\geq$ 90 minutes, the patient will do as well with on-site thrombolytic therapy. Standard practice is to begin TPA if transfer will delay reperfusion by as much as 2 hours. As the doctor providing initial treatment, it is your job to decide how long transfer for angioplasty will take (and to hustle the process along).

Another question is whether to begin thrombolytic therapy before transferring the patient for stenting, or perhaps a combination of low–dose lytic therapy. Most recent trials found a benefit with stenting within 6 hours of thrombolytic therapy. It makes sense, since stenting stabilizes the reperfused vessel, and opens those arteries that did not reperfuse with lytic therapy.

For now, consider the approach outlined in Table 7.2, which is based upon available clinical trials.

Table 7.2 A Triage Strategy for Patients with Acute Myocardial Infarction

1. People in the community, and certainly patients with coronary artery disease, should be aware of the symptoms of MI, and should seek medical attention early. Ideally, they should arrive in the ER less than 1 hour from the onset of chest pain.
2. When possible—certainly in an urban setting—a patient with chest pain and possible MI should be taken directly to a hospital with PCI capability.
3. For patients who reach the ER < 3 hours from the onset of chest pain:

   a.   In a community hospital ER, do not let the ambulance leave until you have done the initial ECG. If it shows ST segment elevation or new BBB, start an IV, begin aspirin and unfractionated heparin, and send the patient on to the tertiary center for stenting. This assumes a transfer time <60 minutes.

   b.   While the patient is en route, notify the tertiary center so that the cath lab is ready.

   c.   If you know that the transfer time for angioplasty will be at least 2 hours, begin thrombolytic therapy, with the goal of starting it within 30 minutes of arrival in the ER. Follow this with transfer of the patient to the interventional cardiology center.

4.   Patients who come to the ER late, > 3 hours from the onset of symptoms, still benefit from stenting, even with transfer delays.

5.   Likewise, those with cardiogenic shock (including the RV infarction syndrome) should be transferred for angioplasty. In such cases, minimizing the time to angioplasty is critical.

Predictors of Outcome with Reperfusion Therapy and the "No-Reflow Phenomenon"

Reperfusion within an hour of the onset of MI usually means a good outcome. Another predictor is the quality of flow after PCI, and there is a grading system: TIMI grade 3 flow in the infarct artery = rapid flow into the artery and rapid washout of contrast from the distal vessel; Grade 2 = sluggish flow and sluggish washout of contrast; Grade 1 = no flow.

In some cases, the infarct artery looks good after initial injection of contrast, but there is delayed washout of contrast from the distal vessel. Injury of the distal microvasculature is responsible for this *no-reflow phenomenon.* In addition to ischemic endothelial injury, distal capillaries and arterioles may have intraluminal platelet and fibrin thrombi. Interstitial myocellular edema may contribute to poor flow by compressing small vessels. The diagnosis of no-reflow is confirmed by the angiographic appearance of the dilated artery, and the pattern of flow.

Interestingly, the surface ECG provides an effective measure of tissue perfusion. No-reflow is often accompanied by persistent ST segment elevation. When there is prompt and sustained resolution of ST segment elevation with reperfusion therapy— e.g., the ST segments come down by 70%—good tissue perfusion is likely. A failure of ST segment elevation to resolve often is associated with persistent chest pain, and is an predictor of poor clinical outcome, even for those with a "successfully" opened infarct artery.

The time to therapy and degree of resolution of ST elevation are the best predictors of clinical outcome.

Here is why: The time to therapy is proportionate to the amount of myocardial necrosis before treatment. Resolution of ST elevation reflects the response to treatment (while the ST segments are elevated, ischemic injury is ongoing).

No-reflow may improve with coronary vasodilators, indicating an element of spasm. Intracoronary adenosine, the most potent coronary vasodilator, is particularly effective. Intracoronary verapamil has been used as well, and both are better than intracoronary nitroglycerin. Intracoronary thrombolytic therapy has not proved useful in treating it.

The response to therapy is determined by the severity of microvascular and interstitial injury. In its most severe form, there is "staining" of the myocardium by contrast that leaks from injured small vessels into the interstitium. This usually is not corrected with treatment and indicates advanced injury. The best way to avoid the no-reflow problem is early reperfusion.

Thrombolytic Therapy

The indication for coronary thrombolytic therapy is STEMI or MI with new bundle branch block and an inability to accomplish PCI within two hours.

You must understand your referral situation. When doctors are questioned about time of transfer and "door-to-balloon" times, they uniformly claim an ability to move the patient and accomplish angioplasty in 45-90 minutes. However, when ER and cath lab logs are carefully reviewed, the reality is closer to 3 hours.

If you are sure that it will take longer than 2 hours to get your patient to angioplasty—to the initial balloon inflation in the coronary artery, not just to the cath lab—begin thrombolytic therapy immediately.

Indications and Patient Selection

The chance of dying with some heart attacks is higher than from others. The early placebo controlled trials of lytic therapy found a benefit with higher-risk MI. As noted, the risk of thrombolytic therapy is justified only when there is obvious coronary occlusion (e.g., ST segment elevation). Those with suspected MI but without ST elevation are better treated with antithrombotic therapy and urgent catheterization when the chest pain does not resolve (see the discussion of acute coronary syndromes including NSTEMI in Chapter 5).

When the ECG does not show ST elevation but you strongly suspect MI, *repeat the ECG*. It is common for ST segment elevation to wax and wane during the early course of MI. In addition, think of other possibilities. Severe pain and diaphoresis may be caused by aortic dissection or esophageal rupture, illnesses where thrombolysis would be a disaster.

Advanced age is not a contraindication to reperfusion. On the other hand, there is not a clear survival benefit with lytic therapy for those over 75 years old. The risk of intracranial bleeding with lytic therapy increases with age. GUSTO-I reported stroke in 0.8% of those < 65 years old, 2.1% between 65 and 74 years of age, and 3.4% over age 75. *While not zero, the risk of hemorrhagic stroke is lower with PCI.* Another issue with age is the patient's ability to handle aggressive and potentially stressful intervention. In community practice, most elderly patients treated with reperfusion therapy are healthy and active. Few doctors use an aggressive treatment strategy for debilitated patients from a nursing home.

Late thrombolysis is of little benefit. Lytic agents are less effective when the clot is older and more organized. Increased fibrin cross-linking makes it harder to disrupt. When given ≥ 12 hours after onset of MI, fewer than half of patients achieve TIMI 3 flow. The LATE study addressed clinical outcomes and found a small benefit when recombinant tissue plasminogen activator (r-tPA) was given between 6-12 hours after the onset of pain but not after 12 hours. Lytic therapy >12 hours from the onset of MI also introduces a new complication: the risk of *myocardial rupture* appears increased.

Stenting is a safer therapy for the patient who arrives late and has persistent pain and ST elevation. It is more effective as well, as increased duration of occlusion—a more organized clot—does not influence outcome with PCI. More than 90% have excellent restoration of flow immediately, even with late stenting. Whether this translates to improved survival is uncertain, but it is preferable to late thrombolysis.

Evolution of Q waves does not mean the infarct is completed. As noted, the infarct artery may open and close. With transient reperfusion, Q waves can develop rapidly. If the ST segments are still elevated and the patient continues to have pain, Q waves are not a contraindication to reperfusion therapy.

Contraindications to Thrombolytic Therapy

The most important consideration is the risk of bleeding. Most bleeding is minor, occurring at vascular puncture sites. As a rule, it can be controlled with local pressure, and a hematoma usually resolves without long-term effects.

The incidence of intracranial hemorrhage in large clinical trials is about 0.75%. An individual's chance of hemorrhagic stroke after thrombolytic therapy increases with any of four risk factors: use of tPA (instead of streptokinase), age >65 years, weight < 70 kg, hypertension on presentation (systolic pressure $\geq$170 mmHg, or diastolic pressure $\geq$95). Note that "uncontrolled hypertension" and prior stroke were contraindications to thrombolysis in the trials that produced these risk data. An even higher risk of stroke would be expected for the patient with a systolic blood pressure above 200 mmHg.

Defibrillation and a brief period of cardiopulmonary resuscitation (CPR) are not contraindications to thrombolysis. When CPR is prolonged more than 10 minutes or there is obvious trauma with chest compression or intubation, the bleeding risk increases.

Pharmacology of Thrombolysis

Clot formation and dissolution are in dynamic equilibrium. Developing thrombus cannot be allowed to propagate indefinitely, and clot within blood vessels or in ureters must eventually be removed to restore patency. This is the role of the fibrinolytic system. As soon as clot forms, the fibrinolytic system is activated.

Plasminogen is the precursor of the active fibrinolytic enzyme, plasmin. Plasminogen is converted to plasmin by "plasminogen activators." These include naturally occurring substances, tissue plasminogen activator (tPA) and urokinase, and the foreign compound, streptokinase. Plasminogen is produced by the liver and is found in the circulation. When clot forms, this free plasminogen is incorporated into the thrombus and is bound to fibrin.

The ideal thrombolytic agent would move into the thrombus and work only on fibrin-bound plasminogen. But most of the thrombolytic agents activate free, circulating plasminogen as well, producing plasmin and the so-called lytic state. Free plasmin digests circulating fibrinogen and other clotting factors, producing a hypocoagulable state.

The major difference among thrombolytic drugs is the degree to which they work on fibrin-bound plasminogen. Tissue plasminogen activator, either native (tPA) or recombinant (r-tPA), relies on fibrin as a cofactor and when bound to fibrin has a 500-fold increase in activity. It is not as potent when free in the circulation (and not bound to fibrin). Streptokinase works on both free and fibrin-bound plasminogen and thus leads to a greater decline in circulating fibrinogen.

The earliest trials showing that lytic therapy is superior to placebo were performed with streptokinase. Comparison studies have shown that r-tPA (Aalteplase) is better than streptokinase, especially when administered using a front-loading protocol. More rapid thrombolysis and earlier achievement of good flow (TIMI grade 3 flow) is the probable explanation. Newer generation r-tPA preparations, tenecteplase and reteplase, have a longer half–life so may be given as intravenous bolus injections, rather than as a continuous infusion. These tPA variants have been shown to produce TIMI-3 flow more rapidly than alteplase, but in comparison trials there has been no improvement in complication rates or in 30-day mortality with the newer agents. Since PCI has been found superior to lytic therapy, we will probably see fewer research dollars spent to develop new thrombolytic agents.

Assessment of Reperfusion and Prognosis

Early resolution of ST segment elevation is the best indicator of good tissue perfusion (note the earlier discussion of the no-reflow phenomenon). Improvement in chest pain is common with thrombolysis and usually accompanies improvement in ST elevation. When the artery first opens, many patients have a run of accelerated idioventricular rhythm (AIVR), and this "slow ventricular tachycardia" is a reliable indicator of reperfusion. It rarely degenerates into ventricular fibrillation, and antiarrhythmic therapy is not needed.

For many patients, ST segment elevation and chest pain do not resolve in a dramatic fashion, so there is uncertainty about the status of the infarct artery after coronary thrombolysis. Lytic therapy is now considered an interval step while the patient is on the way to the cath lab, and used only when there is a delay in transfer.

Other Therapies During the Initial 12 Hours of MI

Reperfusion therapy properly gets top billing as it has the greatest potential for reducing mortality and morbidity (heart failure, serious arrhythmias, etc.). But consider the following.

Beta Adrenergic Blockade

During the acute phase of MI, patients may respond to intravenous beta-blockade with prompt relief of pain and a reduction in ST segment elevation. Randomized trials were performed before the development of reperfusion therapy and demonstrated a reduction in mortality (by 15%), reinfarction (19%), and cardiac arrest (19%). Consider beta blockade for the occasional patient with STEMI for whom reperfusion therapy is not an option.

Oxygen

There is little evidence supporting oxygen therapy for a patient who does not have hypoxemia. It is not identified as a critical therapy by practice guidelines. However, patients often feel better or describe improvement in pain with oxygen treatment. Because there is little risk with nasal oxygen, 2-4 L/minute, there is no reason to omit this traditional treatment.

A common practice has been to continue it for a couple days. In real life, it is usually overlooked, and the patient stays on oxygen until discharge (no harm done, other than the expense). It makes more sense to stop oxygen when the patient is pain free and has normal oxygen saturation on room air, particularly after resuming ambulation.

Control of Pain

The initial treatment of chest pain with sublingual nitroglycerin is fine, even before getting the ECG. If the patient is having angina rather than MI, there may be relief. Hypotension with nitroglycerin usually resolves with recumbency. If it persists, elevate the patient's legs.

Morphine is the preferred analgesic. Like nitroglycerin, it is a venodilator and thus lowers preload. A drop in blood pressure is prevented or treated by placing the patient in a supine position or by raising the legs.

Angiotensin-Converting Enzyme (ACE) Inhibition

Note the following discussion of congestive heart failure complicating MI. Early therapy with ACE inhibitors prevents infarct expansion improving LV function and survival for those with a large, anterior MI. Early treatment—started in the first 24 hours—is best. Angiotensin receptor blockade is a suitable alternative to ACE inhibition for those with prior intolerance.

Complications of Acute MI

The mechanical complications of STEMI have become less common as a result of reperfusion therapy. Nevertheless, we still encounter them in patients who did not get reperfusion therapy or were treated late. And of course, you may see them on board exams…

Cardiogenic Shock

Before the development of reperfusion therapy, cardiogenic shock developed in about 20% of patients with MI, and the 30-day mortality rate was as high as 80%. With modern therapy, the incidence is reduced to 5-7%, and the mortality rate to about 40%. Nevertheless, LV failure remains the leading cause of in–hospital death with MI.

Autopsy studies have shown that the pump loses its ability to maintain blood pressure when 40% of the LV is infarcted, and LV injury is responsible for 80% of cases of shock. Right ventricular infarction, acute ventricular septal defect, mitral regurgitation caused by papillary muscle infarction or rupture, and LV rupture are the other causes of shock. It is important to diagnose these conditions, since the treatment is different.

The hemodynamic definition of cardiogenic shock includes persistent hypotension with systolic blood pressure <90 mmHg, low cardiac index (cardiac output corrected for body surface area), and elevated LV filling pressure (pulmonary wedge pressure >15 mmHg). Most with shock and elevated filling pressure also have pulmonary congestion. The bedside diagnosis is fairly certain when there is low blood pressure, pulmonary edema and clinical evidence of reduced end-organ perfusion (cool clammy skin, low urine output and altered sensorium).

Those with shock with no prior MI are usually having a large anterior MI. A smaller infarction may cause LV failure when there has been prior LV injury; remember that LV injury is cumulative. Shock is more common in older patients and those with multivessel CAD, and both indicate a worse prognosis. The incidence of shock was reduced by about 50% in placebo-controlled studies of thrombolytic therapy. GUSTO-1 found less shock and heart failure with r-tPA, which opens arteries faster than streptokinase. Angioplasty is faster and better than r-tPA and is thus the best therapy for preventing cardiogenic shock.

The only effective treatment for cardiogenic shock is immediate reperfusion. The SHOCK trial tested immediate angioplasty for those with early cardiogenic shock. There was no survival benefit at one month, but the six-month survival was better with immediate angioplasty. The survival benefit was limited to patients less than 75 years old. The one-month mortality of younger patients was 41% with angioplasty, compared with 57% with medical therapy (this is a bad disease). I would suspect even better outcomes with present techniques including stenting and more effective treatment of the no-reflow phenomenon.

For PCI to work, it must be applied immediately. The best results are realized by those with good reperfusion within four hours of the onset of MI, although some benefit is possible up to 12 hours. Thus, a clinical diagnosis of probable cardiogenic shock is an indication for immediate cardiac catheterization and stenting. It is needed even if the patient has received thrombolytic therapy.

While moving toward the cath lab, supportive measures to maintain blood pressure and distal perfusion include catecholamine therapy. Dobutamine is the first choice; it is a pure inotropic agent with few noncardiac effects and low arrhythmogenic potential. Dobutamine may be added to dopamine. When each drug is given at rates as high as 7.5 mcg/kg/min, cardiac output and blood pressure rise without an increase in LV filling pressure. At doses above 10mcg/kg/min, the selective actions of both drugs disappear, and they work as pure vasoconstrictors.

Intra-aortic balloon pump (IABP) counterpulstation is usually started in the cath lab. It raises cardiac output, lowers afterload while raising blood pressure, and improves coronary perfusion pressure. The 40 mL sausage-shaped balloon inflates in the descending aorta during diastole, displacing its volume into the distal circulation, including the coronary arteries (most coronary blood flow takes place during diastole). At a heart rate of 100 beats/min it can boost cardiac output by almost 4L/min. While the IABP is an effective supportive therapy, it is useless unless there is successful reperfusion. A classic study of cardiogenic shock from the 1970s—before the reperfusion era—showed a short-term hemodynamic benefit with IABP counterpulsation but a 91% 1-year mortality. Many of these patients became "balloon dependent." They were stable while the pump was working but slipped back into shock when it was turned off. To definitively treat shock, the infarct artery must be opened.

Right Ventricular (RV) Infarct Syndrome

This usually complicates inferior MI, since the proximal right coronary artery (RCA) supplies branches to the RV (Figure 5.2). About one half of all patients with inferior MI have demonstrable RV dysfunction, but hemodynamically-significant RV failure occurs in less than 10%. This small group has right heart failure (peripheral edema and jugular venous distension without pulmonary congestion), and when severe, can have hypotension, a form of "cardiogenic shock."

LV filling pressure may be normal, but this can be misleading, since LV preload may actually be low. Abrupt dilation of the ischemic RV is limited by the rigid pericardium, and increased pressure in the pericardial space is transmitted to the LV. A common physical finding is pulsus paradoxicus, falsely suggesting tamponade. With animal models of RV infarction, hemodynamics improve when the pericardium is opened, relieving pericardial crowding. Excessive fluid loading as treatment may pericardial pressure, further limiting diastolic filling of the heart.

Many with RV infarction have coexisting LV dysfunction and require an elevated LV filling pressure—above 15-18 mmHg—to maintain stroke volume. LV dysfunction is severe enough in some that shock is the result of both RV and LV failure.

ST segment elevation in both inferior leads (II, III and aVF) and V_1 suggests RV infarction (the infero-posterior MI pattern). More specific is ST elevation in lead V_{4R}, a right precordial lead in the V_4 position. Although most with this finding do not develop shock, the echocardiogram commonly shows dilation of the right atrium and RV, and reduced RV contractility. The echocardiogram is also useful as it excludes pericardial effusion and tamponade as the cause of pulsus paradoxus. Right heart catheterization confirms the diagnosis with elevation of right atrial pressure but minimal or no elevation of pulmonary artery diastolic pressure or pulmonary wedge pressure (e.g., LV filling pressure).

The RV infarction syndrome is prevented by early reperfusion. Even late angioplasty/stenting has been recommended for patients with the RV infarction syndrome. Perhaps because wall RV wall tension is lower, late reperfusion therapy is more effective for RV than LV infarction—at least the rate of progression of injury seems less rapid.

The initial supportive treatment for hypotension is volume expansion. As long as there is no pulmonary congestion, a fluid challenge is safe, giving 200 mL normal saline per hour (or more) for several hours. If this does not correct hypotension, the patient needs hemodynamic monitoring with a pulmonary artery catheter. It is important to keep the pulmonary wedge pressure below 20-22 mmHg to avoid pulmonary congestion. A threshold level of fluid replacement is commonly reached, above which blood pressure and cardiac output no longer increase. At this point, increased pericardial pressure is limiting both RV and LV filling, and further fluid resuscitation will add little.

Intravenous nitroglycerin may aggravate hypotension because it reduces venous return to the heart. On the other hand, arterial vasodilators may help, since lowering left atrial and pulmonary artery pressures reduce RV afterload. When there is LV as well as RV dysfunction, dobutamine is indicated. Increased contractility of the interventricular septum can boost RV stroke volume.

Refractory hypotension often improves with the IABP, particularly for those with LV dysfunction. In addition, balloon pumping improves coronary perfusion pressure, augmenting interventricular septal performance. Spontaneous recovery of RV function is common, and there is less chance of balloon dependence than there is with cardiogenic shock caused by LV injury.

Patients with RV dysfunction do poorly with bradycardia. For this reason, the threshold for pacemaker therapy is lower.

Many with RV dysfunction have spontaneous improvement within four days. But it can be a serious illness, and the mortality rate with RV infarction plus shock is 40%. Without shock mortality is less than 10%. Chronic right heart failure with peripheral edema is rare in survivors. The good prognosis is attributed to good collateral circulation to the inferior wall, and the favorable oxygen supply-demand profile of the RV. Lower right heart diastolic pressure favors the transfer of coronary blood flow from the LV to the RV via collateral vessels.

Congestive Heart Failure

Those with pulmonary congesting during the course of acute MI have a much higher mortality risk (note the earlier description of the Dr. Killip's classification). Early reperfusion therapy has been shown to save LV myocardium and lower the chance of subsequent heart failure.

251

The cause of LV dysfunction after MI is loss of contractile units. Occlusion of a large artery supplying a large myocardial region will have a greater influence on LVEF than occlusion of a smaller side branch. In addition, ischemia increases myocardial stiffness, and diastolic dysfunction adds to elevated pulmonary wedge pressure and congestion.

Infarct expansion may contribute to LV dysfunction. During the week after STEMI, necrotic muscle softens and becomes mushy. This leads to bulging of the infarct zone with expansion and thinning of the LV wall. It is most common with anterior infarction. The most extreme form of infarct expansion is the formation of an LV aneurysm where there is bulging of the apex during systole.

Short of aneurysmal bulging, there is a change in the shape of the LV apex after anterior MI. It loses its normal elliptical, football shape, and becomes rounded, or mushroom-like (Figure 7.4).

As healing takes place, scar is laid down in the mold provided by the altered infarct zone, resulting in a permanent alteration in shape. At that point, the shape of the infarct zone is "cast in scar." This change in LV geometry has a negative effect on LV function. The radius of curvature of the LV is increased. Because of the Laplace relationship (wall tension = pressure x radius), increased radius results in increased in wall tension. This has a negative effect on myocardial energetics, because wall tension is a determinant of myocardial oxygen demand (MVO_2, recall this discussion in Chapter 1). In addition, the bulging segment absorbs some of the contractile energy of the LV that would otherwise have gone toward ejection of blood.

Figure 7.4 Infarct Expansion

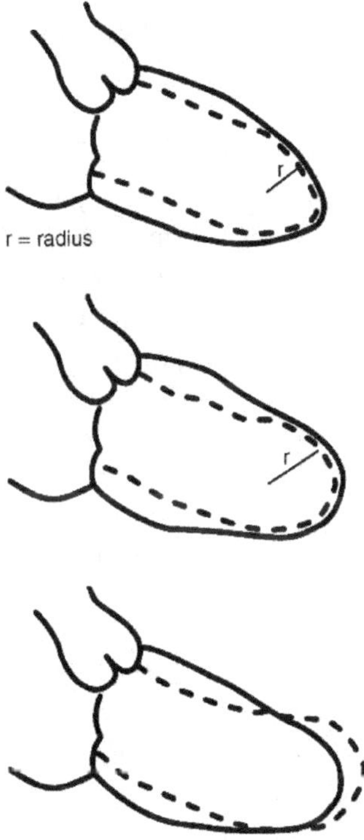

Figure 7.4 Three examples of left ventricular remodeling after MI with a solid line for diastolic contour and a dashed line for systolic contour. **Patient A**: The anterior wall is akinetic, but in diastole the left ventricle still has its ellipsoid shape (there has been no remodeling of LV shape). **Patient B**: In addition to anterior akinesis, the shape of the apex has changed so that it is rounded and more mushroom like. This increases the radius (r) at the apex, and thus increases wall tension. **Patient C**: There is an apical aneurysm. In addition to the rounded apex during diastole, there is aneurysmal bulging of the apex during systole. Notonly is wall tension increased because of increased radius, but contractile energy is also absorbed by the bulging apex. This is the most extreme case of LV remodeling.

Early reperfusion therapy preserves some muscle within the infarct zone and tends to prevent infarct expansion. When viewed in the operating room, the reperfused infarct zone has a marbled appearance, with patches of apparently live tissue mixed with injured muscle.

Box 7.3 Why Does Reperfusion Therapy Work?

The obvious answer is salvaging muscle, e.g., contractile units. However, clinical trials found an interesting disconnect between survival and LV function after reperfusion therapy. Improved survival was obvious, but very few studies demonstrated improved LVEF when comparing thrombolytic therapy to placebo (there have been no placebo-controlled trials with PCI). Another explanation for improved outcome is better LV geometry with reperfusion; said another way, there is a reduction in maladaptive LV remodeling. Saving enough muscle to prevent infarct expansion preserves geometry, lowers LV wall tension and thus may prevent heart failure.

Afterload reduction therapy with ACE inhibition also prevents infarct expansion after anterior MI. This was demonstrated by trials in the pre-thrombolysis era and has not been tested as adjunct therapy with reperfusion therapy. With large anterior MI, it still makes sense and should be started early, within the first day after MI if the blood pressure is stable.

Ventricular Arrhythmias

It is important to distinguish between ventricular arrhythmias occurring during the early hours of infarction and those that occur later (and are chronic). During the early hours of infarction, there is considerable electrical instability, and even a small MI can cause ventricular tachycardia (VT) or fibrillation (VF). With recovery, LVEF may be normal and the long-term prognosis, good. I tell students that resting tachycardia after MI indicates a worse prognosis than VT or VF during the early phase. Resting tachycardia is a marker of low LVEF, whereas the early electrical storm is not.

On the other hand, complex ventricular arrhythmias in the late phase of MI—days after acute MI—are limited to those with large infarction and low LVEF. This is also true of those with a remote history of MI. These patients with ischemic cardiomyopathy have a poor prognosis. Their leading cause of death is VF. Studies in the 1970s found that the best predictor of complex ventricular arrhythmias more than a week after infarction was low LVEF, and a good predictor of low LVEF was complex ventricular arrhythmia. The association is so tight that it is unnecessary to get a 24-hour monitor as a screen for sudden cardiac death. An echo measurement of LVEF is enough. LVEF above 40% indicates low risk.

For decades we chased ventricular ectopy with drug therapy—the goal was to make the 24-hour Holter monitor look better. Then the Cardiac Arrhythmia Suppression Trial (CAST) tested whether suppressing premature ventricular contractions (PVCs) lowers the risk of sudden cardiac death (SCD) in post-MI patients with low LVEF. The surprising result was an increase in SCD with antiarrhythmic drug therapy even though Holter monitoring showed suppression of PVCs. The "proarrhythmia" effect of the drugs apparently outweighs the arrhythmia suppression effect. (CAST was among the earliest multicenter trials leading to "evidence based medicine.")

CAST also suggested that the presence of PVCs does not indicate that there will be progression of ventricular ectopy to VF and SCD. This is further supported by studies showing that beta blockade after MI prevents SCD but does not suppress PVCs on the Holter monitor—there is a disconnect. Membrane-active antiarrhythmic therapy is no longer prescribed for suppression of ventricular arrhythmias after MI. Beta blockade is prescribed to prevent SCD.

The MADIT II trial has changed the approach to SCD after MI: it is now device-based. This randomized study compared conventional medical therapy with prophylactic implantable cardioverter/defibrillator (ICD) treatment. It enrolled 1232 patients >1 month after MI who had LVEF ≤30%. There was no upper age limit although 95% were under 75 years old. Most patients received beta blockers. There was no electrophysiology (EP) testing. The three-year mortality was 28% lower with ICD therapy. The benefit of ICD treatment was independent of advanced age, hypertension, diabetes, left bundle branch block, or other comorbidities.

The survival curves of the two treatment groups did not diverge during the initial 9 months, and at one year the survival benefit with the ICD was minimal. Thus, it would not make sense to recommend an ICD for a patient whose expected survival is less than a year (i.e. because of advance heart failure or another illness). Furthermore, those getting the ICD had more death from heart failure. (At times we are in a choose-your-poison situation. With an ICD, a patient struggling with advanced CHF may lose the option of dying quickly and peacefully. It may not be a decision we should make for a patient, but we may consider it for ourself, or a parent.) Presently, ICD therapy is not indicated for those with Class IV heart failure.

Symptomatic VT may respond to beta blockade. When it does not, consider adding amiodarone. This may be an issue in patients with an ICD, since suppression of VT prevents frequent shocks. And remember that serum potassium is inversely proportional to the risk of VT during and after acute MI.

New Systolic Murmur After MI

Ventricular Septal Defect (VSD)

The incidence of septal rupture with MI was 2% in the pre-reperfusion era, but it is much lower now. It is more common with advanced age, hypertension, and multivessel CAD. Like free-wall rupture, thrombolytic therapy >12 hours from the onset of MI predisposes to rupture of the septum.

The left anterior descending and the posterior descending arteries encircle the septum in the interventricular groove, and both supply perforating branches into the septum (Figure 5.2). Thus, either anterior or inferior MI may cause VSD. The prognosis is worse with inferior MI, possibly because the basal location of the defect makes surgical repair difficult. A VSD caused by anterior MI usually occurs nearer the LV apex. Proximal septal rupture following anterior MI is rare, probably because ischemic injury is so extensive that cardiogenic shock and death happen before rupture can occur.

Most VSDs develop during the first week after MI with about 20% in the first day. A loud, harsh, holosystolic murmur is the rule, and many have a palpable thrill. Biventricular failure follows. With medical therapy, half die within a week, and 85% by 2 weeks.

A new murmur after MI is an indication for an urgent echocardiogram. The Doppler study demonstrates flow across the ventricular septum and excludes mitral regurgitation. The next step is prompt transfer for cardiac cath, then surgery.

Although echo can make the diagnosis, cardiac cath is needed to define coronary anatomy. As part of the procedure, right heart catheterization confirms the diagnosis; the oxygen saturation in the pulmonary artery is higher than it is in the vena cava or right atrium (there is a "step-up" in saturation at the site of left-to-right shunting).

Immediate surgical repair is indicated for the patient who is often dependent on catecholamine and/or IABP support. Success is predicted by good LV function and brief duration of shock. A rare patient stabilizes without developing shock. In such cases, surgery may be delayed 3 to 4 weeks, hoping that partially healed tissue will be easier to repair. During this time, careful monitoring is needed because rapid deterioration is possible.

Mitral Regurgitation (MR)

The incidence of papillary muscle rupture with MI is about 1%. Most cases occur with inferior MI (the papillary muscles are supplied by the right and circumflex arteries). Unlike VSD, a tiny MI may cause mitral regurgitation because infarction of just the tip of the papillary muscle can lead to rupture. The patient may have single-vessel CAD.

The onset of heart failure and pulmonary congestion is abrupt. Many have a loud, holosystolic murmur, but no thrill (which would suggest VSD). When cardiac output and blood pressure are low, the murmur may be soft. Unlike chronic MR, there is no S_3 gallop. In fact, there may be an S_4, since the LV tends to be stiff and is not dilated.

The echo demonstrates MR and often a flail mitral leaflet. LV function may be near-normal. The pulmonary wedge tracing typically shows a tall V wave, analogous to the V wave in the venous pulse in patients with tricuspid regurgitation.

When pulmonary congestion is severe and there is low cardiac output, nitroprusside and the IABP provide a bridge to surgery. Immediate surgery is indicated.

Rupture of the Free Wall of the LV

This is the second most common cause of death in patients hospitalized with MI (following heart failure) and is responsible for 10% of deaths. It occurs 3-7 days after MI at about the same time acute VSD or MR develop. At this time after MI, the necrotic infarct zone is softest.

Rupture commonly happens after a first MI, and it may occur with small or large infarction (usually anterior or lateral in location). Early reperfusion therapy preserves muscle in the infarct zone preventing rupture—as with other mechanical complications of completed MI, this is rarely seen in patients treated early. Single-vessel CAD and poorly developed collaterals are common. Risk factors for rupture are late reperfusion therapy, particularly with thrombolytic therapy >12 hours from onset of MI, hypertension and advanced age. But it is not uncommon in young patients. Steroids and nonsteroidal anti-inflammatory agents may increase the risk of rupture. Because anti-inflammatory therapy may alter healing and scar formation, NSAIDS probably should be avoided for a month after MI.

The clinical picture is one of acute tamponade and death. I have observed a number of cases with the patient still in hospital, and the bedside diagnosis is obvious. A patient with a small, or at least an uncomplicated MI, collapses unexpectedly. There may be mild agitation or other vague symptoms just before cardiac arrest, but no chest pain. Telemetry shows no arrhythmia. After the patient arrests, there is pulseless electrical activity—sinus rhythm may persist for a couple minutes. Resuscitation is unsuccessful and there is no time for emergency surgery. This is a cause of SCD for which there is no effective treatment. There are a couple case reports describing emergency surgical repair and survival, but I have never seen it, even when the clinical diagnosis was made immediately.

Rupture may occur soon after discharge from the hospital and often in a patient with a small, albeit completed MI (e.g., an infarct not interrupted by reperfusion therapy). For this reason, I tell patients with small infarction that the prognosis is good—especially when LV function is normal—but also indicate that there are rare complications of MI during the first month that prevent a guarantee of a benign course.

Psuedoaneurysm

An occasional patient develops rupture that is contained by adherent pericardium, which then expands in an aneurysmal fashion. There is usually clot within the bulge that provides support but that also may embolize. The diagnosis is possible with an echocardiogram; a pseudoaneurysm has a narrow neck where it communicates with the LV, distinguishing it from a true aneurysm. There are no clinical findings indicating its presence, and it is usually an incidental finding on an echocardiogram or chest x-ray. Because rupture of the thin-walled pericardium is possible, surgery is indicated.

LONG-TERM TREATMENT AFTER MI

Risk Stratification and Treatment of Late Complications

A patient preparing to leave the hospital after MI faces the possibility of sudden death, recurrent infarction, heart failure or peripheral embolization during the next year. The standard of care includes laboratory evaluation to identify those at high risk for these late complications and treatment to prevent them.

Sudden Cardiac Death

Normal LVEF indicates a low risk for VF and sudden arrhythmic death. The management of late ventricular arrhythmias has been reviewed. MADIT II recommends ICD therapy for those with LVEF ≤30% at least one month post-MI.

While a normal *predischarge* LVEF indicates low risk, *low* LVEF measured early can be misleading. Remember that MADIT II enrolled patients based on the LVEF at least six weeks after MI. A number of those with low LVEF immediately after infarction have improvement over the next month, especially those who had reperfusion therapy.

The one medical therapy to prevent SCD is beta blockade, and it is indicated for all patients after MI regardless of LV function. Of course, beta blockade is the most useful therapy for heart failure with low LVEF, regardless of the etiology. Clinical trials did not address the duration of beta blockade in patients with normal LV function; like most studies, follow-up did not extend beyond five years. Furthermore, the trials were done before the advent of revascularization therapy for acute MI.

GDMT for ASCVD

At follow-up, perhaps the most important consideration is being sure the patient is on the medicines shown to improve prognosis with stable CAD: aspirin, statin, and ACEI/ARB therapy.

Chapter 8: Cardiac Arrhythmia and Syncope

Abbreviations

AF, atrial fibrillation
AIVR, accelerated idioventricular rhythm
AV, atrioventricular
AVN, AV node
CAD, coronary artery disease
DC, direct current
DCC, DC cardioversion
EP, electrophysiology
ER, emergency room
ICD, implantable cardioverter defibrillator
HOCM, hypertrophic obstructive cardiomyopathy
IHSS, idiopathic hypertrophic subaortic stenosis (also HOCM)
INR, international normalized ratio
LA, left atrium
LV, left ventricle
LVEF, left ventricular ejection fraction
LVH, LV hypertrophy
MI, myocardial infarction
OAC, oral anticoagulants
PAC, premature atrial contraction
PAF, paroxysmal atrial fibrillation
PSVT, paroxysmal supraventricular tachycardia
PVC, premature ventricular contraction
RA, right atrium
RV, right ventricle
SA, sinoatrial
SCD, sudden cardiac death
VA, ventricular arrhythmia
VF, ventricular fibrillation
VT, ventricular tachycardia
WPW, Wolff-Parkinson-White syndrome

SINUS RHYTHMS

Sinus Bradycardia

A rate less than 60 beats/min is usually an indicator of normal cardiac function and rarely causes symptoms. It is common in trained athletes and active young people. Illnesses that may cause sinus bradycardia include hypothyroidism and sick sinus syndrome. Obstructive sleep apnea may cause bradycardia or long sinus pauses while the patient is hypoxic. On the other hand, it is common for the heart rate to slow during sleep, and when a monitor flags a spell of bradycardia, check the time it occurred. Drugs are also a common cause of sinus bradycardia, usually beta blockers, diltiazem and verapamil. This may limit the dose that can be tolerated, although a rate in the low 50s without symptoms is no reason to back away from the medicine.

Beta blocker eye drops given for glaucoma may cause sinus bradycardia or AV nodal block. An aqueous solution of timolol traverses tear ducts to nasal sinuses where 80% can be absorbed within 20 minutes (bioavailability is higher than oral and comparable to intravenous timolol). The effect is magnified when the patient is on another rate lowering drug.

The key question for the patient with sinus bradycardia with an otherwise normal ECG is, "Do you have dizzy spells, or have you blacked out?" In the absence of these symptoms, and especially if exercise tolerance has not changed, further cardiac evaluation is unnecessary.

Sinus Tachycardia

Students and house officers commonly miss the significance of sinus tachycardia as an arrhythmia. It may be an indicator of decompensation in a patient with heart disease.

A rate greater than 100/min may be a benign rhythm, depending on the clinical setting. It is the normal response of a healthy person to exercise, stress or excitement. On the other hand, persistent tachycardia may accompany noncardiac conditions such as anemia, thyrotoxicosis or fever. Arterio-venous malformation is a rare cause, the fast rate suggesting high-output heart failure.

Sinus tachycardia at rest after myocardial infarction (MI) is a marker of low left ventricular ejection fraction (LVEF), and indicates poor prognosis. It also indicates a poor prognosis with congestive heart failure from other causes. On the other hand, ventricular fibrillation (VF) in the first few hours of MI may occur with a small infarction, where LVEF is normal and long-term prognosis is good. Thus, persistent sinus tachycardia in a patient with a history of MI often indicates a worse prognosis than VF at the onset of MI.

Sinus Arrhythmia (*Figure 8.1*)

We occasionally see a young patient in clinic because of irregular heart beat and find that it is sinus arrhythmia. (Check your pulse while taking slow, deep breaths.) The ECG shows normal P waves and PR interval with variation in the R-R interval. It is a parasympathetic (vagal) rather than a sympathetic phenomenon. With inspiration and increased venous return to the heart, stroke volume rises. The vagus is activated and the rate slows for a couple beats, though without a change in cardiac output (recall that cardiac output = heart rate x stroke volume). During expiration there is a decrease in venous return to the chest and heart, and withdrawal of vagal tone leads to a temporary increase in heart rate.

Figure 8.1 Sinus Arrhythmia

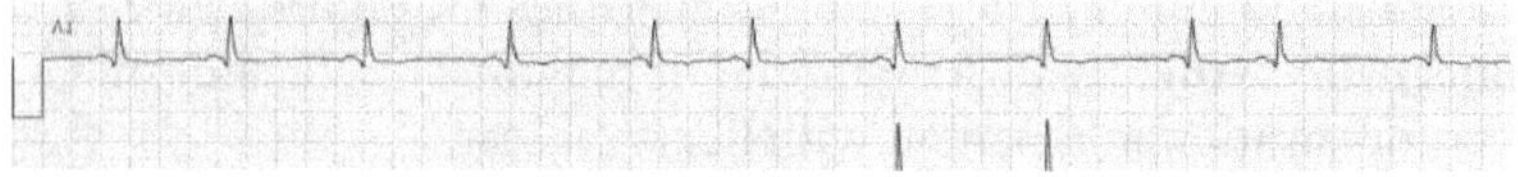

Changes in sympathetic tone also affect heart rate, but this system responds more slowly, over a period of seconds. Increased rate with exercise, stress or pain—the fight or flight response—reflects a rise in serum catecholamines which have a brief half-life. But the catecholamine effect is too slow to produce a beat-to-beat variation in rate. That is a parasympathetic function.

The normal response to reduced cardiac output is to raise heart rate by shutting down the parasympathetic system and increasing sympathetic tone. Turning off the vagus nerve eliminates respiratory variation in heart rate. Thus, an absence of sinus arrhythmia is a marker of LV dysfunction. This has been found to be clinically useful after MI. Heart rate variability can be measured using the mean and standard deviation of R-R intervals. A low standard deviation, meaning little variation in heart rate, indicates low LVEF and poor prognosis.

In clinic, when evaluating a patient with dyspnea who cannot afford an echocardiogram, I check the pulse carefully for sinus arrhythmia as evidence of good LV function. It's a go-to physical finding.

PREMATURE ATRIAL CONTRACTIONS (PACs)

PACs are easy to recognize; the QRS complex is narrow (that is to say, the right and left ventricles are activated simultaneously). An abnormal P wave may be seen before the QRS, possibly distorting the T wave of the preceding beat (Figure 8.2)

Figure 8.2. Premature Atrial Contraction (PAC)

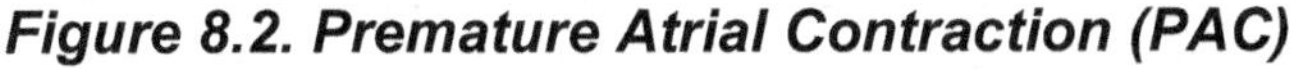

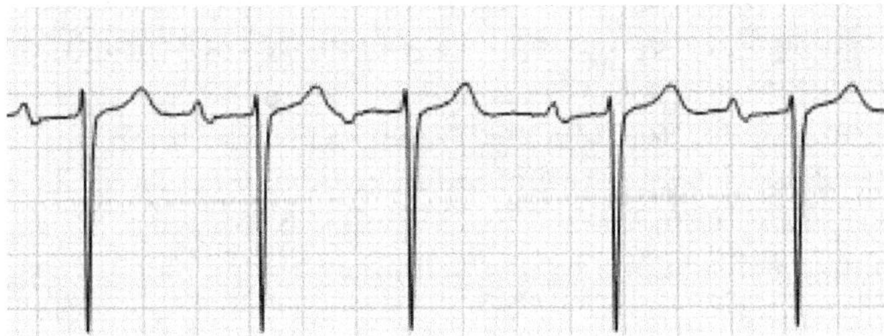

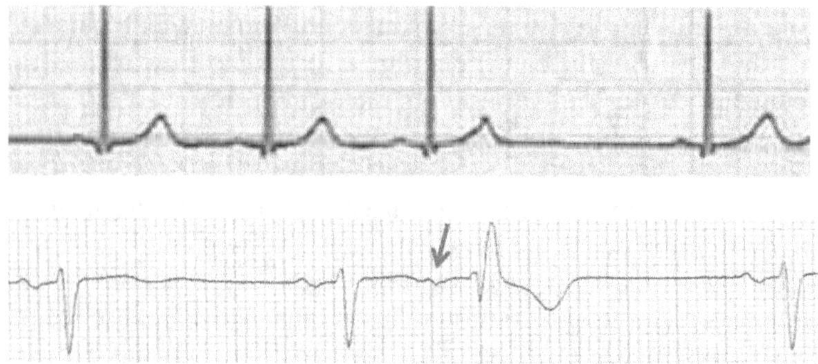

Figure 8.2 Three patients with PACs. <u>Top:</u> The third beat is premature and preceded by a distorted P wave, partially buried in the preceding T wave. <u>Middle:</u> There is a pause after the fourth beat, and the preceding T wave is distorted by a premature P wave. This PAC occurred too early to be conducted through the AV node. A blocked PAC is a common cause of a pause on a rhythm strip; examine the T wave before the pause for evidence of a buried P wave. <u>Bottom:</u> The third beat has a right bundle branch block (RBBB) pattern, and is preceded by a P wave. Because it occurs early, it is conducted aberrantly. The right bundle branch is the 'weakest link' in the infranodal conduction system, so RBBB is a common pattern of aberrancy. It is also identified as an aberrantly conducted PAC because the QRS follows a P wave.

A blocked PAC is a common cause of a pause on the ECG and may be felt as a skipped beat by the patient. It happens when the PAC is early enough that the atrioventricular (AV) node is refractory and will not conduct it. The ectopic P may be buried in the preceding T wave, making it easy to miss. There usually is some distortion of the T wave, but it may be subtle. It is something to look for when telemetry shows pauses (especially on a board exam). PACs are common in healthy people and do not indicate heart disease. If the ECG, cardiac history and examination are normal, no further testing or treatment is necessary.

Paroxysmal Supraventricular Tachycardia (PSVT)

PSVT is a rapid, regular rhythm with a rate of 120 to 200 beats/min (Figure 8.3). Most cases are caused by re-entry within the AV node, and is called AV node re-entrant tachycardia (AVNRT).

Figure 8.3 PSVT

Patient 1

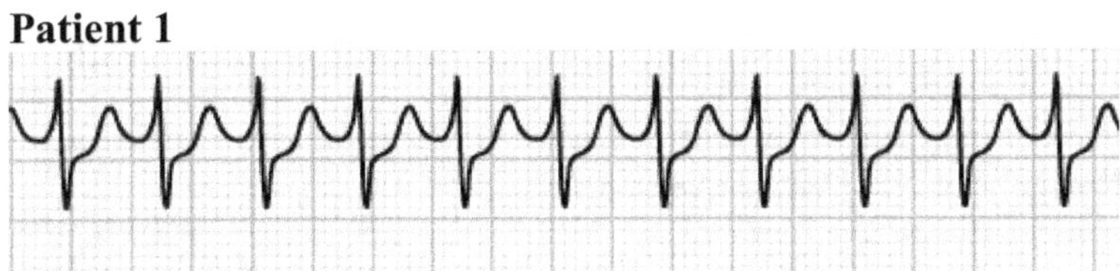

Patient 2

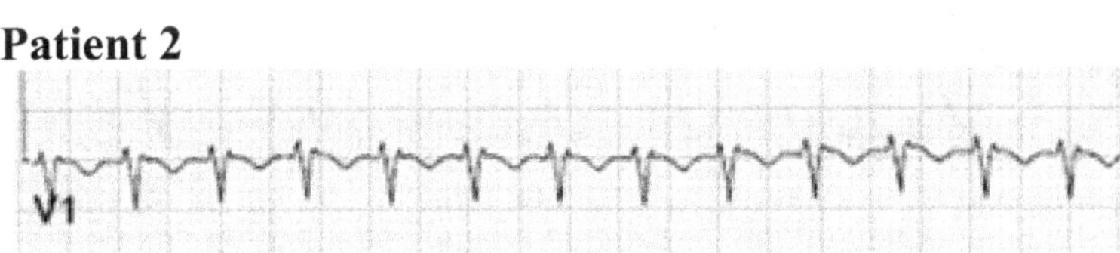

Patient 3 (lead V1)

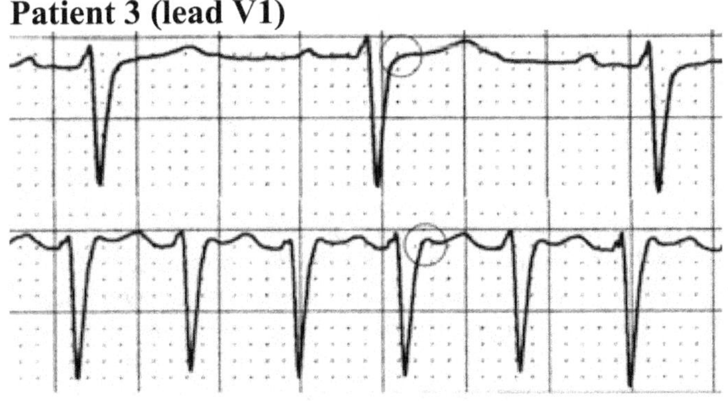

Figure 8.3 Paroxysmal supraventricular tachycardia (PSVT) Patient 1: A rhythm strip showing narrow QRS tachycardia at 160 beats/min. ST segment depression may indicate tachycardia related ischemia. Patient 2: Most SVT involves AV nodal reentry or AVNRT. The retrograde current hits the atrium

creating an "atrial echo," a P wave that may be buried in the QRS, or can appear at the end of the QRS as in this case. The tiny positive deflection at the end of the QRS—giving it the appearance of incomplete RBBB—is the retrograde P wave. <u>Patient 3:</u> This is more apparent with this pair of tracings from the same patient. The retrograde P wave at the end of the QRS is seen with SVT, but not when in sinus rhythm.

Re-entry is a common mechanism of both atrial and ventricular tachyarrhythmias. Although often misunderstood, the concept is fairly simple (<u>Figure 8.4</u>)

Figure 8.4 Re-Entry Sequence

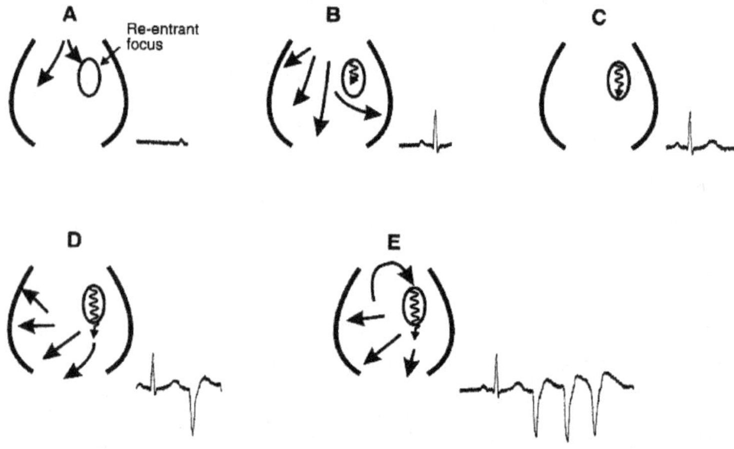

Figure 8.4 This illustrates the concept of re-entry, regardless of the location of the re-entrant focus. Follow the sequence of events. **A:** The wave of depolarization comes from above (the atrium in the case of atrial arrhythmias, the ventricle in this case of ventricular re-entry). **B:** As current moves through the myocardium, it also enters the re-entrant focus, a region that is insulated from the surrounding tissue, **C:** Depolarization of the surrounding myocardium happens quickly, but conduction through the re-entrant focus is slow. **D:** By the time current exits the re-entrant focus, the surrounding tissue has been repolarized and is *vulnerable.* That is to say, the refractory period has ended and it can be stimulated. This produces the

ectopic beat. **E:** If the timing is perfect, current from the ectopic beat re-enters the protected focus, travels through it, and again finds the surrounding tissue vulnerable when it exits. A circuit is established and the result is repetitive ectopic beats. Three characteristics of the re-entrant focus that make this possible: (1) Insulation from the surrounding tissue, (2) unidirectional conduction and (3) slow conduction.

The re-entrant focus is a region that is protected, or insulated, from surrounding tissue. Normally, current enters one end of the focus and exits the other—conduction is unidirectional. Within the re-entrant focus, conduction is slower than conduction in the surrounding tissue. By the time current exits the focus, the surrounding tissue has depolarized and has had time to recover. Thus, the current exiting the focus finds the surrounding tissue vulnerable and ready to be stimulated, and a premature beat is generated. A re-entrant focus in the atrium or AV node causes a PAC, and one in the body of the ventricle causes a premature ventricular contraction (PVC).

If the timing is perfect, the premature beat may slip back into the entrance of the re-entrant focus, leading to another or even to a series of ectopic beats, usually at a rapid rate. A "re-entrant circuit" is created.

AV nodal re-entry is the usual mechanism of PSVT—also called AV nodal re-entrant tachycardia (AVNRT). Current exiting the focus passes normally through the common His bundle, and the resulting QRS complex is narrow. Again, the sequence of ventricular stimulation is normal with simultaneous LV and RV activation. PSVT is therefore a "narrow QRS tachycardia" (Figure 8.3). The P wave is often buried in the QRS; if it comes at the beginning or end of the QRS there may be subtle slurring of the complex creating a pseudo R or S wave. Proof that this is from atrial depolarization requires comparison with a baseline ECG.

It is possible to have a wide QRS with PSVT. A patient may have coexisting bundle branch block with a wide QRS. Alternatively, a diseased infranodal conduction system may be stressed by the fast heart rate, causing aberrant conduction, usually right bundle branch block morphology. The right bundle tends to be the weakest link in the conduction system and the first to fail at high heart rates. Right bundle branch block morphology is a clue that a wide complex tachycardia is SVT with aberrancy rather than ventricular tachycardia (VT).

PSVT is a common arrhythmia in otherwise healthy young people. It is not dangerous, but it can be bothersome, causing palpitations, dizziness and near-syncope. Loss of consciousness is rare. The Valsalva maneuver can terminate spells, and many patients with palpitations learn this on their own. When PSVT occurs infrequently and spells are brief and easily terminated, other therapy may be unnecessary. Drugs that slow AV conduction may control symptoms, including beta blockers, verapamil, diltiazem or digoxin. Intravenous adenosine, a strong AV node blocker, is used to interrupt the tachycardia in the emergency room (always a board question).

When symptoms are frequent and not easily controlled, catheter ablation of the re-entrant focus is possible. An electrophysiology (EP) cure may be preferable to life-long drug therapy for a young person. EP testing is needed to "map" the site of re-entry. An ablation catheter is placed next to the re-entrant focus, and radiofrequency energy is applied to create a mild burn that permanently interrupts conduction through it. The intensity of the burn is about like sunburn; I reassure patients that we do not smell burning flesh or smoke in the catheterization lab.

PREEXCITATION

Preexcitation is the archetypal re-entrant rhythm, and the most common form is the Wolff-Parkinson-White (WPW) syndrome. The mechanism is described in Figure 8.5.

Normally, there is a layer of connective tissue separating the atria and ventricles that serves as insulation, preventing free passage of neural impulses between upper and lower chambers. The AV node is the normal passage through this insulation. Slow conduction (the duration of the PR interval) through the AV node allows time for atrial contraction to augment filling of the ventricle before ventricular systole.

Figure 8.5 Preexcitation of the Left Ventricle Through a Bypass Tract (the Wolff-Parkinson-White Syndrome)

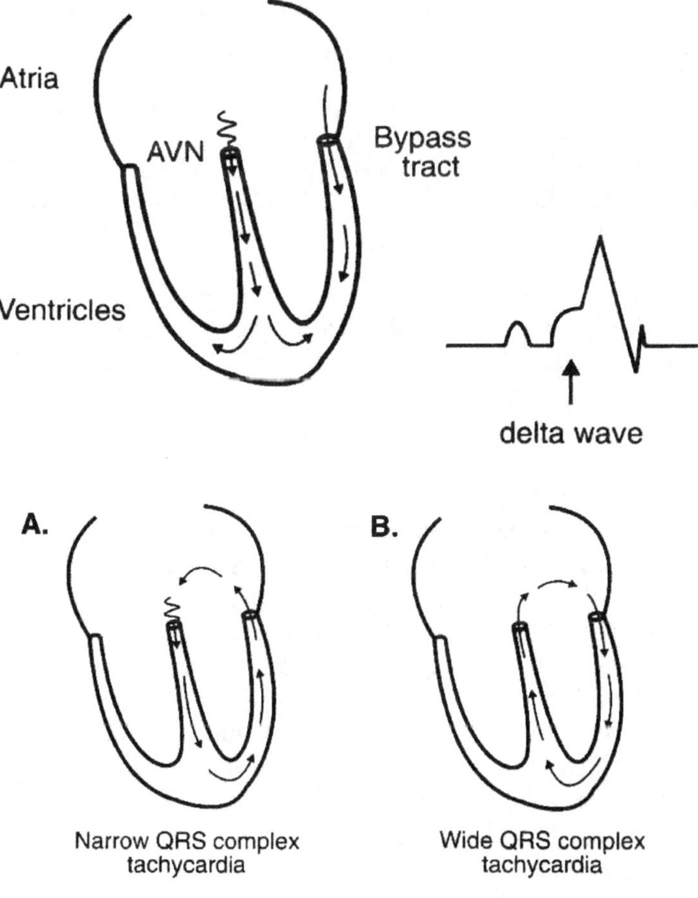

Figure 8.5 This diagram illustrates the construction of a QRS caused by dual conduction of atrial beat through the AV node and a bypass tract between the atria and ventricles. The tract is located on the LV side and near the mitral valve in this particular patient, but bypass tracts may be located at any site where the atria and ventricles come into contact. Simultaneous activation of the ventricles via the bypass tract and the AV node produces a fusion beat, and the morphology depends on the location of the bypass tract. Conduction through the bypass tract is faster than through the AV node. Early activation of the ventricle produces the delta wave and makes the PR interval appear short. A re-entrant circuit can develop between the bypass tract and the AV node, resulting in supraventricular tachycardia. There are two possibilities. **A:** The re-entrant circuit moves antegrade through the AV node, retrograde through the bypass tract. The sequence of ventricular activation is therefore normal, and the QRS is narrow. **B:** The re-entrant circuit is directed retrograde through the AV node and antegrade through the bypass tract. Because activation of the ventricles originates from the lateral wall of the LV, the QRS complex is wide.

The preexcitation syndromes occur because of an additional defect in the insulation between atria and ventricles. (While simplistic, that is how I think of it: a defect or hole in the insulation.) The defect is called a *bypass tract*. As the wave of depolarization passes through the atria, it leaks through the bypass tract as well as through the AV node.

Conduction through the bypass tract is usually faster than AV node conduction. As current exits the bypass tract, it stimulates the ventricle—the ventricle is "pre-excited." An instant later, current exits the AV node and also stimulates the ventricle. The ventricular complex originating from two sites is a "fusion beat." The QRS is wider than normal and starts earlier after the P wave, so the PR interval is short. The initial slurred portion of the QRS caused by preexcitation of the ventricle through the bypass tract is the delta wave (Figures 8.5, 8.6).

Figure 8.6 Preexcitation ECG

Patient 1

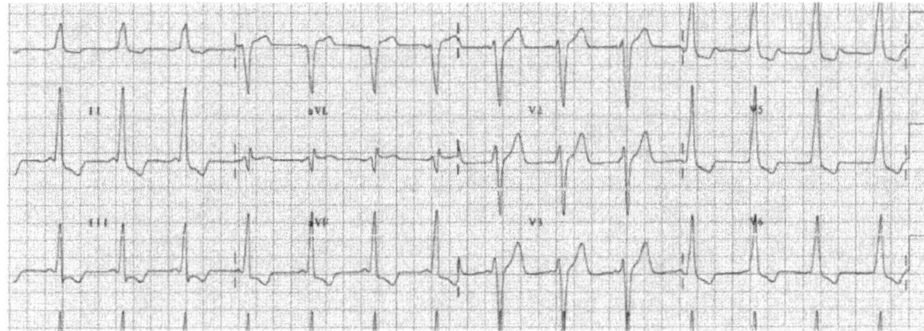

Patient 2

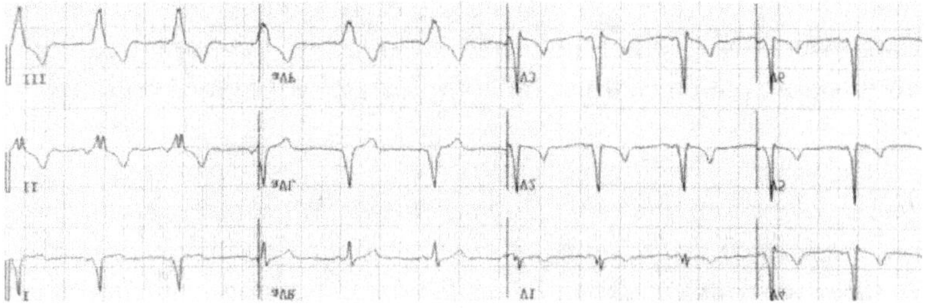

Figure 8.6 Preexcitation syndrome or Wolff Parkinson White (WPW). Both patients have short PR intervals, and the QRS complex is wide. The beginning of the QRS is slurred, the so called delta wave. This distinguishes this from the wide QRS caused by bundle branch block where it is the terminal part of the QRS that is slurred (the result of delayed depolarization of a part of the ventricle), and the QRS upstroke is normal. Patient 2 has an inferior Q wave, which is actually the delta wave. WPW is one cause of "pseudo-infarction" on the ECG.

A bypass tract can conduct both antegrade and retrograde. A PAC that finds the accessory pathway refractory may pass through the AV node, capture the ventricle, conduct retrograde through the accessory (fast) pathway and establish a re-entrant circuit. Because antegrade conduction is through the AV node (slow pathway), the re-entrant rhythm looks like PSVT with a narrow QRS complex. A re-entrant circuit moving in the opposite direction—retrograde through the AV node and antegrade through the accessory pathway—produces a wide QRS complex because the sequence of ventricular activation is abnormal. The resulting wide complex tachycardia looks like VT.

How can you tell whether the wide complex tachycardia is ventricular or supraventricular? At times you cannot, just from the ECG. The clinical setting helps. A young patient with a history of palpitations, no prior heart disease, and no alteration of consciousness is more likely to have PSVT with bypass tract re-entry. An older patient with syncope or near-syncope plus a history of heart failure or MI should be treated assuming a diagnosis of VT. When in doubt, it is hard to go wrong treating an unstable patient with wide complex tachycardia as probable VT.

Immediate direct current (DC) cardioversion is appropriate for any tachyarrhythmia causing hemodynamic instability, even if it is supraventricular. Do not wait for the cardiology consultant or attending; resuscitate the patient.

A diagnosis of PSVT caused by preexcitation affects drug therapy. Digoxin should be avoided because it shortens the refractory period of the accessory pathway and blocks the AV node. If the patient has atrial flutter or fibrillation, these actions may favor antegrade conduction through the accessory pathway and lead to an unusually rapid ventricular rate. Verapamil, diltiazem and beta blockers can do the same thing. On the other hand, membrane active antiarrhythmic drugs tend to slow accessory pathway conduction; intravenous procainamide is a good choice if drug therapy is needed (another board question, and procainamide is always the answer).

Membrane active drugs have been used for long-term management as well. However, catheter ablation of the accessory pathway usually works and is preferable to life-long drug therapy for a young person. Radiofrequency energy is delivered to the region of the bypass tract, burns it and leads to a scar that plugs the defect in the insulation. The indication for ablation is symptomatic tachyarrhythmia. On the other hand, the discovery of a short PR interval and delta wave in an older person without a history of SVT is not in indication for ablation.

You may hear disagreement about this from EP specialists because a rare person with preexcitation has extremely rapid atrial fibrillation as the initial tachyarrhythmia because of fast conduction through the bypass tract. This can degenerate to ventricular fibrillation and sudden cardiac death. This is rare, and standard practice still does not call for ablation of the asymptomatic patient.

JUNCTIONAL (Nodal) RHYTHM

It is recognized by the absence of P waves preceding the QRS, and the rhythm is regular (Figure 8.6). A retrograde P wave following the QRS may be apparent, or it can be buried in the T wave. Since the impulse originates above the bifurcation of the bundle branches, the QRS complex is usually narrow, although patients with pre-existing bundle branch can develop a junctional rhythm.

Figure 8.7 Junctional Rhythm

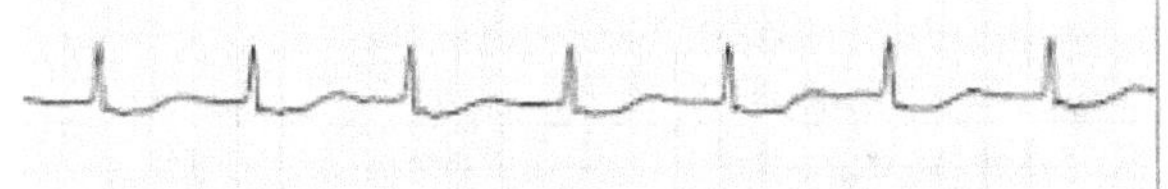

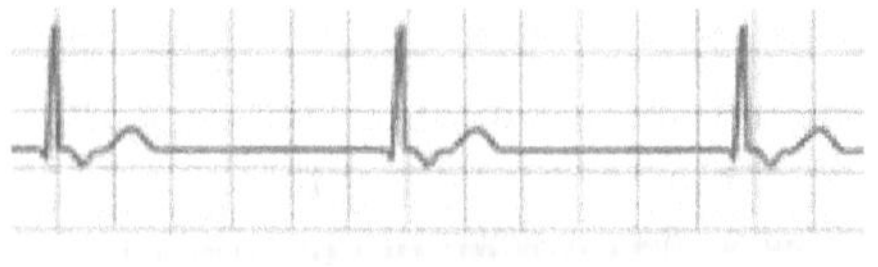

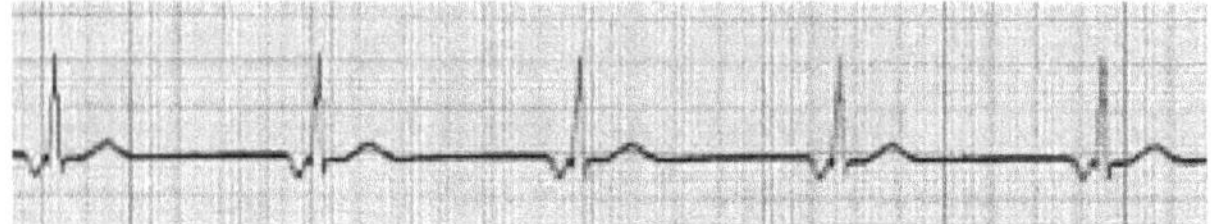

Figure 8.7 Rhythm strips from three patients. The diagnosis is made when the rhythm is regular and there is no P wave, at least no P wave in the usual location. In addition to pacing the ventricle, in some cases the junctional pacemaker stimulates the atria retrograde. Retrograde P waves may occur after the QRS (middle), with distortion of the ST segment, or before the QRS (bottom, a lead II tracing with a short PR, negative P wave and no delta wave). Look more closely at the top tracing; it looks like there is a glitch in the ST segment, probably a retrograde P.

When the rate is less than 60 beats/min, the mechanism usually involves depression of the sinus node, with the AV node assuming the role of dominant pacemaker—it is an "escape rhythm."

An accelerated junctional rhythm above 100 beats/min is less common. In such cases, the mechanism is increased automaticity rather than re-entry; the rate of spontaneous depolarization of the AV node increases, and it becomes the dominant pacemaker. This may be a rhythm associate with digitalis toxicity or acute MI. Junctional tachycardia is common with inferior MI and is unrelated to prognosis. On the other hand, nodal tachycardia with anterior MI—like other supraventricular tacyarrhythmias including sinus tachycardia— is a marker of large infarction, poor LV function and therefore, poor prognosis.

Large acute MI is an exception. Most junctional rhythms are benign, transient, and seldom require treatment. Tachycardia may be controlled with beta blockers, diltiazem or verapamil.

ATRIAL FIBRILLATION (AF)

The incidence of AF has risen for reasons that are not certain, and it is the most common arrhythmia requiring treatment. After chest pain, AF is the most common indication for cardiology consultation in our hospital. It is more common in older people; by age 80 the chance of developing it is about 3% per year.

Pathophysiology

AF may be paroxysmal (PAF) or chronic. Patients with structurally normal hearts may have AF in a setting of electrolyte abnormalities (commonly low potassium or magnesium), alcohol intoxication (the holiday heart syndrome), or thyrotoxicosis. PAF is usually idiopathic, although most with this condition have hypertension, and elevated left atrial pressure is a likely mechanism.

Lone AF refers to the patient with no structural abnormalities on an echocardiogram (and that means a completely normal study), *plus no history of hypertension.* I emphasize hypertension because many do not realize that it is a marker of stroke risk for those with AF, just like left atrial enlargement or mitral valve disease. Lone AF is uncommon, accounting for less than 3% of new AF cases. But it is worth identifying, since this is a benign illness for those ≤60 years old.

One of my mentors (J. O'Neal Humphries) taught that atrial fibrillation is a disease of the left atrium (LA), while flutter comes from the right atrium (RA). In the 1970s he based this on the clinical observation that AF tends to complicate left heart disease, and flutter, right heart disease. AF occurs with mitral valve disease and conditions that raise LV diastolic pressure: hypertension or heart failure. Elevated LV diastolic pressure is transmitted to the LA, and LA enlargement on the echocardiogram is common.

LA contractility and function decline with prolonged AF, but there may be recovery after cardioversion. This mechanical recovery is usually delayed and may take weeks. Think of this as LA myopathy that plays a role in the genesis of AF and LA appendage thrombosis.

We previously believed that recovery of atrial contraction eliminated the risk of thromboembolism. This turns out to be wrong. An important discovery of the AFFIRM trial was that the risk stroke persists long-term after restoration of sinus rhythm. About half of the strokes in this study occurred after stopping warfarin. One explanation is the persistence of paroxysmal AF after cardioversion; this has been documented with extended monitoring. Even brief spells of AF, with duration as short as 6 seconds, can lead to stroke. Additionally, the LA myopathy may persist after cardioversion. In any event, cardioversion cannot be offered in order to stop anticoagulation.

Evaluation of New AF

Hospitalization is not necessary for the hemodynamically stable patient with few symptoms. Those who are symptomatic with a rapid rate or patients with congestive heart failure who have a higher risk of thromboembolism require inpatient stabilization and evaluation. A patient who presents within 48 hours of the onset of AF can have cardioversion in the emergency room, and avoid hospital admission.

The laboratory evaluation includes thyroid function studies. Recall that George H.W. Bush had AF complicating thyrotoxicosis while he was president. In fact, AF is the most common presenting symptom in older people with hyperthyroidism. Other signs of thyrotoxicosis may be absent, and an elderly nursing home patient may even appear sluggish or depressed. This "apathetic hyperthyroidism" is usually discovered during the evaluation of new AF.

In addition to an ECG, the one other cardiac test that is needed is an echocardiogram. You are looking for structural abnormalities including valvular disease, LA enlargement and LV disorders like hypertrophy, enlargement or dysfunction. The house staff often wants to screen for coronary artery disease (inexperienced doctors believe that CAD causes most heart problems). Although AF may complicate a large, acute MI or ischemic cardiomyopathy—conditions that can raise LV diastolic pressure and therefore LA pressure—asymptomatic CAD does not cause it. AF usually occurs in patients with hypertension; consider AF a feature of hypertensive heart disease, not CAD. A history, ECG, echo and thyroid studies are adequate workup unless the patient has angina.

Routine pacemaker interrogation often detects occult, paroxysmal AF. The device clinic may report episodes of "mode switching"—the dual chamber pacer stops pacing the atrium or sensing a normal P wave (the DDD pacing mode), and instead paces just the ventricle (the VVI mode). The usual cause of this is atrial fibrillation with loss of the normal P wave. An asymptomatic patient with mode switching should be presumed to have AF and considered for anticoagulation.

Treatment of AF

At the time of initial evaluation there are three treatment issues: anticoagulation, rate control and cardioversion.

Anticoagulation & Stroke Prevention

The first goal of therapy is to protect the brain. Although the mortality rate with AF is above normal, I generally tell patients that I have known patients who have done well with AF for decades. Morbidity and mortality are usually the result of embolic stroke or the heart condition that caused AF. For example, large populations with AF have reduced longevity but most of them also have hypertension.

Both paroxysmal and sustained AF may cause stroke, and the benefits of oral anticoagulation (OAC) are similar with both clinical patterns. The risk of stroke can be related to the company AF is keeping. With mitral stenosis the stroke risk is as high as 8% per year.

A number of risk factors for stroke have been identified. Greatest among them is prior stroke or transient ischemic attack (TIA). The CHA_2DS_2VASc scoring system awards 2 points for stroke or TIA and age over 74, and 1 point for congestive heart failure, hypertension, age 65-74, female gender, vascular disease, and diabetes (maximum score = 9). Stroke risk is cumulative as seen with these results from one of many validation studies (Table 8.1).

Table 8.1 Annual Risk of Stroke with Atrial Fibrillation: CHA_2DS_2VASc Scoring

CHA_2DS_2VASc_score = 0, annual risk of stroke = 1.9%
Score = 1, risk =1.3%
Score = 2, risk = 2.2%
Score = 3, risk = 3.2%
Score = 4, risk = 4.0%
Score = 5, risk = 6.7%
Score = 6, risk = 9.8%
Score = 9, risk =15.2%

The other side of decision-making is the assessment of bleeding risk with OAC. This can be done with the HAS-BLED scoring system which gives points for hypertension, history of bleeding, abnormal liver or renal function, age > 65, labile INR on warfarin, and alcohol or drug use. CHA_2DS_2VASc and HAS-BLED scoring templates are available online.

When stroke risk with AF exceeds bleeding risk with OAC, anticoagulation is recommended. Practice guidelines have moved toward anticoagulation for more patients with AF.

If the patient cannot or will not take OAC, antiplatelet therapy with the combination of aspirin 81 mg plus clopidogrel was recommended by the ACTIVE trials. In practice, many use clopidogrel alone.

Choice of Oral Anticoagulant

Warfarin, a vitamin K antagonist, has been in use almost a century, and it is the comparison drug in clinical trials of the newer agents. The target INR for non-valvular AF is 2.0-3.0. Warfarin reduces the risk of stroke by 60-70% (data from meta-analysis). Risk reduction with aspirin is less than half that. In one comparison trial, the rate of stroke was 42% lower with warfarin than aspirin + clopidogrel (ACTIVE-W).

Disadvantages of warfarin include INR monitoring, difficulty with control (the best of clinical trials have patients in the therapeutic range less than 70% of the time), poor compliance and patient refusal.

The newer, direct OACs have been approved for AF stroke prophylaxis, but not for patients with mechanical heart valves. Dabigatran is a direct thrombin inhibitor, and rivaroxaban and apixaban inhibit factor Xa. When compared with warfarin, the new agents are at least as good for prevention of stroke. Bleeding risk is the same or slightly better, and all have tended to cause less intracranial bleeding. They have largely replaced warfarin.

The HAS-BLED scoring systems incorporates risk factors have been identified for bleeding with OACs. They include history of bleeding, systolic hypertension, abnormal renal or liver function, history of stroke, unstable or high INRs or poor time spent in the therapeutic range, age > 65 years and drug and alcohol abuse. A number of these are also risk factors for stroke with AF. Of interest "fall risk" is not on this list, and often is an inappropriate excuse to avoid anticoagulation for an older patient. Weighing risk of bleeding with the potential benefits of OAC constitutes 'clinical judgment,' and when there is uncertainty, the rationale for treating or not treating should be in the patient's chart.

Left atrial appendage isolation is an option for the patient with excessive bleeding risk. Most thrombo-emboli originate in the LA appendage, and occlusion of the appendage with the Watchman device is an effective substitute for OAC. The indication is simple: AF plus a contraindication to OAC.

Note that the LA appendage cannot be visualized with trans-thoracic echo. It is clearly seen with the trans-esophageal echo (TEE). In addition, TEE is the proper study to screen for other cardiac sources of emboli, including LV thrombus, infective endocarditis, or cardiac tumor. That said, AF is by far the most common cause of embolic stroke; when evaluating a patient with occult stroke, extended monitoring for AF has higher yield than TEE (although both may be indicated).

Rate Control

An occasional elderly patient has abnormal AV node conduction and has a ventricular rate <100 beats/minute, but most with AF require an AV nodal blocking agent to prevent tachycardia. AF with a rapid ventricular response is a common cause of tachycardia-induced cardiomyopathy, and when rate is controlled or sinus rhythm is restored, LVEF often improves.

Beta blockers, diltiazem, verapamil and digoxin are effective, and your first choice may be influenced by other conditions. For example, if the LVEF is low, a beta blocker would be indicated for both the AF and cardiomyopathy. Verapamil should be avoided when LVEF is low since it depresses contractility enough to precipitate congestive heart failure. Diltiazem should not be used if LVEF is below 45%.

Box 8.1 Choice of Calcium Channel Blocker

1. Verapamil is the most potent for blocking the AV node and depressing contractility but a weak vasodilator. If rate control of SVT or AF is the goal and LV function is normal, it is the best choice. It is well tolerated by elderly patients and those with chronic lung disease.

2. The dihydropyridines (e.g., amlodipine) are pure vasodilators with little effect on contractility or the AV node. They are of no use for rate control with SVT or AF.

3. Diltiazem has intermediate effects, and is not as good as verapamil for rate control of AF. It should not be used with LVEF < 45%.

Patients with a healthy AV node may need two drugs to control the ventricular rate. The goal of therapy is prevention of excessive tachycardia during normal activity, not just at rest. Adding a second drug is preferable to pushing the first to toxicity. At an earlier time, we were taught that there was no upper limit to the dose of digoxin that could be given: the proper dose was the one that controlled the rate. *In current practice, digoxin is seldom used for rate control,* but it can be useful when rate control is difficult (we limit the dose to 0.125 mg/day.

An occasional patient has persistent tachycardia despite multiple drug therapy. Rate control may be achieved with *AV node ablation,* a relatively straightforward EP procedure. Destruction of the AV node creates complete heart block. This requires a permanent ventricular pacemaker for the patient with persistent AF, or a dual chamber pacer with paroxysmal AF. Atrial pacing may prevent recurrence of AF. In practice, the pacer is inserted first, and the ablation is done a week or more later. All rate lowering drugs may then be stopped. Some patients feel better with a more regular rhythm as well as a slower rate, and ventricular pacing provides that.

For a short time after AV node ablation there is an increased risk of sudden death. This is attributed to the slower heart rate leading to a lower threshold for torsade de pointes (see below). To avoid this complication, the pacemaker is initially set at 90 beats/minute, and the rate is gradually reduced over a few months.

Cardioversion and Drug Therapy to Prevent Recurrence of AF

About two thirds of patients have spontaneous return of sinus rhythm within a day of developing AF. After that the rate of conversion is low, and beyond a couple weeks of persistent AF, spontaneous conversion is uncommon. A patient with a first, brief episode of AF may not have a recurrence, and drug therapy to prevent AF is not indicated.

Practice guidelines have allowed cardioversion without anticoagulation if the duration of AF is less than 48 hours, using either drugs or direct current (DC) counter shock. When the duration of AF exceeds two days, the patient should be anticoagulated for three weeks before cardioversion. When the duration of AF is uncertain (often the case with new AF), or the effectiveness of anticoagulation is uncertain, a transesophageal echocardiogram just before cardioversion can exclude left atrial thrombus.

The drugs that block the AV node and slow the ventricular rate are no more effective than placebo in converting AF to sinus rhythm (e.g., beta blockers, verapamil, diltiazem, or digoxin).

However, membrane-active antiarrhythmic drug therapy increases the success of cardioversion. Amiodarone, ibutilide, and dofetilide may be used for cardioversion. Sotalol has poor conversion efficacy but may be effective for maintenance of sinus rhythm after DC cardioversion. Hospitalization and monitoring are not required with amiodarone therapy. With sotalol and dofetilide, treatment is initiated in-hospital for telemetry and monitoring the QT interval on the ECG to prevent pro-arrhythmia (e.g., drug-induced ventricular arrhythmias and sudden cardiac death).

To prevent recurrence of AF, class IC agents, <u>flecainide and propafenone</u>, are approved for those with no structural heart disease, including coronary artery disease. Some recommend stress testing to detect occult coronary disease, but that has not become usual practice. Hypertension is not listed as a contraindication to propafenone or flecainide.

Proarrhythmia is possible but uncommon, and these drugs do not require hospital monitoring when they are started. A "pill-in-a-pocket" approach can be used when paroxysmal AF is infrequent; the patient carries a flecainide pill and takes it with the onset of palpitations.

<u>Amiodarone</u> is the most effective drug for prevention of AF, but there is hesitation to prescribe it for young people because of the duration of exposure to its side effects. On the other hand, it is safe and well tolerated by elderly patients (even those in their 90's). The maintenance dose of amiodarone for AF is 200 mg/day (lower than the dose used to suppress ventricular tachycardia). At this dose pulmonary toxicity is less common. When a patient has been stable on amiodarone for years, we often lower the maintenance dose to 100 mg/day.

Dofetilide and dronedarone are less effective than amiodarone but have fewer dangerous side effects, so they are usually recommended for younger patients. Treatment requires frequent monitoring and includes measurement of the QT interval and serum magnesium.

Both amiodarone and dofetilide can be used when LVEF is low.

For AF that develops in hospital—particularly post-operative AF—intravenous ibutilide is fast acting and about 50% successful. If it does not work, it increases the chance of successful DC cardioversion. Do not forget to check electrolytes, including magnesium (the overlooked cation). Replacing potassium and/or magnesium may lead to cardioversion. Regardless, replacement will increase the effectiveness of drug or DC cardioversion.

Paroxysmal AF (PAF) commonly responds to antiarrhythmic drugs. It may not be abolished, but the intervals between spells lengthen and there is symptomatic improvement. An advantage of sotalol and amiodarone is rate control in addition to prevention so that when AF occurs it causes fewer symptoms.

"Sinus rhythm begets sinus rhythm." With suppression of AF there seems to be a conditioning effect, and the atrium "learns" to stay in sinus rhythm. It is common for a patient to stop having PAF with drug therapy, and there is a question about whether to stop the medicine. Most would agree with a trial off antiarrhythmic drugs after the patient has been symptom-free for months.

Anticoagulation should be continued long term even when the patient is not having symptomatic AF. Extended monitoring often shows brief, asymptomatic bursts of AF, and stroke remains possible. As little as six minutes of AF is associated with increased stroke risk.

AF Ablation

The re-entrant circuit is in the posterior left atrium, near the ostia of the four pulmonary veins. Isolating the pulmonary veins with radiofrequency catheter-induced burn lines works best in patients with paroxysmal AF. Chronic AF does not respond as well. The indication for ablation has been a failure to control symptoms with either rate control or cardioversion/antiarrhythmic drug therapy. Since many with AF are asymptomatic, ablation is not indicated since it does not have a morbidity or mortality benefit. An exception to this is AF ablation for patients with heart failure and low LVEF; small clinical trials have shown that AF ablation improves exercise tolerance, hospitalization, and possibly mortality.

A question patients ask is whether successful ablation eliminates stroke risk and the need for anticoagulation. Presently the answer is that stroke risk persists after ablation. Our EP service will occasionally stop OAC months after successful ablation, and after prolonged monitoring documents an absence of AF.

Post-Operative Atrial Fibrillation

This develops in about 20% of patients after heart surgery, but it may occur after any large operation. It usually increases the length of hospitalization, and some studies have shown an increased risk of perioperative stroke. Beta blockade and amiodarone have been shown to reduce the incidence of AF after heart surgery, but it is not clear that prophylactic therapy reduces length of stay or prevents stroke.

Many with AF in the early post-operative period have hypomagnesemia, and this can develop after any major operation. The mechanism is uncertain, with some suggesting that "cut surfaces either soak up or weep magnesium." Correcting electrolyte abnormalities—usually magnesium and/or potassium depletion—is at least a physiologic approach to rhythm management. Aggressive, prophylactic magnesium replacement was shown to prevent AF in one small study, and there has been no study testing this plus drug therapy.

The general principles of management of AF outlined above apply. It often responds to amiodarone therapy. There is no reason to continue this long term, since late recurrence of AF is uncommon. We usually stop the amiodarone at the one-month follow-up visit.

Likewise, transient post-operative AF is not an indication for long-term anticoagulation. OAC should be considered for those at high risk for recurrence or thromboembolism (e.g., a high $CHADS_2VASC$ score), especially if AF persists for more than 48 hours. For most, AF does not recur, and anticoagulation can be stopped once the patient has been in sinus rhythm for a month.

As noted above, removal or isolation of the LA appendage at the time of surgery lowers the risk of thromboembolism, and extended OAC is unnecessary.

ATRIAL FLUTTER

Although patients with atrial flutter may develop AF, and vice versa, they are quite different in mechanism. AF involves re-entrant circuits in the left atrium (LA). Atrial flutter, on the other hand, is usually a right atrial (RA) rhythm. The recognition of atrial flutter is relatively easy. The rhythm is regular, and the atrial rate is 300/minute or slightly lower in elderly patients. In the absence of AV node blocking agents, 2:1 AV block is the rule, so the patient has a rate of 150/minute. When evaluating a patient at the bedside with abrupt onset of tachycardia that is regular and about 150/min, atrial flutter is a good guess. The ECG shows flutter waves. Vagal maneuvers or intravenous adenosine may abruptly increase the level of AV nodal block, lowering the rate from 150/min to 100 or 75. In that case the flutter waves are more apparent.

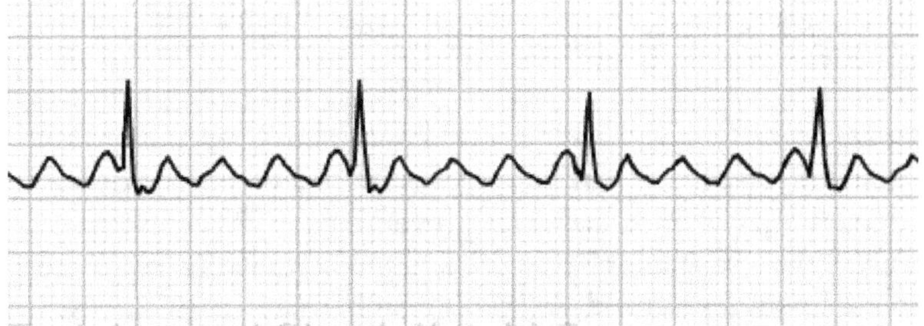

Figure 8.8 The atrial rate is near 300 beats/min, and there if 4:1 AV block, so the ventricular rate is about 75 beats/min. Before the pathoanatomy of atrial flutter was understood, we assumed it was a right atrial illness because of the clinical setting: conditions that raise right atrial pressure cause it. For example, if you are called about new atrial flutter in an elderly, bedridden patient, you should consider pulmonary embolus (this is a common board question). Atrial flutter often accompanies an exacerbation of obstructive lung disease with hypoxia leading to a rise in pulmonary artery pressure, so it may occur with cor pulmonale. It may be resistant to drug therapy until the patient's pulmonary illness improves. Of course, atrial flutter often occurs in patients with left heart disease. That is because elevated LV pressure is transmitted to the pulmonary vasculature leading to elevated right heart pressure (e.g. the most common cause of right heart failure is.....).

The drug therapy of atrial flutter and AF are similar but not identical. Control of ventricular rate with AV node blockade is the same, requiring digoxin, beta blockade, diltiazem or verapamil. Verapamil is commonly overlooked, but it is the preferred drug for the two atrial tachyarrhythmias that complicate pulmonary decompensation: atrial flutter or multifocal atrial tachycardia. Do not use it if LV function is depressed.

Drugs for cardioversion of atrial flutter include ibutilide (best in the acute situation), amiodarone, and sotalol. Sotalol is more effective for atrial flutter than AF.

Preventing a recurrence of atrial flutter requires preventing the premature atrial beat that precipitates it. Beta blockers may work although they are not useful for preventing AF. Also effective are the class IC drugs (flecainide and propafenone), sotalol and amiodarone. Associated obstructive lung disease may limit the use of beta blockers.

A major issue is anticoagulation. Unlike AF, there are no atrial flutter clinical trials to guide us. Observational trials suggest a risk of thromboembolism though not as great as that with AF. Nevertheless, we use the AF anticoagulation guidelines for atrial flutter.

Catheter ablation of atrial flutter is less complicated than AF ablation. The success rate is high, and the cure tends to be permanent. Radiofrequency burns are generated on the right atrial wall to interrupt the re-entrant circuit. Because it is a right atrial procedure it is relatively safe, and it tends to be a quick procedure. Catheter ablation is becoming first-line therapy for chronic or paroxysmal atrial flutter, preferable to long-term drug treatment. Anticoagulation can be stopped 4-6 weeks after successful catheter ablation. While unsupported by clinical trials, it would seem prudent to continue daily aspirin when the risk is low.

VENTRICULAR ARRHYTHMIAS (VA) AND SUDDEN CARDIAC DEATH (SCD)

The clinical setting determines the prognosis in patients with ventricular arrhythmias. Premature ventricular contractions (PVCs, also called ventricular premature beats, VPBs) may be a normal variant in the healthy person with normal LV function.

During the acute phase of myocardial infarction, complex VAs, including ventricular tachycardia (VT) and fibrillation (VF), may occur with minimal LV injury. The re-entrant arrhythmia is purely an electrical event. Long term prognosis—assuming successful treatment of the arrhythmia—is not influenced by the electrical storm during the acute phase of infarction. Rather, prognosis is predicted by LV ejection fraction.

Later after MI, in the chronic stage of coronary artery disease, complex VAs occur in those with severe LV dysfunction and thus indicate poor prognosis. On telemetry or a 24 hour monitor, "complex VA" is defined as high frequent paired PVCs or runs of VT (at least 3 PVCs in a row). The evaluation and treatment of VAs after MI—which applies to all with chronic CAD—are reviewed in chapter 4.

Consider this question: Which would you rather have, VF in the hospital, 3 hours after the onset of a first inferior MI, or sinus tachycardia a week after MI? The answer has to do with LV function and prognosis. With a small MI, and normal LVEF, VF is cardioverted in hospital, and prognosis is good. Sinus tachycardia with chronic CAD is a marker of poor LV function, and poor prognosis.

Pathophysiology

Isolated PVCs may come from either an automatic focus or a re-entrant focus. Repetitive ectopic beats, with three or more defined as VT, are usually re-entrant. That is the case with VF.

An exception to this is accelerated idioventricular rhythm (AIVR, Figure 8.9). The rate may be less than 100 beats/min, and the ectopic focus works like a fixed rate pacemaker. When the sinus rate falls below the ectopic rate, it "takes over" and paces the ventricle until the intrinsic rate increases. AIVR commonly occurs at the moment of reperfusion during MI and is a reliable indicator of successful reperfusion therapy. It is considered benign since it seldom degenerates to VF. It tends to be transient, and is resistant to antiarrhythmic drug therapy (which is not needed, in any event).

Figure 8.9 AIVR

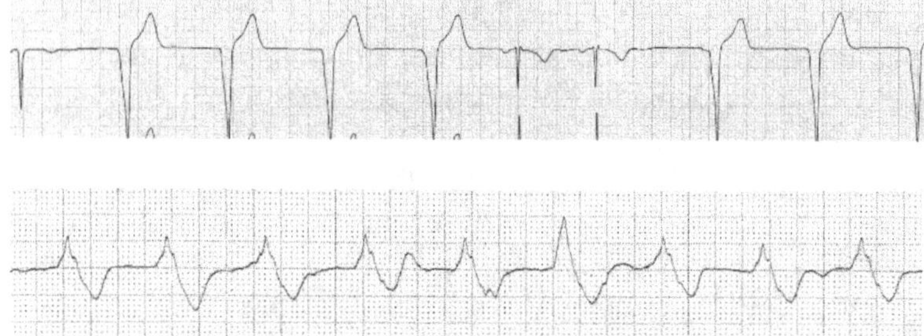

Figure 8.9 Accelerated idioventricular rhythm (AIVR). <u>Top</u>: the baseline rhythm is sinus, and when there is sinus slowing—in this case probably from sinus arrhythmia—the ventricular pacemaker takes over. <u>Bottom</u>: a regular, wide complex rhythm, also AIVR. There is also AV dissociation, with an obvious P wave near the end of the tracing, and probably P waves that distort T waves. Since these P waves are not conducted, the rhythm has to originate below the AV node, confirming that this is a ventricular rhythm.

VAs are exacerbated by low potassium or magnesium. Community-based studies of sudden cardiac death have found that SCD is more common in patients taking diuretics, and that hypokalemia is often present in those who are resuscitated. These patients also have other heart disease, usually LV dysfunction, but the electrolyte abnormality is the last straw. The first step with all rhythm consults is to check electrolytes, an easy problem to fix. If uncorrected, the arrhythmia will be tough to control. Do not overlook magnesium; like potassium it falls with diuretic therapy and also is low after surgery (the earlier discussion of post-operative AF applies to VAs after surgery).

Outside the setting of acute MI, the most common cause of VF and SCD is ischemic cardiomyopathy. Nonischemic dilated cardiomyopathy is only responsible for about 10% of cases. Although re-entry is the mechanism of VF with both diseases, there are some differences. For example, with ischemic heart disease electrophysiologic testing using paced PVCs provokes VT in those at high risk for SCD, and a negative study indicates low risk. Electrophysiologic testing is not as reliable for those with dilated cardiomyopathy and no CAD.

Laboratory Evaluation

Evaluating LV function is the first step. Normal LVEF usually excludes VAs as a cause of palpitations, dizziness or syncope. We used to do a lot of 24-hour ECG (Holter) monitoring. As a screening test, complex VAs on an ambulatory monitor indicates a risk of SCD and occur when LVEF is low. On the other hand, with normal LVEF complex VAs are rarely seen on the ambulatory monitor. Now that LVEF is the indication for defibrillator therapy, we do less monitoring for this purpose.

There are other noninvasive tests that identify high risk of complex VAs. All of them also are markers of low LVEF in patients with prior MI, and they add little to the assessment of risk once LV dysfunction is identified. They include the *heart rate variability (HRV)* test (measuring sinus arrhythmia as discussed earlier), *signal-averaged ECG*, and microvolt *T-wave alternans*. The earlier edition of TCR described these tests at length, but they are no longer in day-to-day clinic use.

Wide QRS Tachycardia

A patient with a rapid rhythm that looks like VT and who has low blood pressure and altered sensorium probably is having VT. Immediate cardioversion is needed. It makes no difference whether the rhythm is ventricular or supraventricular with aberrant conduction—hemodynamic instability mandates cardioversion.

Features of the ECG that suggest a ventricular origin—VT—include a few different features. The most reliable is QRS width, usually >140 msec. Other feature of VT: ventricular beats are monophasic (single R or S wave, not a complex with an RSR pattern), the T vector is opposite the QRS vector, there is QRS concordance in V leads (all positive or all negative). SVT with aberrancy is suggested by a right bundle branch block pattern. The wide complex tachycardia with WPW however looks like VT.

There are some patients with "wide complex tachycardia" who are clinically stable. They may not feel well and may be aware of palpitations, but the blood pressure is stable. How do you determine the origin of the rhythm? Tachycardia stresses the infranodal conduction system and may cause "aberrant conduction"—a bundle branch block pattern with a wide QRS. It is important to distinguish between atrial and ventricular rhythms as the prognosis and treatment are different. If it is supraventricular, it is relatively benign and AV nodal blockers and/or membrane active antiarrhythmic agents may be considered. But if it is ventricular, there is a risk of SCD and an ICD is needed. The right bundle is the weakest link in the conduction system and right bundle branch block suggests aberrant conduction. Monophasic QRS complexes are more likely ventricular in origin.

To make a certain diagnosis requires identification of the relationship of P waves and QRS complexes. A rare patient has identifiable P waves on the surface ECG, and if they are not related to the ventricular (QRS) rhythm, VT is the diagnosis. More commonly, an intracardiac electrogram is needed to magnify the P waves (Figure 8.10). If it shows AV dissociation, the rhythm is VT. If there is a P wave before or after each QRS complex, it is supraventricular tachycardia.

Fig 8.10 Wide Complex Tachycardia

Patient 1

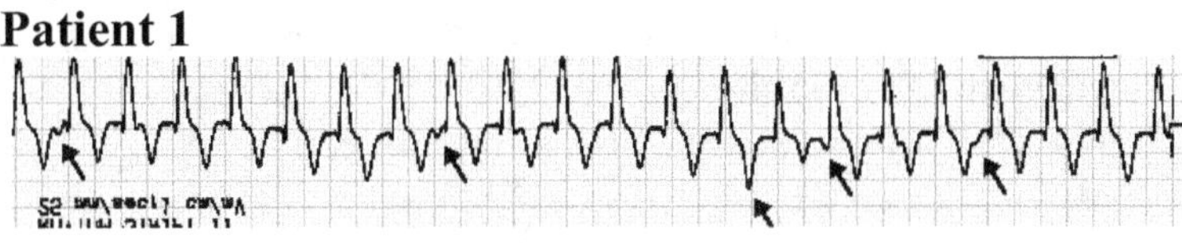

Patient 2

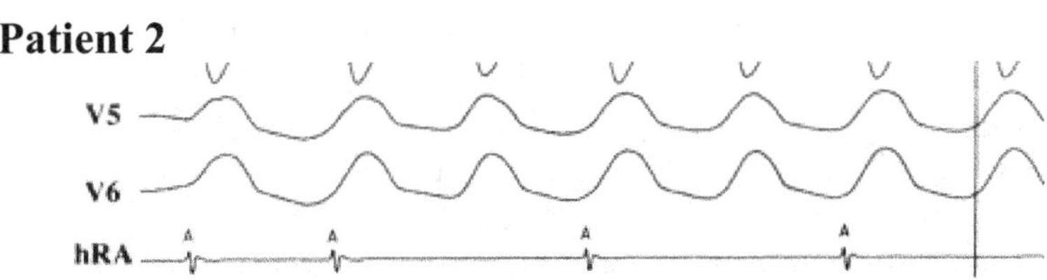

Figure 8.10 Ventricular tachycardia with AV dissociation. <u>Patient 1</u>: P waves can be seen intermittently in this telemetry tracing. Since there is no relation to the QRS complexes—there is AV dissociation—the QRS complexes must be coming from below the atria. <u>Patient 2</u>: In most cases P waves cannot be seen on the surface ECG. In the EP lab a catheter is positioned in the right atrium (RA) to record P waves (here labeled A waves). In this case there is an atrial rhythm that is independent of the ventricular rhythm, and this AV dissociation proves VT as the cause of the wide complex tachycardia. Also note the demonstration of AV dissociation in <u>Figure 8.9</u>.

Another way of guessing the origin of the arrhythmia is the clinical setting. An older person with a history of MI or heart failure or known LV dysfunction is more likely to have VT. SVT is the likely arrhythmia in a young patient with no history of ventricular disease (i.e., past MI). In such cases, a history of palpitations is common.

Treatment of Ventricular Arrhythmias and the Prevention of SCD

We no longer try to suppress PVC's or even nonsustained VT with drug therapy. Beta blockade improves survival with both ischemic and nonischemic cardiomyopathy, and prevention of VF is one way it does this. (Not the only way, of course; withdrawal of adrenergic tone also allows myocardial recovery—Chapter 1.)

Prior to the MADIT-2 trial, EP testing was common. Inducible, sustained VT was the indication for implantable cardioverter-defibrillator (ICD) therapy. MADIT-2 did not use provocative EP testing instead basing treatment on LVEF. Now the indication for ICD insertion is prior MI, LVEF $\leq 30\%$ and an expected survival greater than one year. The trials also required that the patient be six weeks beyond the MI since many with acute MI will have improvement in LVEF during that time, especially when beta blocked.

In ICD trials there was no survival benefit for the first 10 months after ICD insertion. This suggests there is no reason to rush into ICD insertion while instituting therapy for cardiomyopathy. It is common for LVEF to rise to $> 35\%$ with beta blockade. The delay in clear benefit also indicates little point to this treatment for a patient who is not expected to live a year; Class 4 heart failure and terminal illness are contraindications. In fact, at end of life we often turn the ICD off to prevent painful shocks that have little effect on outcome at that stage of illness.

ICD therapy works by first identifying a rapid rate. The device usually incorporates a pacing function to overdrive-pace the ventricle and interrupt the VT circuit. If this does not work, the ICD fires, delivering 15-40 joules to the endocardial surface. It records the rhythm before firing. Later interrogation of the device allows documentation of the arrhythmia. The longevity of the battery is related to the number of discharges, and with average use they last 4 to 8 years before a battery change is needed. The engineering has become quite sophisticated, and modern devices combine ICD and biventricular pacing (Chapter 1).

Management After ICD Discharge

Between 50% and 70% of patients with an ICD have it fire within two years of insertion. Most of these are appropriate, a single shock converting VT. A smaller number have "ICD storm", with multiple discharges. This can be a response to recurrent VT, but an occasional patient is shocked because of rapid AF (misdiagnosed by the ICD as VT), machine malfunction including lead fracture or electromagnetic noise. Table 8.2 provides a rough guide to management:

Table 8.2 Management After ICD Discharge

1. Interrogate the ICD: Determine that firing was an appropriate response to VT,
Exclude AF or PSVT as the inciting tachyarrhythmia,
Detect unit malfunction

2. Exclude treatable cause of VT: Acute MI or unstable angina*, Proarrhythmia from antiarrhythmic drug therapy, Torsade de pointes with a long QT interval, Electrolyte disturbance (low potassium or magnesium)

3. Indications for hospital admission: A broken ICD (lead fracture, etc.),
frequent shocks (ICD storm), or another medical condition that requires admission (MI or unstable

angina, electrolyte abnormality, change in the
arrhythmia, proarrhythmia, etc.)

MI, myocardial infarction; VT, ventricular tachycardia; AF,
atrial fibrillation; PSVT, paroxysmal supraventricular
tachycardia

*Acute ischemia causing increased VT frequency is an
indication for aggressive evaluation, including angiography.

Hospital admission is warranted when there is a change in the
clinical pattern. This would include an increase in the frequency
of discharge, ICD storm, or abnormalities that need correction
(e.g., electrolyte abnormalities or a mechanical malfunction).
Drug therapy may be adjusted to prevent VT, commonly sotalol,
amiodarone or mexilitine. Do not forget the importance of
correcting hypokalemia and hypomagnesemia; an argument can
be made for keeping the potassium above 4.0 mEq/L in patients
with heart failure.

Intermittent cardioversion of VT does not indicate a worse
prognosis or decompensation of heart failure. However, with
severe decompensation and when the patient is near end of life,
frequent ICD discharge—ICD storm—is possible. At that stage
of the illness the ICD does not have a meaningful effect on
survival, and many choose to turn the device off.

Driving After ICD Placement

The American Heart Association currently recommends a 6-
month wait before a patient resumes driving. This restriction
may not be consistent with the data, which show a low motor
vehicle accident (MVA) rate among these patients. In one large
follow-up trial, a few patients had a symptomatic arrhythmia
while driving but were able to control their vehicles despite ICD
discharge. The annual risk of an MVA that could be attributed to
an arrhythmia was 0.4%. Compare that with the 7.1% annual

probability of MVA for all drivers in the United States. Nevertheless, the Heart Association guideline is still the 6-month wait, and your state may have requirements that you should be aware of.

Other SCD Syndromes

Torsade de Pointes

This is a form of polymorphic VT with wide QRS complexes that become larger and then smaller as the axis shifts. It is like the QRS axis is turning about a point, hence the ballet term, torsade de pointes.

Figure 8.11 Torsade de Pointes

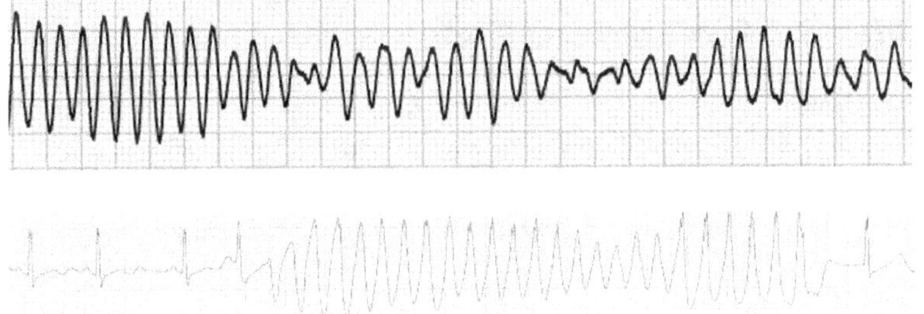

Figure 8.11 The QRS axis revolves about a point. In the second ECG (forgive the poor tracing) note that the QT interval is prolonged before the onset of VT.

It is a triggered arrhythmia, not re-entrant, that occurs in patients with QT interval prolongation. The first case I saw in the early 1970s was a patient with "quinidine syncope" who had been started on the drug for AF. At about that time I encountered another patient with intractable VT who had been on chronic tricyclic antidepressant therapy and had her first episode a couple days after starting antihistamines.

A few years ago, the combination of a popular antihistamine and erythromycin was found to cause SCD, and the mechanism was

Torsade. The antihistamine lengthened the QT interval, and erythromycin competed with the antihistamine for cytochrome P450 binding sites, thus raising the antihistamine level. This complication is less common with azithromycin, which may be preferred over other quinolones.

There are a number of drugs and clinical syndromes that include QT interval prolongation (Table 8.3)

Table 8.3 Prolonged QT Interval

Familial:
Jervell and Lange-Nielsen syndrome (congenital deafness, autosomal recessive)
Romano-Ward syndrome (normal hearing, autosomal dominant)

Acquired:
Drugs
Sotalol (common, and follow-up requires QT measurement)
Dofetilide (follow-up requires QT measurement)
Quinidine
Procainamide and its metabolites
Amiodarone (uncommon)
Disopyraminde
Phenothiazines and derivatives (including many antihistamines)
Tricyclic antidepressants
Erythromycin (when combined with antihistamines)
Pentamidine
Some antimalarials
Cisipride (Propulsid)
Ranoloazine

Electrolyte abnormalities
Hypokalemia and hypomagnesemia (diuretics, extreme diets, diarrhea, surgery)
Hypocalcemia (a less common cause of VT; the T wave is delayed but the T wave duration is not prolonged as it is with other causes of long QT)

Others
Acute myocardial ischemia
Central nervous system lesions
Hypothermia
Bradycardia

The conditions and drugs that cause QT prolongation and VT are synergistic. For example, a patient who is on sotalol who develops low magnesium and potassium because of diuretic therapy may develop QT prolongation and torsade de pointes. Torsade is thus a common form of proarrhythmia—or drug-induced VT—and it tends to develop early after starting a new drug. It can be idiosyncratic as well as dose dependent.

Lability of the QT interval is a predictor of sudden cardiac death in those with long QT. The QT interval may lengthen after a pause, and Torsade may be triggered by a pause. Treatment may include increasing the heart rate with temporary pacing or with isoproterenol. This prevents pauses, and at higher rates the QT shortens.

First line therapy for torsade is intravenous magnesium which shortens the QT interval. Other antiarrhythmic drugs are avoided. VT that is hemodynamically unstable requires DC cardioversion.

Note the cardiac drugs that can prolong the QT interval, including ranolazine and dofetilide. Our hospital pharmacy now requires measuring the QT interval and serum K and Mg before starting these drugs. Dofetilide must be started with the patient monitored in the hospital, and follow-up includes QT interval measurement.

Proarrhythmia without QT Prolongation

The class IC antiarrhythmic drugs, flecanide and propafenone, slow intraventricular depolarization and widen the QRS, but have little effect on repolarization (the QT interval). The mechanism of arrhythmia is re-entry, and it is dose-dependent. This complication of therapy may be avoided by getting an ECG a couple weeks after starting therapy to check the QRS duration. QRS prolongation may be present only with exercise, and treadmill testing may be considered for the patient who is having dizzy spells or palpitations.

Unlike torsade, which occurs soon after starting the medicine, this drug-induced monomorphic VT may occur late. VT is more common when LV function is depressed so class IC drug therapy is limited to those with normal LVEF.

Arrhythmogenic Right Ventricular Dysplasia (ARVD)

This rare familial disorder causes fatty infiltration of the right ventricle with some loss of muscle. The ECG usually is abnormal with T wave inversion in precordial leads. The VT has a left bundle branch block pattern. The RV may appear abnormal on the transthoracic echocardiogram, and the MRI demonstrates increased thickness of the RV wall. The diagnosis is confirmed with endomyocardial biopsy.

Beta-blockade, class IC antiarrhythmic agents, calcium blockers or amiodarone may prevent VT. Ablation of an arrhythmogenic focus has been described, but ICD therapy is often needed. Markers of poor prognosis include exercise-induced VAs or syncope, a dilated RV and sustained VT.

Brugada Syndrome

This is an autosomal dominant disorder that is characterized by ST segment elevation right precordial leads (Figure 8.12). The heart is structurally normal, the work-up for ischemia is negative, and electrolytes are normal. The diagnosis of Brugada syndrome requires the ECG changes plus clinical evidence of ventricular arrhythmias, or a family history of the syndrome.

The usual arrhythmia is polymorphic VT, which may degenerate to VF. SCD occurs most commonly in early morning hours, during sleep. The illness is endemic in Southeast Asia and more common in men at about age 40 (although cases have been reported at all ages, including infancy). SCD may be the initial symptom. VT may cause syncope, and many who develop VF have a history of syncope.

Figure 8.12 Brugada Syndrome

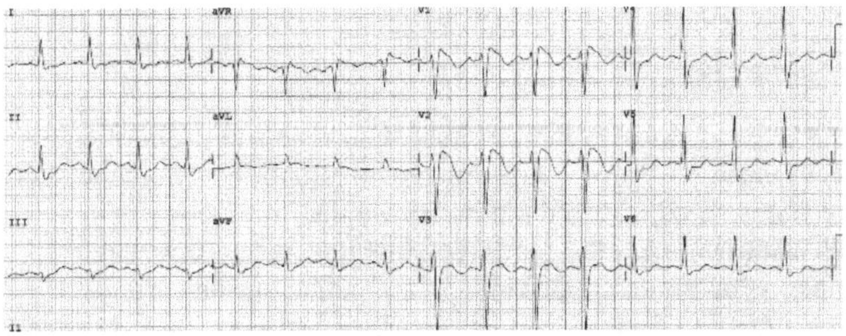

Figure 8.12 At first glance, this could be right bundle branch block with an RSR pattern in V2 and wide looking QRS. However, QRS duration is normal in most other leads, and the apparent widening is actually elevation of the ST segment, most notable in V1-2. The 'coved' ST can be variable. Some with the syndrome have less prominent ST changes (Brugada types 2 and 3), and provocative testing may be needed for diagnosis.

The molecular disorder is a defect in the membrane's sodium channel. Sodium channel blockers—including flecainide and procainamide—cause a worsening of the right precordial ST segment changes. These drugs may also trigger VT. When right precordial ST changes are not diagnostic, intravenous procainamide may elicit the typical ECG findings. Ajmaline and flecainide have been used for provocative testing as well.

Hypertrophic Obstructive Cardiomyopathy (HOCM, Chapter 2)

Predictors of sudden death with HOCM include a family history of SCD and a history of syncope. SCD may be the presenting symptom, but this is rare. The severity of outflow tract obstruction is not related to arrhythmia or sudden death risk. Reducing outflow tract obstruction with alcohol infusion or surgical ablation has not been shown to lower the risk of death. There have been observational trials suggesting that amiodarone may help those with documented VT, but the current approach is ICD therapy for high-risk patients.

Sudden Death in Young Athletes

HOCM is the most common cause. Collapse and death often occur during exertion. Outflow tract obstruction is worse when the LV is small, so a reduction in vascular volume—dehydration—may trigger SCD (Chapter 2). Limiting water intake as an aid to conditioning—a practice during spring training a few decades ago—is clearly a bad idea.

A systolic murmur that is heard during the Valsalva maneuver suggests LV outflow tract obstruction. If there is uncertainty, listen during squatting, then after standing; the murmur usually increases dramatically. Doing this doesn't take long, and it is a good move when you hear a soft murmur doing school physical exams. Sudden death in young athletes is rare enough that guidelines do not support routine echocardiographic screening.

An *anomalous coronary artery* is the second most-common structural abnormality that causes SCD in young athletes. Usually this involves a left main artery that originates from right cusp, and then courses between the pulmonary artery and aorta. With exercise, the great vessels swell and pinch the left main artery, creating ischemia. Consider it when there is a history of chest pain or syncope with exertion. Stress testing may not be positive, since ischemia may be episodic. Rather, evaluate with CT or MR angiography. If there are symptoms, particularly VT, bypass surgery is indicated.

The variety of other cardiac conditions that may cause sudden death in young people include acute myocarditis, Marfan's syndrome with rupture of an aortic aneurysm, long QT interval syndromes, occult mitral or aortic valve disease, infiltrative cardiomyopathies (i.e., cardiac sarcoidosis), dilated cardiomyopathy, a tunneled (bridged) coronary artery and premature atherosclerotic CAD. There are non-cardiac causes that show up in most series, but account for small numbers of the deaths: drug abuse, asthma, heat stroke, and ruptured cerebral artery.

Commotio cordis is a recently described cause of death in young athletes. VT is caused by an apparently minor blow over the sternum, not severe enough to cause chest wall injury. For example, the shortstop is hit by a ground ball. Energy from the blow is transmitted to the heart, provoking VT and VF. Animal studies indicate that contact must be just before the peak of the T wave at the so-called vulnerable phase of repolarization. Mechanical energy stimulates an "R on T" PVC which precipitates VT. This is a freak accident since the vulnerable phase occupies just 1% of the cardiac cycle. Strategies to prevent it include softer baseballs and chest protective devices for some youth sports (hockey, lacrosse, baseball).

Hypertrophic cardiomyopathy is the usual reason for avoiding high-intensity sport (that would not include golf or bowling).

Exercise-induced VAs with any other condition would also contraindicate intense exercise. Myocarditis is an indication for temporary withdrawal from sports, with resumption based upon recovery. While there are no guidelines defining recovery, it would require the passage of time, normal LV function and sedimentation rate, and no symptoms with resumption of normal activity. A stress ECG would be useful.

BRADYARRHYTHMIAS

Heart Block

The term "block" often confuses patients, not to mention medical students. We glibly refer to blocked arteries, blocked valves and blocked nerves, and these can be unrelated illnesses. The term, heart block, is usually reserved for nerve conduction disorders. It may occur at any level of the cardiac nervous system. Block is possible though uncommon within sinoatrial (SA) node or in the body of the atrium. It is most common in the atrioventricular (AV) node and the nerves below it. These infranodal nerves include the His-Purkinje system.

Blocked conduction may alter intervals on the ECG and may cause bradycardia and syncope. When block is complete there is no transmission to distal structures, but the heart rarely stops. Instead, an auxiliary pacemaker below the level of block takes over. The intrinsic rate of the backup pacemaker is incrementally slower the farther it is from the SA node. Control of heart rate reminds me of the children's game, King of the Mountain. Pacers highest on the mountain, beginning with the SA node, get the first chance to rule because they have the fastest rate of spontaneous depolarization. When conduction beyond that pacer is blocked, one just below takes over. As you go lower on the mountain, the pacers have a slower intrinsic rate. In addition, these lower level pacers are less influenced by the autonomic nervous system.

As an example, when complete block develops in the AV node, a pacemaker in the bundle of His just below the node paces with an intrinsic rate of 35-45 beats/min. It might be hard to exercise with a rate that slow, but at that rate syncope is still uncommon. If complete block occurs farther down, within the interventricular septum and beyond the division of the two bundle branches, the backup pacer is in the body of the ventricles. The ECG complex it generates looks like a PVC with a wide QRS. These deeper, ventricular pacers have a much slower intrinsic rate, occasionally as slow as 10-20 beats/min. In this case, syncope and even sudden death are possible.

Furthermore, a backup pacer in the body of the ventricle is unresponsive to the autonomic nervous system. A higher pacer, near the AV node, may respond to catecholamine stimulation or atropine with an increased rate of firing.

From this outline of general principles, you begin to see that the level of block determines prognosis, and identification of this level is critical.

First-Degree AV Block

The site of conduction delay is the AV node, and the PR interval is prolonged, measuring at least 0.22 seconds. Increased vagal tone, hyperkalemia, digitalis, diltiazem, verapamil and beta blockers all may slow AV conduction. It is common in elderly patients who may have a sick AV node with no associated CAD. Right coronary artery occlusion—acute inferior MI—may also cause first degree heart block because the AV nodal artery is a branch of the vessel supplying the inferior wall (usually the right coronary artery).

Second-Degree AV Block

Second degree block is the failure of some beats to reach the ventricles—the ventricles are not activated. On the ECG some P wave are not followed by a QRS complex.

Second-degree block is classified as two types, *Mobitz I or II* (also called Type I or II block). *Mobitz I block* occurs within the AV node and is associated with the Wenckebach phenomenon. The dysfunctional node tires with each succeeding beat until it is so tired that a P wave is completely blocked. On the rhythm strip there is progressive lengthening of the PR interval until a P is not followed by a QRS (Figure 8.13). The PR interval of the cycle following the blocked beat is shorter, reflecting recuperation of the AV node. In some cases, progressive lengthening of the PR is subtle. However, if the PR following the blocked beat is obviously shorter, the diagnosis is Wenckebach (Mobitz I).

Figure 8.13 Mobitz I HB

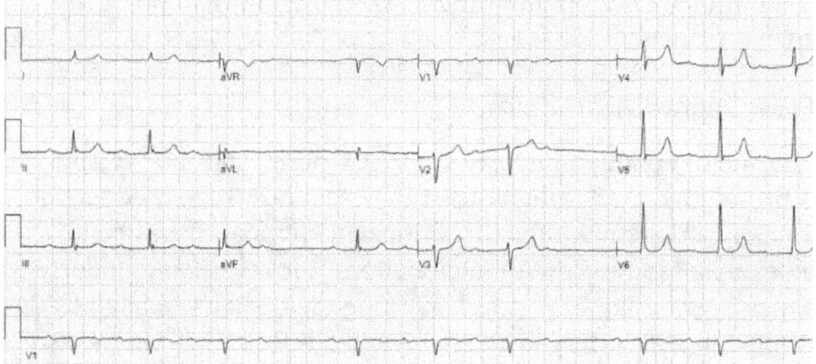

Figure 8.13 Progressive lengthening of the PR, and a shorter PR after the blocked beat

The conduction system below the AV node is usually normal in patients with Mobitz I, so the QRS complex is narrow. In fact, a *narrow QRS* excludes block below the AV node. On the other hand, a wide QRS does not guarantee that block is infranodal, since it is possible for a patient to have conduction abnormalities in the node and below it (e.g., a person with bundle branch block may develop delayed conduction in the AV node). Most cases of drug induced heart block are nodal, not infranodal.

Mobitz II block is caused by block below the AV node. It does not cause progressive prolongation of the PR in the beats before the blocked P wave. Because the infranodal conduction system is diseased, the QRS is usually wide. Mobitz II block often precedes symptomatic complete heart block and is an indicator for pacemaker therapy. Most who have it are symptomatic, but pacing is justified even in the absence of symptoms.

2:1 block: is it Mobitz I or II? Block in the AV node (Mobitz I) can be severe enough that every other beat is blocked. This eliminates progressive lengthening of the PR interval as a diagnostic marker of AV nodal rather than infranodal block. It is a common digitalis toxic rhythm.

There are a couple ways to determine the level of block. The easiest is QRS duration. If narrow, the block is nodal. If wide, it may be infranodal. Check an old ECG; a narrow QRS previously but a wide one now suggests new infranodal conduction disease. The response to exercise and increased heart rate can be helpful; if there is more transmission through the AV node (e.g. block improves), then block is nodal rather than infranodal.

A long rhythm strip may help. At times the block is less severe, and the 2:1 block is replaced by 3:2 or 4:3 conduction. During these times the typical variation of the PR interval indicates Mobitz I. With Mobitz II there is no PR variability.

When in doubt, a His bundle electrogram in the EP laboratory is diagnostic (Figure 8.14). A long H-V interval identifies infranodal conduction disease and is an indication for pacemaker therapy. This is a simple, low-risk study. An electrode catheter is advanced from the femoral vein to the right atrium—it takes about 10 minutes to complete.

Figure 8.14 His Bundle Recordings from 3 Patients

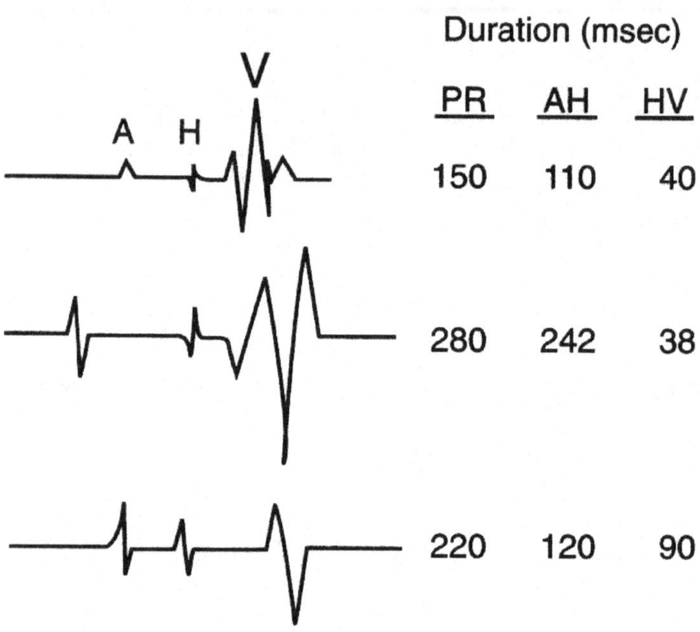

Figure 8.14 The goal of EP study when evaluating heart block is to determine the anatomic level of conduction delay. The HIs (H) spike is generated by depolarization of the His bundle, just below and adjacent to the AV node, and is recorded with a bipolar catheter positioned next to the tricuspid valve. The H spike essentially divides the PR interval into its AV nodal (the AH interval) and infranodal (HV) portions. Top: the PR interval is normal as is the HV interval (<55 msec). Middle: A patient with first-degree AV block (long PR). Marked prolongation of the AH interval indicates that the level of block is the AV node. Infranodal conduction (the HV interval) is normal, so there is no delay in the conduction of the AV node. Bottom: The prolonged HV interval indicates infranodal conduction delay. With infranodal disease, there is a higher risk of developing symptomatic heart block.

Third-Degree, Complete Heart Block

Nothing gets through. There are P waves and QRS complexes, but they are unrelated (Figure 8.15). This is an example of AV dissociation (another is VT with an unrelated atrial rhythm). How can you tell whether complete block is at the level of the AV node or below it?

Figure 8.15 Complete Heart Block

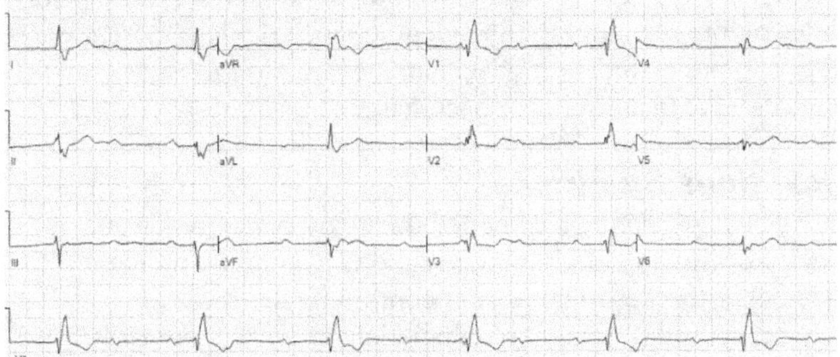

Figure 8.15 There is AV dissociation. The atrial rate is about 80/minute, the ventricular rate, 30/minute, and the two are unrelated. The wide QRS indicates a ventricular backup pacemaker, and this elderly patient had bundle branch block on previous ECGs.

The principles are those discussed above with 2:1 heart block. When block is nodal, the takeover pacemaker is high in the His system, before its bifurcation, so the QRS is narrow and the rate is above 40 beats/minute. The rate increases with catecholamine stimulation. Congenital heart block is usually AV nodal, and young people with this condition are often asymptomatic and feel they have good exercise tolerance. With exercise the heart rate rises since the take-over pacer in the His bundle responds to catecholamines. (The condition is often discovered when a young person has an initial ECG; there is a history of low heart rate, but normal exercise tolerance.)

Infranodal complete heart block is more common with elderly patients. It may cause syncope (Stokes-Adams attacks) but frequently presents as fatigue or heart failure. Even if it is asymptomatic it is an indication for pacemaker therapy because sudden death is possible. The etiology is often misunderstood. Senile heart block is not caused by ischemia. Instead, a degenerative, fibrotic process involving the cardiac nerves below the AV node is the usual cause—think of them as frayed wires. Most of these patients have bundle branch block on prior ECGs before developing third-degree block. Unless there are other symptoms indicating ischemia, evaluation for CAD is unnecessary. Just put in the pacemaker.

Sick Sinus Syndrome

Sick sinus syndrome, also called the tachy-brady syndrome, usually occurs in elderly patients and is a common indication for pacemaker therapy. The patient commonly has atrial tachyarrhythmias, which may include paroxysmal AF or PSVT, alternating with spells of marked sinus bradycardia. There may be disturbingly long sinoatrial pauses with syncope. An EP study is rarely needed to make the diagnosis. When performed it involves rapid atrial pacing, then determining how long it takes the SA note to fire when pacing is terminated (the "sinus node recovery time").

The rapid atrial rhythms are controlled using the therapies described earlier. Most patients need beta blockade, diltiazem, verapamil or digoxin. However, these medicines aggravate the bradyarrhythmia—hence the need for both drug treatment and cardiac pacing.

Pacemaker Therapy

The most common indication for cardiac pacing is a symptomatic bradyarrhythmia. It is important to document the slow rhythm while the patient is having symptoms. When there are no symptoms, pacemaker therapy is indicated for complete heart block, Mobitz II block (the patient usually has symptoms) or asystolic pauses at least 4 seconds in duration.

As noted in Chapter 4, permanent pacing is rarely needed for third-degree block caused by inferior MI. The level of block is the AV node, and spontaneous recovery is the rule.

Pacemaker Nomenclature

A three-letter code is used. The first letter refers to the chamber paced, the second to the chamber sensed, and the third to the "mode of response" (inhibited or triggered). Single chamber, VVI pacing is the simplest pacing system: a lead in the right ventricle paces the heart, and the same lead is the sensor. If the heart rate is adequate, the pacer senses this and is inhibited for a preset period. If it senses no ventricular beat (there is a pause), it paces the ventricle.

For some time, dual-chamber pacers had a pacing electrode in the ventricle and only a sensing electrode in the right atrium. This sensed a P wave and triggered a ventricular beat (VAT pacing).

The modern dual chamber pacer is DDD: it paces both the atrium and ventricle and senses with both electrodes. When the atrial lead senses a P wave, it inhibits atrial pacing. If the ventricular lead does not sense a QRS on time, it paces the ventricle.

Physiologic Pacing

Single chamber ventricular pacing protects against a slow heart rate. However, it bypasses atrial contraction, and the atrial contribution to diastolic filling is lost. This may be intolerable for the patient with LV diastolic dysfunction. In such cases, stroke volume may fall 25% or more. This is common problem for elderly patients who tend to have stiff left ventricles (and who are the major consumers of cardiac pacing).

The "pacemaker syndrome" is one consequence of VVI pacing and loss of atrial contraction. The patient describes spells of fatigue or weakness caused by an abrupt fall in cardiac output whenever the ventricular pacemaker turns on. The solution is dual chamber pacing which preserves atrial contraction.

DDD pacing is thus useful when there is abnormal LV function. Note that DDD pacing is not possible when the underlying rhythm is AF. Intermittent AF leads to "mode switching;" the DDD pacer switches to the VVI mode. When interrogation in the device clinic documents mode switching, you will be notified that your patient probably is having paroxysmal AF and should be treated—anticoagulation, rate control, etc.

Pacemaker Follow-Up and Troubleshooting

All patients should be enrolled in a device clinic. Regular telephone monitoring using a fingertip electrode and a transmitter allows remote troubleshooting. Pacemaker leads and batteries may fail unexpectedly, and failure is easily detected with telephone telemetry. A drop in the pacing rate indicates that the battery is reaching end-of-life.

If the pacer is not firing at all because the patient has a normal rhythm and rate, it is still possible to check pacemaker function. The patient places a magnet—which comes with the pacemaker—over the battery pack. This temporarily turns the sensing function off and the pacer fires at its fixed rate, documenting that it is able to pace the heart. You may use a magnet in the emergency room to establish fixed rate pacing; usually there are pacemaker magnets stuck on a cabinet.

Patients ask about electrical interference, but the shielding of contemporary pacemakers is effective. Household appliances, microwave ovens, cellular telephones, and airport security scanning are not a problem, although it makes sense to avoid direct contact of the electrical device and the pacemaker battery.

More powerful electromagnetic devices such as arc welding equipment may be a threat, and the pacemaker company should be consulted when there is a doubt about safety.

Direct current cardioversion, electroconvulsive therapy, lithotripsy and electrocautery during surgery are safe as long as they do not direct energy to the region of the pacemaker battery. On the other hand, magnetic resonance imaging subjects the pacemaker to intense magnetic fields and is generally contraindicated (MRI compatible pacemakers are now available, though used infrequently). Radiation therapy may alter pacer function if the battery is directly in the radiation beam. In both cases, if absolutely needed, contact the device clinic.

SYNCOPE

The sudden loss of consciousness may occur when systolic blood pressure falls below 70 mmHg (and usually much lower). A drop in cardiac output or arterial dilation are the usual causes, and common etiologies are reviewed in Table 8.4. As a rule, syncope caused by heart disease conveys a worse prognosis, while vasovagal syncope is benign.

This is a rough outline of the cause of syncope. Because of the long list it would seem to be a complicated evaluation. However, as you read through the text, you will see that the history, physical exam, ECG and echocardiogram are adequate work-up for most patients.

Table 8.4 Syncope

Cardiac Causes
Slow heart rate: Heart block (Stokes-Adams attacks), asystole, atrial fibrillation with a slow ventricular rate (common in elderly patients, and a feature of the tachy-brady syndrome). Most

bradyarrhythmias may be aggravated by digoxin, beta blockers, verapamil and diltiazem.

Rapid ventricular rhythms: The echocardiogram and ECG exclude most causes of VT (low LVEF, prolonged QT interval, HOCM, RV dysplasia)

Mechanical causes of low cardiac output: Left heart: aortic stenosis, hypertrophic cardiomyopathy with LV outflow tract obstruction, atrial myxoma, prosthetic valve malfunction. Rarely syncope complicates mitral stenosis and aortic regurgitation. Right heart: RV dysplasia, pulmonary embolism, primary pulmonary hypertension, pulmonic valve stenosis, Eisenmenger's syndrome, tetralogy of Fallot (pulmonary outflow obstruction), pericardial tamponade.

Pacemaker failure: Loss of pacing and severe bradycardia.

Noncardiac Causes (disorders of blood pressure control)
Volume depletion or overshoot with blood pressure therapy (often in combination): Syncope immediately upon standing.

Neurocardiogenic, vasovagal syncope: The most common cause of syncope, with the diagnosis based on clinical history (see text). Syncope is delayed, a few minutes after standing.

Carotid sinus syncope: Usually elderly patients. About 25% report symptoms with stimulation of the carotid sinus (sudden turns, shaving, a tight collar). A few have pathologic conditions of the neck (tumor, prior radiation, large lymph nodes, prior trauma or surgery).

Situational syncope: Micturition, cough or sneeze, defecation and straining, swallowing and Valsalva syncope. Vagal activation is the usual mechanism, and is treated like other vasovagal syndromes (text).

<u>Migraine syndromes:</u> Syncope is possible, but other features of migraine are usually present.

<u>Metabolic:</u> Hypoglycemia, hypoxia, hyperventilation (with associated finger and circumoral tingling, and suggestive history).

<u>Hysterical syncope:</u> A diagnosis of exclusion.

The patient's other cardiac or medical history may point to an etiology. Thus, a history of MI or heart failure would be consistent with VT as the cause. An elderly person with no history of heart disease but with left bundle branch block may have intermittent complete heart block.

The evaluation and treatment of cardiac arrhythmias has been reviewed. Arrhythmias are uncommon in otherwise healthy young people. Think instead of neurocardiogenic or carotid sinus syncope, and screen for other cardiac lesions that may not be apparent on physical examination.

I find that the house staff is quick to order carotid Doppler studies when evaluating new syncope. It is a waste of time; carotid disease causes TIA or stroke, both with lateralizing neurologic symptoms. Ischemia of both cerebral hemispheres would be required for loss of consciousness. Basilar artery ischemia can cause dizziness or syncope, and it is accompanied by other brainstem, cranial nerve symptoms. Furthermore, the basilar arteries cannot be evaluated with noninvasive studies in the vascular laboratory (this is not a part of the "carotid Doppler study").

Neurocardiogenic (Vasodepressor, Vaso-Vagal) Syncope

Before the discovery of this illness, most cases of syncope were labeled idiopathic. Neurocardiogenic syncope is responsible for most of these, and it is the single most common cause of syncope.

The pathophysiology is related to the autonomic reflexes that control blood pressure with changes in posture. It goes something like this: the initiating event is venous pooling with a shift to upright posture. Reduced venous return leads to lower cardiac output, which activates arterial baroreceptors. They send a signal to the central blood pressure regulating center, which in turn sends a signal to increase adrenergic tone. Both heart rate and LV contractility increase. So far, all this is the normal response to the change in position.

There are stretch receptors in the LV that sense the increase in contractility. For uncertain reasons, patients with neurally-mediated syncope have an overshoot of the LV stretch-receptor response to the increase in contractility. These receptors are connected to the central vasomotor center, and there are two responses to its excessive activation: *vagal discharge*, leading to decreased heart rate and vasodilation (and rarely, asystole), and *withdrawal of sympathetic tone*, aggravating vasodilation and hypotension. In most cases, hypotension is the predominant mechanism leading to syncope.

This complex series of signals between peripheral stretch receptors, and the blood pressure control center in the mid-brain takes some time, leading to a characteristic delay in syncope after the change in posture. Most patients are upright for 2 to 5 minutes before dizziness begins, but the symptom may be delayed as much as 15 min.

A typical history is, "I got up, walked to the kitchen to fix a cup of tea, and fell while standing at the sink." Syncope can occur while sitting as well as with standing.

On the other hand, when a patient describes dizziness immediately upon standing, think of drug-induced hypotension (too much BP medicine), hypovolemia, or both.

That's it. The diagnosis is based on the history, and the key is whether syncope occurs immediately on standing or is delayed.

You may try to elicit neurocardiogenic syncope at the bedside, having the patient stand while monitoring blood pressure, but you must monitor for 10-15 minutes. A more formal approach is the *tilt-table test* which monitors arterial pressure even longer. One study reported a mean time to syncope of 12 minutes after upright tilt. Strapping the patient to the tilt table avoids muscular activity that may prevent the initial vagal response. Repeating it with isoproterenol infusion may increase the sensitivity of this test, although this reduces specificity (more false positives).

That said, enthusiasm for tilt table testing has waned. False negatives are common. With a negative tilt study but typical symptoms—syncope after rising with some delay—there is little point in pursuing an alternative diagnosis.

POTS: the postural orthostatic tachycardia syndrome is a variant of the neurocardiogenic syndrome that is most common in young women. It is defined by an orthostatic rise in heart rate more than 30 beats/min. This may add palpitations to the combination of symptoms described. The diagnosis is occasionally made for a young person with persistent tachycardia, and autonomic dysfunction may be a cause (a gene related to norepinephrine metabolism has been identified in a small subset of patients).

Treatment of Vaso-Vagal Syncope

Increasing vascular volume is the basis of most treatment. Diuretics should be stopped if possible, and extra dietary salt allowed. Hydration with water alone is less effective than electrolyte containing drinks; Gatorade is a commonly prescribed CV treatment. Fludrocortisone, a salt retaining mineralocorticoid, is occasionally used for volume expansion. Elastic stockings may help to prevent venous pooling.

Patients taking antihypertensive medicine may improve if the dose is reduced and blood pressure is allowed to rise. A number of other medicines may be tried, although the results are variable. Beta blockers have been used to block the inappropriate increase in LV contractility that is a part of the reflex loop. Midodrine, an alpha-adrenergic agonist, may help, although our personal experience is disappointing. SSRI's have been used, as have other medicines. With any therapeutic trial, stop the medicine if it isn't helping.

An occasional patient has vagal symptoms as a prodrome—clamminess, mild nausea, contracting vision, a closed-in feeling—and this makes the diagnosis more certain. In such cases where there is warning, isometric exercise may abort the attack. Isometric exercise—even hand grip—prompts an immediate increase in alpha adrenergic tone, raising blood pressure within a few seconds.

A young person with neurocardiogenic syncope may have long periods of asystole. It is quite alarming to witness 4-8 second pauses on telemetry, and such pauses usually cause a loss of consciousness. These spells often respond to beta blockade (oddly enough), and pacemaker therapy may not be needed.

Aerobic exercise—a walking program—often helps.

Chapter 9: Hypertension, Aortic Disease and Cor Pulmonale

Abbreviations

AAA, abdominal aortic aneurysm
ACEI angiotensin converting enzyme inhibitor/inhibition
ARB, angiotensin receptor blocker/blockade
BP, blood pressure
CTA, CT angiography
CAD, coronary artery disease
CHF, congestive heart failure
CPAP, continuous positive airway pressure
CVD, cardiovascular disease
ECG, electrocardiogram
HTN, hypertension
JNC, Joint National Committee providing blood pressure
treatment standards
LDL, low density lipoprotein (cholesterol)
LV, left ventricle (ventricular)
LVEF, LV ejection fraction
LVH, LV hypertrophy
MFS, Marfan's syndrome
MI, myocardial infarction
MRFIT, Multiple Risk Factor Intervention Trial
MRA, magnetic resonance angiography
P_2, pulmonic second heart sound
PA, pulmonary artery
PPH, primary pulmonary hypertension
PVR, pulmonary vascular resistance
RAA, renin-angiotensin-aldosterone (system)
RA, right atrium
RBBB, right bundle branch block
RV, right ventricle
SCD, sudden cardiac death
TR, tricuspid valve regurgitation

HYPERTENSION

The reason to treat HTN is to prevent end organ damage, primarily cardiovascular (CV) and kidney disease. Declining mortality rates from stroke and coronary artery disease (CAD) over the last 40 may be attributed in part to more effective antihypertensive therapy. The Framingham study in the 1960s identified hypertensive heart disease as the most common cause of congestive heart failure (CHF); now CAD dominates, probably because of better therapy for HTN. In clinical trials, antihypertensive treatment lowered the rate of stroke by 40%, myocardial infarction by 25% and CHF by more than 50%.

Yet we are not doing as well as we should. In the 1990s, a "rule of halves" was described for the United States and Western Europe based on population surveys: half the hypertensive population was undetected, half of those diagnosed were untreated, and half of those treated had inadequate control. It is slightly better now; but 30% with HBP are not aware they have it.

Evaluating Hypertension

Blood pressure should be measured with the patient seated, at least 30 minutes after exposure to coffee or cigarettes. Smokers often stop for a last drag before coming into the office. An elevated pressure should be reconfirmed in 5-10 minutes in the other arm. If still elevated, HTN should not be diagnosed until elevated pressure is confirmed with two subsequent visits. Have the office nurse check the pressure with the patient not scheduled to see the doctor; this may help avoid "white coat hypertension." You and your staff should tell the patient what the blood pressure is.

Blood pressure is a continuous variable with CVD risk beginning to increase when blood pressure rises above 115/75. The incidence of CVD doubles for each incremental increase of 20/10 mm Hg. Furthermore, those in the prehypertension category have twice the risk of developing HTN. At lower levels, lifestyle modification may be adequate. Both systolic and diastolic hypertension are indications for treatment, although *elevated systolic pressure is the more potent risk factor for CVD*.

While a systolic pressure of 115 mmHg might seem ideal, there have been no trials testing whether *drug treatment* to push it to that level improves outcome. In fact, guidelines for management of HTN have raised the treatment target to a systolic pressure of 150 mmHg for those ≥ 60 years old, and 140 mmHg for younger patients, even those with diabetes or azotemia. That decision has been controversial, since we have targeted a systolic pressure of 130 mmHg for diabetic patients for years.

Examination and Laboratory Studies

The goal of the initial evaluation is to gauge the risk of CVD, detect end-organ disease, and screen for correctible cause of HTN. Risk factors for CVD, particularly the metabolic syndrome, have been reviewed in Chapter 4.

Abnormalities on physical examination that are noteworthy include retinal arterial narrowing, depressed lower extremity pulses or blood pressure (coarctation of the aorta), a forceful cardiac apical impulse or S_4 gallop, and an abnormal abdominal exam (bruit, enlarged aorta, masses). Retinal artery narrowing (A/V < 2/3) gives some idea about long term BP control, much like Hgb-A1C with diabetes, and I consider it a go-to physical finding.

As an exercise, try to justify each of the following laboratory tests commonly recommended for newly diagnosed HTN. Do it before reading our explanation (and let us know if we missed something obvious).

Urinalysis. Urine glucose is a crude screen for diabetes. Albuminuria is a diagnostic criterion for kidney disease, even when serum creatinine is normal. Like other indicators of end-organ disease it signals a need for more aggressive treatment. Proteinuria has also been identified as a risk factor for early CVD. Trace albumin should be followed-up with a 24 hour urine exam.

Chemistries. Serum *potassium* is especially important. When low and off diuretics, it may indicate hyperaldosteronism (Conn's syndrome) as the cause of hypertension. Hypokalemia is a dangerous complication of diuretic therapy and seems worse with thiazides than loop diuretics. Out-of-hospital cardiac arrest can complicate hypokalemia and thiazide use. The MRFIT trial showed no mortality benefit with risk factor modification with early follow-up (there was a benefit later). An excess of sudden cardiac death (SCD) in the treated group was ascribed to thiazide therapy and hypokalemia.

Sodium measurement is less useful in patients with mild hypertension and who are otherwise healthy. In those with CHF, low sodium indicates poor prognosis and is a marker of high plasma renin activity (and increased sensitivity to ACE inhibition—start with low dose therapy).

Creatinine and blood urea nitrogen are important as screens for underlying renal dysfunction and is also an indication for more aggressive therapy. Elevated glucose can indicate diabetes when measured in a fasting state, but elevated hemoglobin A1c makes the diagnosis. Hyperglycemia may also be associated with secondary causes of HBP including Cushing's syndrome, pheochromocytoma, and primary aldosteronism.

Lipid analysis is a part of the CVD risk assessment. High tryglycerides and low HDL cholesterol are features of the metabolic syndrome (along with abdominal obesity, glucose intolerance and hypertension). In this case, the LDL cholesterol level may be normal, but the LDL particles tend to be small and dense and are more atherogenic.

Calcium and phosphate measurement is a screen for hyperparathyroidism, a potential cause of HTN. *Uric acid* may rise with diuretic therapy, and a baseline is useful. The *hematocrit* has little direct relationship to HTN, but it is cheap and reasonable to screen for anemia if the patient is to have blood drawn.

Electrocardiogram. The ECG is a crude tool. Its sensitivity for detecting left ventricular hypertrophy (LVH) is less than 50%. The earliest sign of hypertensive heart disease may be left atrial abnormality, usually a biphasic P wave in V_1 (Figure 9.1). Suspicion of LVH is a reasonable indication for an echocardiogram. Making that diagnosis also confirms hypertensive heart disease—e.g. end-organ disease—and reinforces a need for aggressive BP control.

Figure 9.1 Left Atrial Abnormality

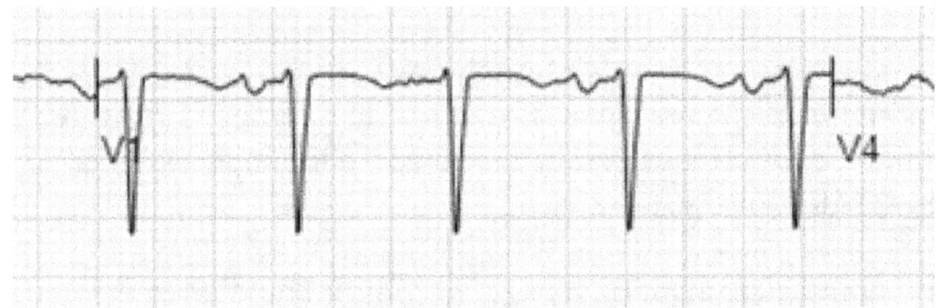

Figure 9.1 The diagnostic criterion is a biphasic P wave in V_1, and the terminal, negative deflection should be a box wide and deep.

A *chest x-ray* is another sensible and relatively inexpensive screen for a middle aged person. It is relatively unreliable as a test for cardiac enlargement. Patients with LVH have "concentric" hypertrophy with little chamber enlargement. Coarctation of the aorta may cause rib notching (by collateral vessels) and a "3"sign (dilated ascending aorta).

Secondary Hypertension

Hypertension is a complication of a number of illnesses, many of them apparent from the screening evaluation. There is an element of uncertainty when deciding how much farther to go when looking for a correctible cause of HTN. Current guidelines suggest testing for identifiable causes if BP control is difficult.

About 5-10% of HTN is secondary (Table 9.1). That does not seem like much, yet HTN is so common that we all see cases. In some series, renovascular hypertension accounts for 5%. Primary aldosteronism (0.5%), coarctation of the aorta (0.5%), pheochromocytoma (0.2%) and Cushing's syndrome (0.1%) are much less common. Sleep apnea and excessive alcohol use are often overlooked, and BP control may depend on their correction.

Table 9.1: Secondary Causes of Hypertension (with Signs and Evaluation)

1. Renal artery stenosis: HTN under age 20; new onset HTN + a recent increase in creatinine (Cr); a rise in Cr after starting ACEI treatment; abdominal/flank bruit. Screen with renal Doppler studies, MRA or CTA.

2. Hyperaldosteronism (Conn's syndrome): Hypokalemia (especially if the patient is on ACEI/ARB therapy). Measure renin/aldosterone ratio; if abnormal, a CT scan for adrenal adenoma. This is the cause of drug resistant HTN in more than 20%. It usually is overlooked; the hypokalemia is attributed to diuretic therapy.

3. Sleep apnea: Snoring, day-time somnolence, thick neck. Sleep study.

4. Pheochromocytoma: Paroxysmal HTN, headache, flushing, tachycardia. Urinary catecholamine metabolites (metanephrines, VMA).

5. Hypothyroidism: Diastolic HTN, fatigue, weight loss, weakness. TSH and free thyroxine level.

6. Hyperthyroidism: Systolic HTN, heat intolerance, weight loss, tremor, new AF. TSH and free thyroxine level.

7. Hyperparathyroidism: Kidney stones, osteoporosis, weakness, lethargy. Serum calcium and parathyroid hormone levels.

8. Chronic renal disease

9. Coarctation of the aorta: Decreased or delayed femoral pulses, low leg BP. Chest xray (rib notching, 3 sign), CT scan of the aorta.

10. Excessive alcohol intake: Take this history when BP control is a problem, and evaluate with a trial of abstinence.

11. Cushing's syndrome: Typical physical findings. Dexamethasone suppression test.

12. Drug side effects: NSAIDs, estrogen birth control pills, appetite suppressants, pseudoephedrine, monoamine oxidase inhibitors (Nardil), nicotine, amphetamines, testosterone, erythropoietin, cyclosporin.

NSAID, non-steroidal anti-inflammatory drug; Cr, creatinine; CT, computed tomography; TSH, thyroid stimulating hormone; ACEI, angiotensin converting enzyme inhibitor; ARB, angiotensin receptor blocker; MRA, magnetic resonance angiography; VMA, vanillylmandelic

---

Treatment of Hypertension

Practice guidelines emphasize lifestyle modification, including weight loss, sodium restriction, physical activity and reduced alcohol consumption. The Dietary Approach to Stop Hypertension (DASH) diet lowers the systolic BP about 10 mm Hg; it is rich in fruits and low-fat dairy products (and thus is high in potassium and calcium), and is low in saturated fats. The DASH diet plus a 1.6 gm sodium limit is as effective as single drug therapy in reducing BP. We have little information about the long-term effects of popular low carbohydrate diets (e.g., the Atkins diet).

Drug Therapy

The JNC (the Joint National Committee) 8 targets for systolic and diastolic pressure follow:
$\geq$60 years old, 150/90
< 60 years old, 140/90, or $\geq$ 60 in patients with diabetes or chronic kidney disease

Thus, if treatment brings the BP to 130/95, additional treatment is warranted to push the diastolic pressure below 90 mmHg.

Clinical trials evaluating CVD outcomes have found no drug class superior to thiazide diuretics as initial treatment. Furthermore, diuretics enhance the actions of other drugs. One reason for failure of vasodilator therapy is inadequate diuresis. Sodium retention is a normal response to vasodilatation—it is perceived by the kidney as hypovolemia. Control of pressure requires correction of the consequent hypervolemia.

Table 9.2 The JNC 8 Treatment Recommendations

1. <u>General, nonblack population</u>: thiazides, calcium channel blockers (CCB), ACEI or ARB as initial therapy.

2. <u>General black population</u>: thiazides or CCB initially

3. <u>Chronic kidney disease:</u> treatment should include ACEI or ARB (slows progression of disease)

4. <u>Uptitrate or add therapy</u> at one month intervals until target is reached.

5. <u>ACEI and ARBs</u>: do not use together

6. <u>If 3 drugs are needed</u>, refer to a hypertension specialist (nephrologists, not cardiologists are HTN specialists)

The most notable change with drug recommendations is exclusion of beta blockers from the list first or second drugs to use. There are some additional principals that guide treatment:

Most patients require multiple drugs to reach the BP goal. Combination pills simplify treatment and lower cost.

A common reason for treatment failure is omission of diuretics. Vasodilators alone may prompt salt and water retention so diuretics should be added early. Thiazides work better than loop diuretics when renal function is normal, probably because the duration of action is much longer than loop diuretics. Note that the half-life of hydrochlorthiazide is 4-12 hours, but that of chlorthalidone is > 24 hours. Loop diuretics are indicated when creatinine is elevated.

Other illness influences the choice of therapy. Thus, a patient with vascular disease, congestive heart failure, chronic kidney disease or diabetes should be on an ACEI, since there is a survival benefit. Beta blockers improve prognosis in those with a history of MI, or heart failure with low LVEF.

The incidence of cough with ACEI drugs is about 10%, and angioedema is common. A student asked why we don't start with an ARB—a good question. The answer is that the two drug classes do not produce identical effects. ACE (the enzyme) contributes to the breakdown of both bradykinin and substance P so the ACE inhibitors lead to increases in both substances. This is the mechanism of ACEI induced cough and angioedema, since both can cause bronchoconstriction as well as vasodilation.

Chronic Kidney Disease (CKD)

Patients with kidney disease (creatinine >1.5 mg/dL for men, >1.4 mg/dL for women) tend to have a steady decline in creatinine clearance. The rate of decline is slower when BP is lowered to ≤130/80. Multidrug therapy is usually needed and should include blockade of the rennin-angiotensin-aldosterone system (RAAS) with an ACEI or ARB. The renal protective effect of RAA blockade applies to both nondiabetic and diabetic patients, and it is most pronounced for those with proteinuria. ACE inhibition reduces proteinuria. Those with mild renal dysfunction also have a higher incidence of CVD, and ACEI therapy lowers the rate of cardiac events.

Medical residents often avoid ACEI therapy when creatinine is elevated. On the contrary, RAAS blockade is *indicated,* since it slows the progression of CKD with both diabetic and hypertensive nephropathy; the only contraindication is renal artery stenosis. Recheck a creatinine a couple days after starting RAAS blocking therapy. A rise in serum creatinine > 0.3 mg/dL suggests co-existing renal artery stenosis, which should be evaluated. Renal dysfunction plus *hyperkalemia* is a contraindication to ACE inhibitors or ARBs.

Diuretics and reduced sodium intake are especially important since sodium retention is a common feature of renal dysfunction. Nonsteroidal anti-inflammatory drugs may provoke renal vasoconstriction and further lower glomerular filtration leading to salt retention and possibly to hyperkalemia. They and potassium containing salt substitutes should be avoided.

African-Americans

As a group they have earlier onset HTN and are more likely to have end-organ disease. For years we thought that the RAAS played a minor role when compared with other racial groups. This was based upon the relative ineffectiveness of ACE inhibitors as monotherapy when compared with diuretics and calcium channel blockers. The critical observation, however, is that monotherapy with any drug is ineffective for this group, especially with ACE inhibitors or beta blockers.

With appropriate combination therapy, both ACE inhibition and beta blockade are effective for black patients. The African-American Study of Kidney Disease (AASK) trial compared ramipril, metoprolol and amlodipine plus diuretic therapy in patients with moderate renal dysfunction (glomerular filtration rate 20-60 mL/min). The BP response was identical in the ramipril and amlodipine arms, but the rate of decline of renal function was substantially better with ramipril therapy. Thus, for Black patients, 1) ACE inhibition is as effective as calcium channel blockade in lowering BP when used as part of a multidrug regimen, 2) it provides the best protection of renal function and thus should be the first choice of therapy. The study underscores an important management principle: drug therapy is about more than lowering blood pressure. The other actions of drugs independent of BP effects—renal or vascular protection—are at least as important.

That sound good, but the latest JNC recommendation for Black patients favored CCBs as initial therapy, not ACEI. On the other hand, when there is elevation of creatinine, RAAS blockade is indicated.

Elderly Patients

About two thirds of people older than 65 years has HTN; this is a group that is undertreated. The work-up and choice of drugs is no different than with younger patients, although new guidelines suggest a more lenient target: 150/90. An abrupt rise in BP suggests atherosclerotic renal artery stenosis, especially when there is an increase in creatinine.

Postural hypotension is more common in older patients, and you should start with lower dose therapy to avoid this side effect. Volume depletion is a common cause. For this reason, targeting therapy to an upright blood pressure makes sense for older patients. If the blood pressure is borderline, measure it after a walk down the hall and while standing. Also be aware of the BP lowering effect of other drugs, especially those used to treat older men with prostate disease.

Women

Oral contraceptives raise blood pressure, and this effect increases with the duration of therapy. Hormone replacement therapy, with its lower dose of estrogen, has no effect on BP.

During pregnancy, ACE inhibitors and ARBs should not be used because of fetal toxicity (avoid them if there is a chance of pregnancy). Methyldopa and nifedipine are safe. Beta blockers may be used late in pregnancy but can slow fetal growth. Thiazides may be used, but furosemide may be embryotoxic.

Resistance to Drug Therapy

The incidence of drug resistant hypertension is about 20% and this should prompt reconsideration of secondary hypertension (Table 9.1), or noncompliance with the medicine regimen. In the absence of these illnesses, common causes of drug resistance are outlined in Table 9.3. The most common of these are noncompliance, inadequate diuretic therapy, use of nonsteroidal anti-inflammatory drugs, excessive alcohol intake, hypokalemia, and sleep apnea. More recently, hyperaldosteronism has been found in more than 20% of those resistant to multidrug therapy. Spironolactone usually works, but the possibility merits diagnostic testing (measure renin/aldosterone ratio; if abnormal, a CT scan for adrenal adenoma).

Table 9.3 Treatment Resistant HTN (in addition to causes of secondary HTN, Table 9.1)

Pseudo resistance
1. White coat hypertension
2. Use of a regular cuff on an obese arm

Noncompliance to therapy
1. Excess salt intake

Drug-related causes
1. Dose too low or incorrect dosing schedule
2. Failure to add a diuretic
3. Wrong diuretic (loop diuretic is needed with high creatinine)
4. Hypokalemia, thiazide induced (correction can lower BP; but think about hyperaldosteronism)
5. Other drugs: nasal decongestants, appetite suppressants, cocaine, oral contraceptives, steroids, cyclosporine, erythropoietin, antidepressants, nonsteroidal anti-inflammatory drugs

Associated conditions
1. Sleep apnea
2. Increasing obesity
3. Insulin resistance/hyperinsulinemia (metabolic syndrome)
4. Alcohol intake >1 oz per day (often overlooked, and changing this can help!)
5. Chronic pain

It is common for primary care providers to send problem hypertension to cardiology clinic, but it is probably the wrong choice. Nephrology does a better job. Most cardiologists have less hands-on experience with management of HTN than the general internist.

DISEASES OF THE AORTA

Abdominal Aortic Aneurysm (AAA)

About three fourths of aortic aneurysms are limited to the abdomen, originating below the renal arteries and usually sparing the visceral circulation. The size of the AAA determines the chance of rupture. There is a 50% chance of rupture in one year with a diameter >6 cm, 15-20% when the AAA measures 5-6 cm, and less than 2% with a diameter <4 cm. Without surgery, the 5-year mortality with an aneurysm larger than 6 cm is about 90%.

Most AAAs are detected during abdominal examination or with ultrasound screening studies. Because of the high mortality risk with undetected, large aneurysms, routine screening with abdominal ultrasound has been recommended for men 60 years old, especially smokers.

AAA is an atherosclerotic illness, and cigarette smoking, male sex and family history are the major risk factors. Recall that wall tension = intraluminal pressure x radius (LaPlace's law). Thus, hypertension—high intraluminal pressure—contributes to aneurysm growth. As expansion occurs in 80% of patients, time is another risk factor for rupture. Gradual expansion is the rule with 20% enlarging rapidly (more than 0.5 cm per year).

Randomized trials compared surveillance vs. early surgery for small AAA and found no advantage with surgery for aneurysms less than 5.5 cm. In addition to AAA size, the patient's general medical condition also influences the timing of surgery. When the general health is good, surgery is recommended for an AAA ≥ 5.5 cm. On the other hand, a patient with multiple medical problems who is considered a poor surgical candidate may have repair delayed until the aneurysm approaches 6 cm. Mortality with elective surgery in the ADAM trial was just 1.8%, substantially better than a decade earlier. Surgical mortality is higher with rapidly expanding aneurysms (5-15%), while surgery during acute rupture has a mortality risk closer to 40%.

The newest approach is endovascular aneurysm repair using stents. The first devices were introduced in the early 1990s, and current models have been tested in more than 1000 patients. With proper patient selection, stenting works well and appears a durable solution to AAA. Its role in treating rupture is uncertain.

The medical therapy of small AAA begins with risk factor modification and blood pressure control. Beta blockade has not been found to have special benefit for abdominal aneurysm. Reducing vascular inflammation may help, and GDMT for atherosclerosis is indicated: statin, aspirin, ACEI/ARB therapy.

Thoracic Aortic Aneurysm

In young patients the usual cause is Marfan's syndrome (MFS) or other connective tissue disease, while older patients have atherosclerotic disease. Bicuspid aortic valve is associated with ascending aortic aneurysm and dissection, and current guidelines call for treating this like MFS. Expanding aneurysms may cause pain or compression symptoms—hoarseness, cough, dysphagia, or the superior vena cava syndrome.

A diameter greater than 7 cm indicates a high risk of rupture. Surgery is recommended when the diameter of the thoracic aneurysms reaches 5.5 cm when atherosclerosis is the cause. For patients with Marfan's syndrome, other connective tissue disease, or bicuspid aortic valve, repair is indicated at 4.5 cm. Small patients possibly should have repair earlier, as should those with rapid expanding aneurysms base on serial imaging. A family history of aneurysm and dissection at an early age would lead to repair of an aneurysm in the 4.5 cm range. High surgical risk would favor delaying surgery in the absence of symptoms. Expansion tends to be slow with aneurysms smaller than 5 cm, and annual CT or MRI imaging is adequate. Above 5 cm the expansion rate increases four-fold, and twice-yearly imaging is needed.

Medical therapy includes risk factor modification and control of hypertension. Beta blockade is indicated for thoracic aneurysm. Reducing the velocity of LV ejection protects the ascending aorta. This has been proven for those with Marfan's syndrome, and beta blockade makes sense as initial antihypertensive treatment for all with thoracic aneurysm. (AS noted earlier, studies of AAA showed no benefit with beta blockade; the shearing force of the LV ejection wave apparently dissipates by the time it reaches the distal aorta.)

Losartan, an ARB, has been found to lower the rate of dilation of the aortic root in adults and children with MFS. The basic defect in Marfan's is deficiency or malformation of the fibrillin-1 protein. This affects the structural integrity of the extracellular matrix in the aortic wall, which in turn causes the release of transforming growth factor-beta (TGF-beta). TGF-beta contributes to aortic media degeneration. Losartan inhibits the expression of TGF-beta. The effect is limited to the proximal, and there is no apparent effect on the mid and distal ascending aorta. The therapeutic approach is new, and the initial, small randomized trial showed no survival benefit. It has not been tested as adjunctive therapy to beta blockade.

Pregnancy is high risk with MFS and should be avoided if the proximal aorta is larger than 4.0 cm.

Thoracic Aortic Dissection
Risk factors for dissection are poorly controlled hypertension, advanced age, and medial disease. A number of inherited aortic diseases may cause it including Marfan's, Loeys-Deitz, and Ehlers-Danlos syndromes, coarctation, bicuspid aortic valve, arteritis and Turner and Noonan syndromes. Men are more commonly affected. Over age 50, hypertension is the usual etiology, and under age 40, Marfan's syndrome is the most common cause. While those with an aneurysm are at increased risk for dissection, not all dissections begin with a large aneurysm.

The standard classification of dissection is based on location: Type A dissection begins in the proximal aorta, just above the aortic valve, and accounts for three fourths of cases. A Type A dissection may extend all the way around to the distal aorta (DeBakey class 1), or may be limited to the proximal aorta (DeBakey class 2). Type B dissection (formerly called DeBakey class 3) begins distal to the left subclavian artery and involves the distal aorta (25% of cases).

Dissection causes chest pain. The diagnosis is often missed, since this is an uncommon cause of chest pain. The pain may be mid chest, and radiation to the back occurs in less than half of cases. *The most useful diagnostic feature is that the pain is at maximum intensity at its onset* (more than 80% of cases, and this figures into board questions routinely). In contrast, the pain of MI or angina starts slowly and crescendos.

The dissection may occlude major branches of the aorta. For example, chest pain plus stroke (carotid occlusion) suggests dissection. On physical examination, indications of limb ischemia, including diminished pulses or unequal blood pressures is evidence for dissection. Acute inferior MI with ST segment elevation on the ECG may occur if the dissection occludes the right coronary ostium. Occlusion of the left coronary ostium is possible, but most with this complication die suddenly. Proximal dissection may cause aortic regurgitation. Neck vein distension suggests rupture into the pericardium and tamponade.

Diagnosis requires a transesophageal echocardiogram or CT or MRI imaging. All are sensitive and specific, and the choice of technique is based on speed and availability. Abdominal ultrasound is a screening test for AAA, and it is not useful for the evaluation of possible dissection of the aorta (nor is transthoracic echocardiography). The mediastinum and/or aorta appear widened on chest x-ray in 80-90% of patients with thoracic dissection, making this a useful but not diagnostic test.

Management is aimed at stopping the progression of dissection. Medical therapy includes: 1) lowering the systolic blood pressure to 100-120 mm Hg if there is adequate perfusion of vital organs (nitroprusside is the intravenous vasodilator of choice); 2) beta blockade to counter the shearing force of LV ejection which may increase with vasodilator therapy; 3) pain control.

Indications for emergency surgery are severe aortic regurgitation, threatened rupture, occlusion of a branch artery and persistent, uncontrollable pain. In addition, surgery improves survival for those with proximal, Type A dissection. It is no better than medical management for those with stable distal dissection. With Type B dissection, a patient who has survived the acute phase and has no indication for emergency surgery has a 1-year survival rate; with both medical and surgical therapy that is about 90%.

Operative mortality ranges from 5% to as high as 70%, with highest risk predicted by cardiac tamponade, renal or visceral ischemia, the site of the tear, coexisting lung disease and delayed time to surgery. Tissue adhesives are now used to join the separated layers of aorta, eradicating the false lumen in more than half the cases. "Glue aortoplasty" results in less bleeding, fewer postoperative complications and probably improved survival (there have been no randomized studies, as there seldom are when a new surgical technique clearly makes things better).

Endovascular stenting has been tested in small numbers of patients who were poor surgical candidates, usually with descending aortic dissection (Type B). Predictably, outcomes have been poor, and at this time stenting is considered a palliative procedure for those whose symptoms are from lower extremity ischemia.

Residual aortic disease requires surgery within 10 years in 20% to 30% of patients who survive aortic dissection, with or without initial surgical therapy. Aggressive medical therapy is needed (risk factor and blood pressure control, beta blockade, statins).

AORTIC TRAUMA

The most common cause is sudden high-speed deceleration during a motor vehicle accident. This creates shearing forces that are greatest where mobile and fixed portions of the aorta meet, most commonly, the aortic isthmus, where the ligamentum arteriousum inserts (the former ductus arteriosus just beyond the left subclavian artery).

The diagnosis may be masked by other injuries. Localized hematoma can cause dyspnea or stridor, dysphagia or the superior vena cava syndrome. There may be an interscapular bruit on exam. The chest x-ray is abnormal in 90% (opacification between the aorta and pulmonary artery or mediastinal widening). Contrast CT or MRI confirms the diagnosis. Surgical correction is usually successful and may prevent sudden death.

CARDIAC COMPLICATIONS OF OTHER MEDICAL ILLNESSES

Chronic Lung Disease (Cor Pulmonale)

Lung disease can cause pulmonary hypertension, leading to right heart failure. Think of it when a patient with lung disease develops peripheral edema. The three mechanisms are *hypoxic vasoconstriction* (especially with chronic bronchitis, cystic fibrosis, obesity hypoventilation—sleep apnea—and other hypoventilation syndromes), *obstruction of the vascular bed* (pulmonary embolism, pulmonary artery hypertension (PAH), sickle cell disease), and *obliteration of lung parenchyma* with loss of vascular surface area (emphysema, bronchiectasis, cystic fibrosis, interstitial lung disease).

Hypoxia is a potent pulmonary vasoconstrictor. When prolonged, there is an increase in the thickness of the walls of small pulmonary artery (PA) branches. With time these changes become permanent. A patient with chronic lung disease plus hypoxia, typically the "blue bloater" with bronchitis, is more prone to cor pulmonale than another with emphysema who has equally severe airway obstruction but normal arterial oxygen saturation (the "pink puffer"). One of the indications for home oxygen therapy is right heart failure, since correction of hypoxemia relieves pulmonary hypertension.

Not everyone with bronchitis develops cor pulmonale. Some patients are susceptible, but most are not. That also appears to be the case with a number of cardiac illnesses where a minority of patients, perhaps 20%, develop pulmonary hypertension and right heart failure, including mitral stenosis, atrial septal defect and cardiomyopathy.

This may be the percentage of the population having hyper-reactive pulmonary vasculature. When stressed with hypoxia or hemodynamic overload. these patients develop pulmonary hypertension. Because the PA clamps down, the left heart is protected, and the clinical picture is isolated right heart CHF.

Clinical and Laboratory Findings

Cor pulmonale is right heart failure—peripheral edema—in a patient with lung disease. The chest x-ray shows no pulmonary congestion, and the echocardiogram confirms normal LV function. Dyspnea is usual but is caused by the lung disease. Palpitations and atrial arrhythmias are common, especially atrial flutter and multifocal atrial tachycardia (Figure 9.2).

Figure 9.2 Multifocal Atrial Tachycardia (MAT).

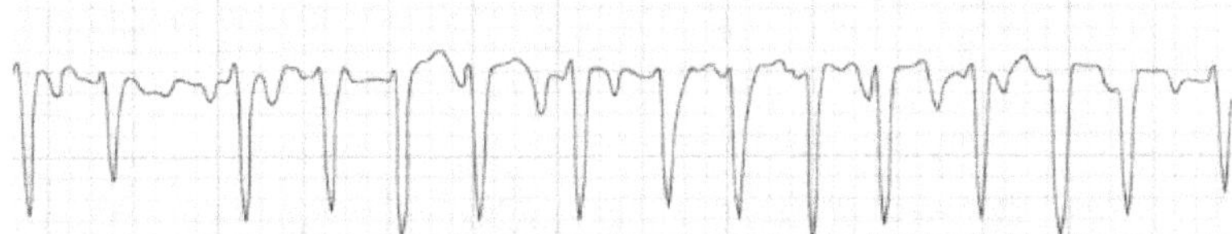

Figure 9.2 This is an irregular rhythm, like atrial fibrillation. It is tachycardia since the rate is above 100/min (with a normal heart rate, it would be called wandering atrial pacemaker). The diagnosis is made from the rhythm strip showing multiple P wave morphologies.

There are a variety of ECG findings with chronic lung disease. The "pulmonary disease pattern" (Figure 9.3) results from a change in the position of the heart in the chest. The rightward shift in the P wave axis is seen as a negative P wave in lead AVL, a finding that indicates emphysema.

Figure 9.3 ECGs with Chronic Lung Disease

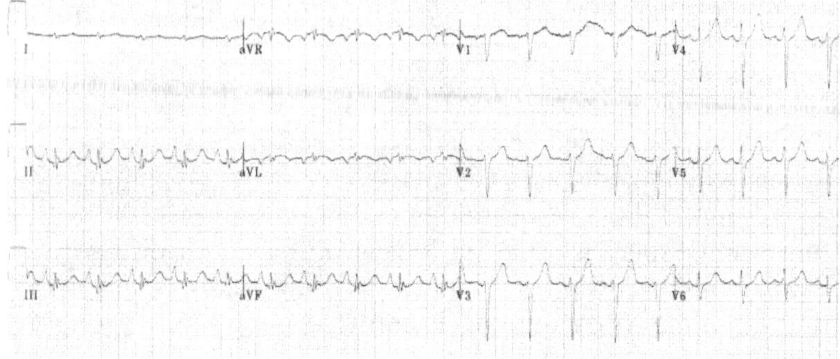

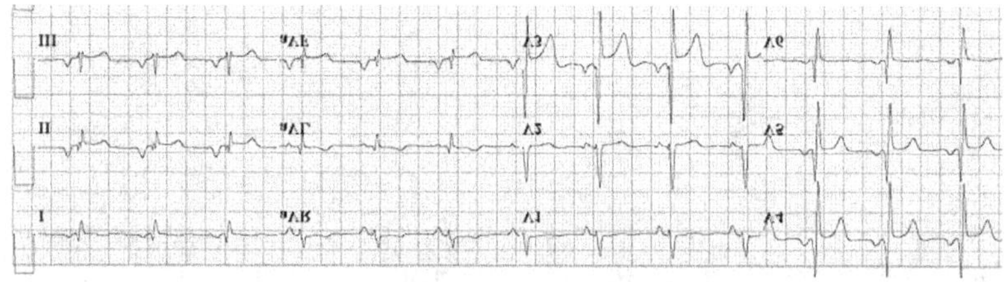

Figure 9.3 <u>Top:</u> There are features suggesting emphysema: low voltage, poor R wave progression, and a negative P wave in aVL which may be diagnostic. In addition, right atrial abnormality (tall P waves in inferior leads), the vertical axis, and persistent S wave in V6 are findings seen with RV hypertrophy. <u>Bottom:</u> Right ventricular hypertrophy with tall R in V_1 and persistent deep S in V_6. Supporting the diagnosis are right axis deviation, right atrial abnormality and T inversion in right precordial leads, the RV strain pattern. If the patient has lung disease and edema, this ECG confirms a diagnosis of cor pulmonale.

Other cardiac findings of right heart failure are subtle and may be hard to detect when the chest exam is grossly abnormal. P_2 is accentuated with pulmonary hypertension. There may be an RV lift and a right side S_3 gallop (audible during inspiration). Jugular venous distension is a prominent finding, and if there is a prominent V wave, consider tricuspid regurgitation. With RV failure there may be an inspiratory rise in jugular venous pressure (Kussmaul's sign) and pulsus paradoxus.

Although the chest exam is abnormal with lung disease, a normal exam does not exclude cor pulmonale. Other causes such as sleep apnea, primary pulmonary hypertension (also called PAH), and recurrent pulmonary embolus may not affect the chest examination.

The chest x-ray findings of PAH and cor pulmonale are enlargement of the RV and central pulmonary arteries. Decreased vessel markings at the periphery in contrast to the large central vessels produce a "pruned tree" appearance. Right ventricular hypertrophy on the ECG indicates pulmonary hypertension and RV overload, making cor pulmonale the likely diagnosis (Figure 9.3). However, there are patients with the disease who do not have RVH on the ECG.

The echocardiogram is the key test, showing RV and possibly right atrial (RA) enlargement. Most with pulmonary hypertension have mild tricuspid regurgitation (often without a murmur), and the TR jet is used for Doppler estimation of PA pressure. The echocardiogram also excludes other causes of pulmonary hypertension such as occult mitral stenosis or left heart failure (systolic or diastolic). In many patients with advanced lung disease, increased air between the echo transducer and the heart prevents good imaging. The clinical diagnosis of cor pulmonale usually is sufficient.

Patients are commonly referred for right heart catheterization. The major finding is elevated PA pressure. The pulmonary wedge pressure—the surrogate for LV filling pressure—is normal unless there is LV dysfunction. Normally the PA diastolic pressure is equal to the wedge pressure, since during diastole the PA, pulmonary capillary bed, pulmonary veins, left atrium and LV are in open communication. With an increase in pulmonary vascular resistance (PVR), PA diastolic pressure is higher than LA or pulmonary wedge pressure.

The hemodynamic diagnosis of cor pulmonale is pulmonary hypertension in the face of normal LV diastolic pressures; it is the lung disease and not left heart failure that causes right heart failure. Smokers get CAD and have MIs, so many with cor pulmonale also have left heart disease. In such cases pulmonary wedge pressure is high, but the PA diastolic pressure is even higher. This transpulmonary gradient defines elevated PVR and is the constant finding of cor pulmonale.

Other diagnostic testing may be needed to determine the etiology. When there is no apparent lung disease, evaluate the patient for pulmonary embolus. Chronic thrombotic pulmonary hypertension—CTEPH—is best diagnosed with a ventilation-perfusion lung scan. A sleep study may be needed to diagnose sleep apnea. In such cases, bradyarrhythmias during sleep are common. Last month the consult team saw a 70 year old patient with edema who had 5 second sinus pauses on telemetry while asleep. The QRS duration and PR intervals were normal. Rather than an urgent pacemaker, we documented sleep apnea and treated his arrhythmia and right heart failure with nocturnal positive pressure ventilation (CPAP).

Treatment

Improving oxygenation relieves pulmonary vasoconstriction. The usual indication for home oxygen therapy with COPD is hypoxemia, an O2 saturation <85%. Cor pulmonale is an indication for home oxygen therapy in those with borderline oxygen saturation. Pulmonary hypertension may improve with part-time, overnight oxygen therapy. However, clinical trials have shown improved survival with 24-hour therapy for patients needing oxygen for chronic lung disease, and those results would apply to patients with cor pulmonale. Supplemental oxygen must be used cautiously when there is chronic hypercarbia and respiratory acidosis. Vigorous treatment of the lung disease is critical.

Specific treatment of the heart failure is of limited benefit. Edema requires diuretic therapy. When there is splanchnic congestion, common with right heart failure, absorption of oral furosemide may be limited; consider using the loop diuretics that are more effectively absorbed (torsemide and bumetanide).

Our pulmonary colleagues occasionally request right heart catheterization to see if vasodilator therapy will lower PA pressure. This often works PAH but seldom does when there is parenchymal lung disease. Afterload reduction therapy using ACEI is not indicated, and beta blockade does not help.

Atrial tachyarrhythmias are common, particularly atrial flutter. Those with cor pulmonale are more susceptible to digitalis toxicity, and beta blocker therapy may exacerbate bronchospasm. For these reasons, verapamil is a better choice for rate control (and is often overlooked). The successful treatment of atrial arrhythmias, like heart failure, requires control of the lung disease. Cardioversion may be considered for atrial flutter, but maintaining sinus rhythm is unlikely unless pulmonary function improves. On the other hand, atrial flutter ablation can be effective, and is relatively low risk.

Pulmonary Artery Hypertension (PAH)—Formerly Known as Primary Pulmonary Hypertension

This uncommon illness is marked by pulmonary vasoconstriction, intimal proliferation and thrombosis in situ. It is probably caused by endothelial dysfunction. It usually affects young women who present with dyspnea; other symptoms include chest pain, edema (right heart failure), light-headedness and syncope. It is a fatal illness, with survival determined by the response to vasodilators.

Anticoagulation is recommended. Vasodilator therapy is critical. Calcium channel blockade works for some patients; in one study a favorable response led to a 94% 5-year survival, compared with 36% in those who did not respond.

Prostacyclin is a vasodilator produced by the endothelium that is deficient in some patients with PAH. It has been shown to increase survival and relieve symptoms, even in those with advanced PAH (functional Class 3-4). On average, patients have at least a 50% reduction in PVR, and the effect persists with chronic therapy. Epoprostenol (Flolan) is given by constant infusion through a permanent central catheter using an ambulatory pump. A few patients have been on it 10 years. Oral and subcutaneous prostacyclins are being developed. More recently, bosentan, an endothelin receptor blocker, has been approved and is the first oral medicine available for PPH. Some respond to sildenafil and other PDE inhibitors.

Other Medical Conditions and Their Cardiovascular Effects

This review focuses on the big picture, and what is included requires picking and choosing. To flesh it out—perhaps to jog your memory—Table 9.4 summarizes cardiovascular effects of a variety of medical illnesses, some that we have not reviewed in detail.

Table 9.4 Cardiovascular Effects of Some Noncardiac Illnesses

Endocrine Disorders:

Cushing's syndrome: HTN in 80%, diagnose with dexamethasone suppression test. Clinical diagnosis is based on body habitus, moon facies, stretch marks.

Hyperaldosteronism (Conn's syndrome): Expanded extracellular volume, moderate diastolic HTN and hypokalemia resistant to replacement therapy. Treat HTN with spironolactone (or resection of an adrenal adenoma).

Adrenocortical insufficiency: Chronic (Addison's disease): asthenia, fatigue, hypotension and a small heart on x-ray. Low morning cortisol level, and failure to respond to stimulating hormone. Acute (Waterhouse-Fredrichsen's syndrome with sepsis): shock.

Hyperparathyroidism: HTN common in elderly patients. Hypercalcemia and hyperphosphatemia. Thiazides may aggravate the hypercalcemia.

Hypoparathyroidism: Hypocalcemia, with long QT interval.

Pheochromocytoma: HTN, sustained in 60% of cases, although labile. Half have paroxysms of flushing and HTN that can resemble anxiety attacks.

Diabetes insipidus: Polyuria and polydipsia, an inability to concentrate the urine. If the patient cannot drink, volume depletion and hypotension soon develop.

Hyperthyroidism: Atrial fibrillation, a common presenting sign, especially in the elderly. Also, sinus tachycardia with decreased systemic vascular resistance, high systolic BP and low diastolic BP (wide pulse pressure), high-output heart failure.

Hypothyroidism: Low heart rate, reduced LV contractility (though CHF is rare and function improves with treatment), increased diastolic BP in 20% but low systolic BP (a narrow pulse pressure), slowly accumulating pericardial effusion that can be massive.

Connective tissue disease:
Systemic lupus erythematosus (SLE): Pericardial effusion (tamponade and constriction are possible). Atypical endocarditis

(Libman-Sacks endocarditis, with valve nodules at autopsy that rarely cause valvular dysfunction). High incidence of acute MI that is unrelated to usual risk factors but instead is caused by systemic inflammation.

Rheumatoid arthritis (RA): Fibrinous pericarditis occurs in 30% with RA. Usually clinically silent, but constriction is possible. Effusions can be large. Rheumatoid nodules can affect myocardium, valve or conduction system. As with SLE, high incidence of MI secondary to inflammation.

Polyarteritis nodosa (PAN): Segmental, necrotizing arteritis of small-medium vessels, including coronary arteries. MI and conduction system disease are possible but uncommon. Renal arteritis causes HTN and renal failure, ultimately causing heart failure in 60% of patients with PAN.

Ankylosing spondylitis: 10% have aortic root inflammation, then sclerosis, then aortic regurgitation (usually with chronic disease). Conduction abnormalities are possible.

Scleroderma (systemic sclerosis): Raynaud's phenomenon is an early symptom. Fibrosis possible in heart, lungs and kidney. CHF, ventricular arrhythmia, or conduction disease occurs in 1/3 of patients. Fibrosis can lead to pulmonary hypertension and cor pulmonale, or there may be PAH (vasospasm without lung fibrosis).

Polymyositis and Dermatomyositis: 40% have cardiac involvement: conduction abnormalities, tachyarrhymias, pericarditis with effusion or dilated cardiomyopathy. Coronary arteritis is possible but rare.

Ehlers-Danlos Syndrome: Multiple genotypes with variable cardiac involvement. Mitral valve prolapse and aortic aneurysm (with rupture or dissection) are the major problems.

Marfan's Syndrome & Loeys-Dietz Syndrome: see text.

Osteogenesis imperfect: Fragile bones, blue sclera. Aortic and/or mitral regurgitation possible, plus large artery fragility.

Neoplastic diseases and treatments:
Metastatic tumors: 30 x more common than primary malignant tumors of the heart. Lung, breast, lymphoma, leukemia and melanoma are most common. Most clinical disease is pericardial, with myocardial or intracavitary disease less common.

Atrial myxoma: Can mimic mitral valve disease. Thromboembolism (stroke) is common. Most have constitutional symptoms (fever, weight loss, fatigue) with an elevated sedimentation rate (high ESR is a great board question).

Rhabdomyoma: Benign tumor of myocardium in young children, often accompanies tuberous sclerosis. Surgically resectible.

Carcinoid (and hypercosinophilic syndromes): Carcinoid tumor and eosinophils secrete serotonin, leading to endocardial fibroelastosis. Fenfleuramine, a diet pill and serotonin agonist, also was found to cause this form of endocarditis. Restrictive cardiomyopathy may develop. It can cause isolated right heart failure with TR or pulmonic stenosis.

Angiosarcoma: Malignant, usually in the RA or pericardium. Right heart failure or pericardial pain. Death within a year.

Rhabdomyosarcoma: Malignant, in any cardiac chamber, and may alter valve function. Death within a year.

Complications of Radiation: Pericarditis is the most common and may lead to constriction, possibly years later (remember to

get that history when there is isolated right heart failure).
Accelerated coronary atherosclerosis is possible. Radiation or
surgery to the neck can cause carotid sinus syncope.

Adriamycin: Cardiomyopathy may occur when the cumulative
dose is >450 mg/sqm. Surprisingly, an excessive dose is
commonly used when treating breast cancer.

5-Fluorouracil: Coronary artery spasm and angina have been
reported.

Cyclophosphamide: At high doses (pre-bone marrow
transplant), hemorrhagic myopericarditis is possible.

Neuromuscular and neurologic disease:
Duchenne muscular dystrophy: Cardiac involvement common:
cardiomyopathy, conduction disorders, mitral valve prolapse
(from papillary muscle disease), narrow and deep Q waves.

Myotonic dystrophy: 80% have cardiac involvement, usually
conduction disorders and other arrhythmias. Myocardial disease
is rare.

Friedreich's ataxia: Dilated cardiomyopathy (CHF is the most
common cause of death). The degree of LV dysfunction does
not parallel severity of the neuromuscular disorder; this is true
of most neuromuscular diseases that may also affect the
myocardium.
There is a hypertrophic variant as well.

Stroke: Deep and symmetrical T wave inversion with troponin
elevation (subendocardial myolysis); atrial and ventricular
arrhythmias; hypertension in the initial stages, especially with
hemorrhagic stroke (usually back to baseline in 10 days);
noncardiac pulmonary edema (adult respiratory distress
syndrome) is possible.

End-stage renal disease--complications:
Hypertension: HTN develops in most patients, regardless of the etiology of renal failure (see text).

Heart failure: Multiple complications of ESRD contribute: hypertension, hypervolemia, anemia, lipid abnormalities, disordered calcium metabolism, dialysis shunts (high output failure), thiamine and other vitamin deficiencies. On the other hand, patients with ESRD and edema may be erroneously diagnosed with HFpEF, when fluid retention is from the kidney disease.

ASCVD: The process is accelerated, and MI is the most common cause of death in patients on dialysis. Interestingly, it is not prevented by treating the usual risk factors for CAD (there may be another mechanism of disease).

Nutritional disorders:
Obesity: The metabolic syndrome, LVH plus LV dilation (elevated preload and afterload, the cardiomyopathy of obesity), obstructive sleep apnea, premature CAD, SCD.

Alcohol: HTN resistant to therapy, AF ("holiday heart"), cardiomyopathy (incidence in alcoholics is 10%-40%).

Thiamine deficiency (beriberi): Vasodilatation, biventricular failure, edema. Common in alcoholics, and routine administration of thiamine on admission for detox makes sense. It can be aggravated by diuretic therapy (excretion of thiamine parallels increased excretion of potassium and magnesium). CHF may improve with replacement, with LVEF recovering like magic over a period of a week. Consider this in a frail patient with CHF who is not eating well.

Protein/calorie malnutrition: A decrease in body weight is accompanied by smaller heart size, slower heart rate and QT interval prolongation. LVEF is normal. SCD is possible with electrolyte disturbances.

HTN, hypertension; LV, left ventricle; LVEF, LV ejection fraction; CHF, congestive heart failure; CAD, coronary artery disease; AR, aortic regurgitation; MR, mitral regurgitation; ARDS, adult respiratory distress syndrome; SCD, sudden cardiac death (usually ventricular fibrillation); ASCVD, atherosclerotic cardiovascular disease, AF, atrial fibrillation, ESR, erythrocyte sedimentation rate.

Chapter 10: Cardiology Consults

Abbreviations

ACC, American College of Cardiology
AHA, American Heart Association
ASD, atrial septal defect
CAD, coronary artery disease
CHF, congestive heart failure
CV, cardiovascular
DC, direct current
ECG, electrocardiogram
LA, left atrium
LMW, low molecular weight (heparin)
LV, left ventricle (ventricular)
LVEF, LV ejection fraction
MI, myocardial infarction
PA, pulmonary artery
PDA, patent ductus arteriosus
Periop, perioperative
PFO, patent foramen ovale
RA, right atrium
RV, right ventricle
VSD, ventricular septal defect

This chapter touches on other clinical problems encountered by the cardiology consult team. Drop us a note if you feel there are other subjects that deserve review.

PREOPERATIVE CARE OF THE PATIENT HAVING NONCARDIAC SURGERY

The Screening Protocol

Coronary artery disease (CAD) is ubiquitous, and myocardial ischemia is the most dangerous cardiac problem that can occur during anesthesia and surgery. Primary care doctors and cardiologists are asked to assess a preoperative patient's

cardiovascular (CV) risk and to "clear the patient for surgery."
That is a phrase we generally don't use. Rather than "clearing"
the patient, we instead provide an estimate of risk so that the
patient and family and surgeon can approach surgery "with their
eyes open"—a useful phrase when talking with patients.

The preoperative screening approach is outlined in Figure 10.1,
and it is based on current practice guidelines.

Figure 10.1 Assessment of Cardiovascular Risk with Non-cardiac Procedures

<u>**Preoperative Screening Protocol**</u>

Step 1: Emergency surgery (i.e. trauma, acute illness)
→ Surgery
Step 2: Unstable heart disease (angina, HF, arrhythmia)
→ Treat the heart disease first
Step 3: Minor or low risk procedure (below)
→ Surgery as planned
Step 4: Functional capacity > 4 METS and asymptomatic
→ Surgery as planned
Step 5: Functional capacity poor or unknown: Calculate the
Revised Cardiac Risk Index (below)
    a. Risk Index = 0   → Surgery as planned
    b. Risk Index = 1-2 & High risk or Intermediate risk
surgery: consider stress testing*

    c. Risk Index > 2 & High risk surgery: cardiology consult,
can risk can be decreased?

    d. Risk Index > 2 & Intermediate risk surgery: consider
stress testing*
If the stress study is abnormal, refer to cardiology.

*Consider stress testing *if it will change management.*

Cardiac risk of non-cardiac procedures:

High risk (> 5% MACE): vascular surgery, emergency surgery, long operations with large fluid shifts or blood loss
Intermediate risk (1-5% MACE): minor vascular surgery, head and neck, orthopedic, urologic, thoracic or abdominal surgery, long operations
Low risk (<1% MACE): superficial surgery, endoscopic surgery and endoscopy, cataracts, derm surgery, breast surgery

MACE: major adverse cardiac event

Functional capacity in METS (metabolic equivalents)

1 MET: sitting at rest
2 METS: household activities, dressing
4 METS: Walking to the second floor, brisk walking on level ground
4-10 METS: short run, moderate sports, scrubbing floors (heavy housework)
10+ METS: strenuous activities or sports

Revised Cardiac Risk Index (RCRI)

One point for each of the following:
Congestive heart failure
Coronary artery disease
Cerebrovascular disease
Creatine > 2
Diabetes, insulin dependent
Intermediate risk surgical procedure

Most of us dislike algorithms, but in this case the algorithm clearly defines the standard of care; without it you will err. Make a copy from the original for your clinic bulletin board and refer to it when you see a preoperative consult. After a few uses, the process will become clear.

Most of the data used to define the patient's risk come from the history and physical examination. These are the stages of screening, taken from this algorithm:

1. Emergency surgery: a patient needing emergency, life-saving surgery requires no special cardiac testing. Examples would include trauma, an acute abdominal process, etc. In such cases, your assessment of cardiac risk is based on the history and physical exam; the patient and family should understand CV risk, especially when it is high.

2. Active cardiac problems: for example, unstable angina, or an unstable rhythm such as atrial fibrillation with inadequate rate control. Treating the urgent cardiac problem must be done before elective surgery. If coronary stenting is needed for ACS, there will be a delay because of the antithrombotic therapy needed to prevent stent thrombosis. The required wait-time is shorter with some of the newer drug eluting stents, and just six weeks is needed when a bare metal stent is used.

3. The next and often most important step is assessment of exercise tolerance. If an asymptomatic patient can exercise at the 4 MET level without cardiac symptoms, no other testing is needed preop. That is the equivalent of walking up one flight of stairs.

4. If the patient is unable to exercise or clearly has poor exercise tolerance, the algorithm becomes more complicated. It requires calculation of the *Lee Cardiac Risk Index*, which you can remember as the "4 C's and a D," assigning 1 point for each.

5. At this point there is an interaction between the patient's risk, the risk index score, and the risk of the operation (Figure 10.1). Stress testing may be used to refine risk assessment when the Lee Index score is high and surgical risk is intermediate or high. On the other hand, if surgical risk is low, or the Lee Index score is low (zero or one), the guidelines do not suggest stress testing.

Note that the guidelines also state that stress testing may be considered "if it will change management." What that means can be illustrated with a couple examples: 1) An elderly man with a long-standing hernia is tired of it but has a high Lee risk score. A stress study indicating active ischemia would argue for conservative treatment rather than surgery, although the patient and surgeon may decide on surgery regardless. 2) A patient with peripheral arterial disease, diabetes and chronic kidney disease has a non-healing foot ulcer; a negative stress study would be reassuring. But a positive study would favor a simple low-risk operation, amputation, rather than a long and perhaps low-yield vascular procedure.

On the other hand, when a high-risk patient must have an operation, stress testing may not change management. It does allow better assessment of prognosis, since a negative stress study does identify lower risk. But for most patients that is not that important: high risk is high risk and putting a number on it does not make a difference.

Occasionally the anesthesiologist—who is used to applying the RCRI—or surgeon insists on a stress test, and that is fine. But more commonly, when the cardiologists says that stress testing isn't needed they agree. What they want is the cardiologist's note that clearly defines risk and that the patient and family understand.

Making the Operation Safer

Why not fix the coronary artery disease to make the operation safer? If that worked, there would be a rationale for more stress testing preoperatively.

Unfortunately, it doesn't work. A series of Dutch studies, the DECREASE trials, tested a strategy of no testing vs. stress echo, then coronary revascularization for those found to have high risk ischemia. They did not find lower perioperative MI or mortality with this screening protocol.

The largest study was done in the VA medical system, the CARP trial. High risk patients having high risk vascular surgery were screened and then had cardiac cath. The 510 patients with disease suitable for PCI were randomized to stenting or no stenting. The result: revascularization did not lower the risk of perioperative MI or death. These results from multiple studies are reminiscent of COURAGE trial results: for clinically stable patients with CAD, fixing the blockage does not prevent MI or death. CARP found this to be true for those having non-cardiac surgery.

Stress Test of Choice

The AHA/ACC practice guidelines indicate that the stress ECG is the test of choice for patients able to complete a symptom limited treadmill study; a negative study with good exercise tolerance indicates low risk. Of course, the guidelines also indicate that any person with good exercise tolerance does not need stress testing as part of the preop evaluation. But if there is a decision for stress testing, the stress ECG is a good choice.

Many who are to have stress testing are not able to walk on the treadmill and require pharmacologic stress testing with imaging. Adenosine perfusion scanning and dobutamine stress echocardiography are equally effective. Intermediate risk patients with active ischemia on the stress study have as much as

10-fold increase in CV risk. When the imaging study shows no active ischemia, risk of MI is less than 3-5%.

If the perfusion scan shows a small area of ischemic, with < 5% of the LV affected, risk is much lower than it would be with a large perfusion abnormality. In the case of extensive ischemia, many cardiologists recommend angiography (despite the CARP result).

A person with prior MI may have a fixed perfusion abnormality, a scar but no reversible ischemia; this is not active ischemia, and additional testing is not needed. An occasional scan shows "scar with peri-infarct ischemia." Peri-infarct ischemia is the watershed zone adjacent to the scar that has enough collateral flow to avoid injury. It does not indicate another stenosed artery that is on the brink of occlusion with new infarction and does not indicate increased perioperative risk.

Measurement of left ventricular ejection fraction is not part of routine preoperative screening protocols. An echocardiogram may be helpful in sorting out dyspnea of uncertain cause or to support a diagnosis of heart failure. A previously undetected heart murmur also would be an indication for echo.

Management of the High Risk Patient

Revascularization

As noted, it is not indicated for a stable patient. But it is surprisingly common to discover new onset, and therefore unstable angina when taking a preoperative history. In that case, the patient has unstable heart disease, and the elective operation is delayed until the heart disease is addressed.

Beta Blockade

There were multiple, small studies with variable results, some showing a protective effect. The POISE trial was designed to answer the question about perioperative beta blockade and found higher mortality in the treated group. This was driven by a high rate of stroke with metoprolol. Unfortunately, the protocol was flawed. Patients not previously on beta blockers were given remarkably high dose, long-acting metoprolol, as much as 400 mg, in the 24 hours before and after surgery. Resulting hypotension probably accounts for the increased rate of stroke.

So there remains uncertainty about prophylactic beta blockade. Most feel that if a patient is on a beta blocker, it should be continued perioperatively. If you want to start beta blockade before surgery, it should be done far enough in advance to regulate the dose.

Other Therapies

There is no single anesthetic technique or drug that provides the best cardiac protection. Spinal anesthesia is not necessarily safer for the heart. It is rare, but sudden cardiac death is possible with spinal anesthesia or with epidural nerve block at the T1-4 level, where the preganglionic sympathetic nerves exit the spine. Blocking them can lead to lower blood pressure and reduced blood return to the heart. That sets off the reflexes that end with vagal discharge (see the description of neurocardiogenic syncope in Chapter 8). Most have a benign vaso-vagal spell, but there are reports of extreme reaction with asystole and death.

Observational studies have found less CV risk with laparoscopic surgery compared with open procedures. That has not been tested in randomized trials.

Other Cardiac Illnesses

Valvular Heart Disease, Antibiotic Prophylaxis

Current guidelines are in Table 10.1. A trend in recent years is a narrowing of specific indications for antibiotic prophylaxis

Table 10.1 Antibiotic prophylaxis to prevent infective endocarditis (IE)

Prophylaxis <u>is recommended</u> for the following:
Drainage of an infected site, or for oral, lower gastrointestinal, gallbladder, or genitourinary procedures, <u>plus</u> any of the following conditions.
   Prosthetic cardiac valves (mechanical valves)
   Previous IE
   Congenital heart disease (CHD)
   Cyanotic CHD, including those with palliative shunts and conduits
   Repaired CHD that included a device (foreign body), for the first six months post-op
   Repaired CHD with a prosthetic device that cannot endothelialize
   Heart transplant patients with valvulopathy

Prophylaxis <u>is not needed</u> for the following:
Anesthetic injection through non-infected tissue
Routine dental procedures including orthodontic placement or adjustment
Presence of
   Pacemakers or cardioverter-defibrillators
   Prosthetic vascular grafts or patches
   Hemodialysis shunts or prosthetic grafts
   Coronary artery stents
   Peripheral vascular stents
   Devices for closure of atrial septal or ventricular septal defects

---

Congestive Heart Failure

CHF increases the mortality of noncardiac surgery, and it is associated with longer hospitalization. The rate of readmission to hospital during the month after surgery is much higher.

Experience suggests this often is because the patient is managed by the surgeon after the operation and is discharged without his/her heart failure medicines. A patient with CHF might do better if an internist was actively involved, but that is not the usual pattern of practice in most hospitals (nor will Medicare pay for the service).

A patient with CHF should be at dry weight and well compensated at the time of surgery. Careful monitoring of fluid status and electrolytes is needed after surgery and fluid overload avoided.

That is the essence of perioperative management. Remember that low magnesium as well as potassium increases the risk of atrial and ventricular tachyarrhythmias after surgery. Magnesium often falls after large operations. The reason is uncertain, and there has been speculation that cut tissue either soaks up or weeps magnesium. Magnesium and/or potassium deficiency may be aggravated by diuretic therapy.

There has been controversy about the use of pulmonary artery pressure monitoring in general, and none of the available trials has documented any benefit in the perioperative setting. In some studies, patients having right heart catheterization fared slightly worse than those managed using clinical parameters. Patient selection issues cloud interpretation of these results, but at least there was no clear benefit. The practice guidelines allow their perioperative use in high-risk patients but do not require it. Our heart failure team often uses hemodynamic monitoring and "tailored therapy" to tune a patient with decompensated CHF before noncardiac surgery. This includes aggressive treatment with vasodilators, inotropes, and diuretics, and rarely, mechanical assist devices.

ISOLATED RIGHT HEART FAILURE

The following have been discussed in previous chapters, but are gathered together for review, since this is a common consult: the patient with marked peripheral edema but no rales.

Left Heart Failure

It is a conundrum: the patient with systemic congestion and altered LV function who has never had pulmonary congestion. How can the cause of right heart failure be left heart failure if (clinically) there is no left heart failure? But it can occur in patients with a variety of left heart disorders, including low LVEF, LV diastolic dysfunction or valve disease (most commonly with mitral stenosis).

One explanation is that there is a percentage of the population with hyper-reactive pulmonary vasculature. When stressed with hypoxia or hemodynamic overload, these patients develop pulmonary hypertension. High PA pressure protects the pulmonary capillary bed, and congestion develops proximal to it. The clinical picture is "isolated" right heart failure.

Another explanation is increased lymphatic flow. In animal studies of heart failure, pulmonary lymphatic flow increased 5-fold. The occasional patient with especially efficient lymphatic drainage may not have pulmonary interstitial congestion.

Cor Pulmonale

When thinking of reactive pulmonary hypertension, remember cor pulmonale (Chapter 9). Not everyone with chronic lung disease gets it, and developing it requires lung disease plus susceptibility—e.g., a touchy pulmonary vasculature. The extreme example of this is PAH, a vasospastic disorder possibly caused by endothelial dysfunction.

Pericardial Disease

Both pericardial tamponade and constriction limit cardiac filling (Chapter 2 for a longer discussion of pericardial disease). Consider them "external" causes of right heart failure. The right atrium (RA) and ventricle (RV) are compressed and just cannot accommodate normal volume. This inadequate preload, since that is what it is, results in reduced stroke volume.

Acute tamponade causes a precipitous fall in blood pressure. An example is cardiac rupture after MI. Subacute pericardial tamponade presents with symptoms of low cardiac output such as fatigue or weakness and peripheral edema. On the other hand, when the pericardial effusion develops slowly the pericardium has time to stretch, and there may be no compression of the heart. That is often the case with the pericardial effusion of hypothyroidism, which can be massive.

Constrictive pericarditis develops slowly with symptoms of low cardiac output and right heart failure. We see one or two cases a year of "cryptogenic cirrhosis" and massive ascites on the liver transplant that turns out to be constriction. Stripping the pericardium may cure the liver disease.

CONGENITAL HEART DISEASE SEEN IN ADULTS

This is a large subject and will review three topics: Eisenmenger's syndrome, because management can be tricky and primary care practitioners often follow patients with this condition; atrial septal defect (ASD), because it is common, easily missed and often encountered on board exams; and patent foramen ovale (PFO), as there has been renewed interest in it as a cause of peripheral embolism and stroke.

Eisenmenger's Syndrome
Adults with congenital heart disease who are cyanotic have Eisenmenger's syndrome: pulmonary hypertension causing right

to left shunting. The most common causes are ventricular septal defect (VSD), patent ductus arteriosus (PDA), transposition of the great vessels, and rarely, atrial septal defect (ASD). About half of those with large VSD or PDA develop Eisenmenger's syndrome.

Lesions that transmit both high pressure and volume to the PA tend to provoke pulmonary hypertension, explaining why VSD and PDA are common causes. With these high-pressure lesions, pulmonary hypertension becomes fixed in infancy. ASD, which delivers high volume but not high pressure to the PA, infrequently causes Eisenmenger's syndrome. When it happens, it develops later in life. As with other causes of isolated right heart failure, a susceptible pulmonary vasculature seems a requirement.

High pulmonary blood pressure leads to irreversible microvascular changes. Endothelial dysfunction, growth factors and platelet aggregation appear to contribute to intimal proliferation and progressive occlusion of small arterioles. Once these anatomic changes are present, high pulmonary vascular resistance is irreversible.

Eventually pulmonary resistance exceeds systemic resistance. The direction of shunting reverses, becoming right to left. Desaturated blood reaches the left heart, and the resulting arterial hypoxemia stimulates erythrocytosis.

Most patients have symptoms of low cardiac output including fatigue and poor exercise tolerance. Right heart failure is common, and there may be an element of left heart congestion as well. The patient's appearance is striking with central cyanosis and clubbed fingers. The cardiac exam reflects the underlying condition.

Erythrocytosis causing hyperviscosity is the major day-to-day management issue. Formerly we used frequent phlebotomy to keep the hematocrit under 65%. Targeting the hematocrit is not the current practice. Rather, the indication for phlebotomy is symptoms of hyperviscosity, including headache, irritability, lethargy, fatigue, dizziness and visual disturbances. Most develop symptoms when the hematocrit approaches 70%, and the goal of phlebotomy is to reduce it below 65%. Simultaneous volume replacement with saline is needed.

Iron deficiency and microcytosis are common, especially with recurrent phlebotomy. The small red blood cells are rigid, do not deform normally, and thus do not pass through capillaries as easily. This contributes to sludging. When red cell indices indicate microcytosis or there is low serum iron, iron therapy is needed (an apparent paradox in a patient with an elevated hematocrit).

There are a number of other complications of Eisenmenger's syndrome. With right-left shunting, paradoxical embolus is a possible cause of stroke. For the same reason, brain abscess may be a consequence of transient bacteremia. Stress is poorly tolerated. With pregnancy, maternal mortality is about 50%, and pregnancy is inadvisable. The perioperative mortality is high with noncardiac surgery. High altitude travel should be avoided, and commercial air transportation is best tolerated with the patient on supplemental oxygen.

The prognosis with Eisenmenger's syndrome is better than it is with other causes of pulmonary hypertension. Survival is 80% at 10 years, 77% at 15 years, and 42% at 25 years. Predictors of early mortality include syncope, elevated RV filling pressure and right heart failure, and more severe hypoxemia (oxygen saturation less than 85% at rest). The location of the right-to-left shunt does not affect prognosis. Causes of death include ventricular fibrillation, heart failure, hemoptysis, stroke, brain abscess, thromboembolism and complications of surgery or pregnancy.

Atrial Septal Defect (ASD)

There are three possible sites of communication between the
right and left atria. The most common defect (more than 80% of
cases) is the ostium secundum ASD, located in the mid-septum,
well above the atrioventricular valves.

The ostium primum defect (15% of cases) originates in the
endocardial cushion, a structure in the center of the fetal heart
that also contributes to the formation of the mitral and tricuspid
valves and the upper part of the interventricular septum. The
most extreme form of endocardial cushion defect is the absence
of these structures, resulting in a single-chambered heart. With
primum ASD, there may be cleft mitral or tricuspid leaflets and
regurgitation. The interventricular conduction system also is
affected, and left axis deviation (usually left anterior fascicular
block) is a marker of primum rather than secundum ASD (a
cardiology board question—how to diagnose primum ASD from
the ECG).

The sinus venosus defect is the least common ASD, occurring at
the entrance of either the superior or the inferior vena cava.

The usual ASD is large, close to 2 cm in diameter. Because of
its size, there is no jet effect and little turbulence. Thus, the ASD
itself does not generate a murmur. The large defect also means
that pressures in the two atria are equal. Blood flows toward the
right atrium because the RV is more compliant than the LV
during diastole.

The major hemodynamic effect is volume overload of the RA,
RV and PA. When the catheterization report indicates a 2:1
shunt, it means that the pulmonary blood flow is twice the
systemic blood flow, and that the RV is handling twice as much
volume as the LV.

Increased pulmonary blood flow may provoke a rise in PA
pressure, and a form of Eisenmenger's syndrome occurs in

about 10% of patients, usually appearing in adolescence. The incidence of Eisenmenger's reaction with VSD or PDA is higher and the onset is younger. These conditions also increase flow to the PA, but they also transmit arterial pressure. The combination of high pressure and high flow is a stronger stimulus of pulmonary vascular reactivity.

Clinical Presentation, Laboratory Evaluation and Treatment

ASD is often diagnosed late in life. Young adults are rarely symptomatic; the diagnosis may be made with routine physical examination or chest x-ray. Middle-aged patients usually present with atrial arrhythmias. Heart failure may develop as the initial symptom in older people. It would seem that the LV would be protected, but a common pattern is biventricular failure rather than just RV failure.

This probably has to do with how the interventricular septum works. It has to "choose sides" to work as a part of either the LV or RV. It chooses the side with the greater workload, normally the LV. With chronic RV overload, it works instead with the RV, moving away from the lateral wall of the LV rather than toward it during systole. This is the so-called "paradoxical septal motion" described by the echocardiogram when there is RV overload. Loss of septal function may contribute to the eventual failure of the LV when there is chronic RV overload. In this case, "chronic" may mean five or six decades of abnormal cardiac loading before symptoms develop.

The physical findings of ASD are obvious. S_2 is widely split, with no respiratory variation. Because of volume overload, emptying of the RV is delayed, and P_2 is late. The large ASD distributes the increased venous return to the heart during inspiration equally to both atria. Fixed splitting of S_2 is a reliable finding, and its absence excludes ASD.

There is usually a systolic murmur at the left base. This is not caused by flow across the ASD but rather by high flow across the normal pulmonic valve (with a 2:1 shunt, the pulmonic valve has twice the normal flow). With a primum defect, a cleft mitral or tricuspid leaflet causes the typical regurgitant murmur.

The typical pattern of RV volume overload on the ECG is incomplete right bundle branch block, a usual finding with ASD. The primum defect causes left anterior fascicular block, and checking the QRS axis in a patient with ASD is a mark of clinical sophistication. Pulmonary plethora on the chest x-ray is always present, and experienced radiologists claim that it is not subtle (though I have a hard time seeing it). *A normal chest x-ray and ECG exclude significant right-left shunting and ASD.* I emphasize this point as many doctors naively assume that the echocardiogram is needed to diagnose or exclude structural heart disease.

The echocardiogram confirms RV enlargement and paradoxical septal motion. The ASD is easily visualized and flow across the defect may be documented with echocardiographic contrast agents and Doppler. In addition, the echo-Doppler study allows estimation of PA pressure.

Surgical repair of ASD is recommended when the pulmonary to systemic blood flow is above 1.5:1, especially when the RV size is increased. Surgery is not done to prevent pulmonary hypertension, a rare complication that develops before age 30 when it does occur. In middle age, repair is done to prevent atrial arrhythmias and eventual heart failure. There is a survival benefit with surgery even for patients older than 50 years, most of whom are symptomatic.

Patent Foramen Ovale (PFO) and Embolic Stroke
Most *arterial emboli* originate from the left heart (atrial fibrillation or flutter, mitral stenosis, valve vegetations, dilated cardiomyopathy, atrial myxoma) or from aortic or large artery

atheroma. With the Eisenmenger syndrome and right to left shunting across a cardiac lesion (i.e. VSD, PDA or ASD), clot from leg veins may cross to the arterial circulation—so-called paradoxical embolization. One of the worst complications of Eisenmenger's is the passage of infected material from the venous circulation leading to brain abscess.

About 25% of us have incomplete closure of the foramen ovale at birth. This communication between RA and LA is small and functionally insignificant. Higher pressure in the LA should cause any shunting to be left-to-right. The PFO can be an exception to this. Those of us who worked in the cath lab in the '70s used green dye to test for shunts: with PFO, injection of the dye into a femoral vein results in the early appearance of a small amount of the dye in the arterial circulation (right-to-left shunting). Dye injected from the arm vein does not cross from right to left. The PFO seems to work as a baffle, shunting a tiny amount of the return from the inferior vena cava, from the RA to the LA (but it does not catch blood from the superior vena cava). It is possible for this baffle to catch small venous emboli, sending them to the arterial circulation.

Case controlled studies have shown that the incidence of PFO is somewhat higher than usual in young patients who have had "cryptogenic stroke," e.g. stroke despite normal carotid arteries. The highest risk anatomy is PFO plus an associated atrial septum aneurysm. The aneurysm either increases the chance of interatrial shunting or provides a locus for thrombus formation. In a European study of patients who had cryptogenic stroke, those with PFO plus aneurysm had an almost four-fold increase in recurrent stroke during follow-up.

The other element of the equation is a source of embolus. The diagnosis of paradoxical embolus is more believable if venous stasis or a hypercoagulable state is demonstrated.

Medical therapy for acute paradoxical embolism and stroke is thrombolysis with tissue plasminogen activator. Long-term therapy is anticoagulation. Thus, it is treated like other illnesses where an embolus originates from the heart, including atrial fibrillation and left ventricular mural thrombus. One exception to this is bacterial endocarditis; anticoagulation does not prevent thromboembolism.

Many advocate PFO closure for all patients who have had stroke, arguing that the catheter-based repair of PFO is safer than life-long anticoagulation.

PREGNANCY AND HEART DISEASE

Normal pregnancy leads to hemodynamic changes that increase the workload of the heart. There is a 40% increase in maternal blood volume and a similar increase in cardiac output. There is vasodilatation with a decline in both systemic vascular resistance and diastolic blood pressure. Pulse pressure and heart rate increase. These changes peak in the second trimester.

The cardiovascular system is thus hyperdynamic. With volume overload and increased rapid filling of the LV in early diastole, there may be an S_3 gallop. A heart murmur is a common reason for cardiac referral. An echocardiogram showing no structural abnormality provides reassurance that the murmur is "physiologic," usually from high flow across the pulmonic valve. Or what you think is a murmur may be a bruit from the breast. One of my teachers commented that the cardiac exam in a normal pregnant woman can sound like a washing machine. Murmurs with valve stenosis become louder with increased flow. On the other hand, the physical findings of mitral valve prolapse or hypertrophic subaortic stenosis may disappear with increased LV volume.

There are a number of cardiac illnesses that increase *maternal mortality* (Table 10.2,). The risk increases with worsening functional class. The highest risk conditions are considered contraindications to pregnancy. The usual medical indications for terminating pregnancy are pulmonary hypertension (PA pressure >50 mm Hg, either primary pulmonary hypertension or Eisenmenger's syndrome), dilated cardiomyopathy, Marfan's syndrome with marked aortic root dilatation, pulmonary ateriovenous fistulae and any cardiac disease that cannot be corrected with class 3 or 4 symptoms that are refractory to medical therapy.

Table 10.2 Mortality Risk Associated with Heart Disease in Pregnancy

Low risk (<1%)
Septal defects
Patent ductus arteriosis
Pulmonic, tricuspid valve lesions
NYHA classes I and II

Moderate risk (5%-15%)
NYHA class III or IV mitral stenosis
Aortic stenosis
Marfan's syndrome with a normal aortic root
Uncomplicated coarctation of the aorta
Prior myocardial infarction

High risk (25%-50%)
Eisenmenger's syndrome
Pulmonary hypertension
Marfan's syndrome with a dilated aortic root
History of peripartum cardiomyopathy

There is concern about inheritance. The risk of transmitting the Marfan's syndrome to the child is about 50% (it is autosomal dominant), and that is the case with familial hypertrophic cardiomyopathy as well (although the familial form is uncommon). For other congenital heart diseases with polygenic inheritance, the chance of a fetal abnormality is about 13%, roughly 12-times the risk in the normal population. This estimate is higher than the 5% that we quoted a decade ago, and it varies with different conditions. There are about 200 inherited conditions with associated heart disease, and 85 of them allow survival to the reproductive age. Genetic counseling is important when considering pregnancy.

Management

Arrhythmias may develop or worsen during pregnancy. However, most with preexisting arrhythmias tolerate pregnancy well. The first step in management is exclusion of correctible causes: electrolyte abnormalities, thyroid disease, alcohol, other drugs, caffeine and smoking. Try to avoid drug therapy unless the arrhythmia is symptomatic, hemodynamically important or life threatening. Digoxin, metoprolol, and diltiazem may be used during pregnancy. Amiodarone is not safe (intrauterine growth retardation, thyroid dysfunction, fetal distress). Animal studies with high drug doses have raised concerns about most of the available drugs. We are reluctant to begin antiarrhythmic therapy in the first trimester unless it is absolutely necessary. Low-moderate dose DC cardioversion is relatively safe for the fetus.

The usual indications for *anticoagulation* apply for those with atrial fibrillation and *valve prostheses*. Heparin is safer for the baby while warfarin is safer for the mother. Warfarin crosses the placenta and may cause a variety of defects, including cerebral hemorrhage, fetal wasting, optic atrophy, and other developmental disorders. The highest risk is from conception to the 14th week, and risk increases with the dose of warfarin. There are no clear guidelines for management, and some recommend subcutaneous heparin during the first trimester, then switching to warfarin.

Severe LV dysfunction is a contraindication to pregnancy. Those with advanced heart failure—functional class 3 or 4—have a significant mortality risk, and termination of pregnancy should be considered. The usual treatment principles for heart failure apply. The one exception is angiotensin converting enzyme (ACE) inhibitors (and probably receptor blockers); fetal renal dysfunction is common. In fact, ACE inhibitor therapy during early pregnancy may be an indication for therapeutic abortion. Calcium channel blockers and/or hydralazine are preferred for afterload reduction.

Endocarditis prophylaxis is suggested as "an option" during vaginal delivery for highest risk patients, although most prescribe it for these conditions: complex congenital disease, a prosthetic valve, prior endocarditis, a surgically created arteriovenous shunt, valve disease including mitral valve prolapse with regurgitation and/or thickened leaflets. It is not required for ASD, previously repaired ventricular septal defect, patent ductus arteriosus or a functional heart murmur (with a no apparent structural abnormality on the echocardiogram.

For most patients, vaginal delivery at the 38th week is safer than cesarean section. The one exception may be Marfan's syndrome. Immediately after delivery, pressure on the inferior vena cava is relieved increasing venous return to the heart. This auto-transfusion effect may aggravate cardiac symptoms. Cardiac output may remain above pre-pregnancy levels for weeks, especially if the mother is breast-feeding.

Peripartum Cardiomyopathy (PPCM)

This form of dilated cardiomyopathy affects women with no previous heart disease. It may occur in the last month of pregnancy or during the first 6 months postpartum; peak incidence is 1-2 months postpartum.

The cause is unknown. It is more common in black women, and it is more common in Africa. Other risk factors for developing cardiomyopathy are maternal age >30 years, multiparity, twin pregnancy, malnutrition, hypertension or pre-eclampsia. It recurs in 50% with subsequent pregnancies, even when LV function has returned to normal. A second episode often is worse than the first, and possibly fatal, especially for those who do not have complete recovery of LV function. Most consider postpartum cardiomyopathy a reason to avoid future pregnancy.

The treatment includes standard therapy for heart failure. An exception is angiotensin converting enzyme inhibitors and angiotensin receptor blockers, which affect the fetal kidneys and should be avoided during pregnancy. Hydralazine and/or calcium channel blockers are safer afterload reducers prepartum.

More than half of the patients recover. The prognosis is good for those with normalization of LV size and ejection fraction within six months. Clinical features indicating a worse prognosis are onset of symptoms late after delivery, severe depression of LVEF, marked LV enlargement and new left bundle branch block.

END-OF-LIFE (EOL) DECISIONS AND PALLIATIVE CARE FOR PATIENTS WITH HEART DISEASE

You will observe a general reluctance to "give up" on the patient with heart disease. There is always the possibility of one more interventional procedure. Scientific medicine's central ethic is prolongation of life, and aggressive therapy often is life-saving. But there is a dilemma when life-prolonging surgery seems too aggressive for an elderly or severely disabled person. This is especially true for the patient who has had multiple cardiac procedures in the past.

The first step in resolving the dilemma is considering the patient's wishes. The central principal of medical ethics is patient autonomy. As doctors we do not have unquestioned control over what happens to patients. Instead, our responsibility is to inform, recommend alternatives, and then to respect and support the patient's decision. This means that when we are old and sick no one can make us do something we do not want. It is what we want for ourselves, and it should be what we want for our patients.

Even so, surveys of elderly patients and their families document concern about inappropriate and aggressive care at the end of life. Old people often feel that they are convinced to have procedures they do not want.

Peaceful Death, Another Goal of Medicine

In addition to prolonging life and relieving suffering, at some stage of our lives the goal of medical care is a peaceful death. We wince at the spectacle of the hopelessly ill old person subjected to a prolonged intensive care unit death.

The trend in scientific medicine has been the elimination of illnesses that are rapidly fatal. What remains are conditions like dementia, stroke and heart failure. I occasionally encounter a chronically ill, elderly person who has decided to reclaim the traditional "old man's friends" by declining curative treatment for acute illnesses such as pneumonia, heart attack or urosepsis. This usually meets resistance from the doctor. However, an autonomous person has the right to refuse any treatment, whether it is antibiotics for pneumonia, chemotherapy for advanced cancer.

This is not an argument against life-prolonging therapy for older patients. Indeed, treatment shown to prolong life by clinical trials should be applied irrespective of age, *if that is what the patient wants*. Instead, you should support your patient who has decided to avoid possibly life-prolonging but *unwanted* therapy. (That would include surgical correction of aortic stenosis, an implanted defibrillator after myocardial infarction, or any cardiac intervention.)

If you do not convince your patient to accept a cure, are you are in some way responsible for the resulting death? If you believe that you are, you have fallen prey to the doctor's delusion of control over life and death. In matter of fact, a terminally ill patient dies of a disease. Our intervention affects only the timing and the amount of suffering. By avoiding life-prolonging therapy at the patient's direction, the doctor is not responsible for death, nor is the patient.

Palliative Care

Those with terminal heart failure or coronary artery disease should have aggressive medical therapy, since it relieves symptoms. When usual drug therapies become ineffective, it helps to involve hospice.

Current federal regulations provide for hospice care if survival is estimated to be less than 6 months, and patients with advanced heart disease meet this criterion. Hospice nurses are good at regulating heart failure therapy. Their day-to-day adjustment of diuretics and other medicines may allow the patient to remain at home, out of the hospital. For those with heart disease, hospice care often leads to dramatic improvement of symptoms, so much so that it is possible to discontinue hospice (at least for a while). This has been observed for those with advanced lung disease as well.

Morphine

Morphine is the key addition to EOL care when standard therapy no longer controls cardiac symptoms. It is a venodilator that reduces blood return to the heart and relieves pulmonary congestion. In addition, it blunts the anxiety that comes with dyspnea. Morphine is also effective for control of angina when other therapy has failed.

There is concern that morphine may depress respiration. In practice, this is rare for patients on chronic therapy for pulmonary congestion or severe dyspnea from advanced lung disease. Tolerance develops, and even high dose therapy is safe if an abrupt escalation of the dose is avoided.

Morphine is palliative care for advanced heart disease, and we require hospice management when prescribing it. As noted, hospice nurses are skilled with its use, and hospice enrollment prevents the appearance of opioid misuse.

Extreme Symptoms in the Terminal Patient

What can we do for a patient who comes to the ER with extreme and probably end-of-life symptoms, usually pulmonary edema refractory to intravenous furosemide? It is unfortunate when the ER doctor offers (or demands) intubation and mechanical ventilation, despite a previous decision to avoid it. A desperate patient and family will have a change of mind when this is offered as the only chance for relief.

An effective alternative is high dose morphine, titrated to relieve dyspnea. There may be depression of respiration with a dose sufficient to relieve symptoms. In this case, the moral imperative is to relieve suffering for the dying patient, even if high-dose opioids hasten death. There is no culpability. It is not assisted suicide or euthanasia, but rather necessary treatment for extreme symptoms.

www.ingramcontent.com/pod-product-compliance
Lightning Source LLC
Chambersburg PA
CBHW072004170726
47999CB00013B/26